Cambridge History of Medicine
EDITORS: CHARLES WEBSTER AND CHARLES ROSENBERG

The cultural meaning of popular science

The cultural meaning of popular science

PHRENOLOGY AND THE ORGANIZATION OF CONSENT
IN NINETEENTH-CENTURY BRITAIN

Roger Cooter

*The University of Manchester Institute of
Science and Technology*

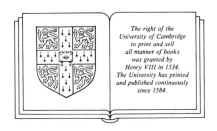

*The right of the
University of Cambridge
to print and sell
all manner of books
was granted by
Henry VIII in 1534.
The University has printed
and published continuously
since 1584.*

CAMBRIDGE UNIVERSITY PRESS

CAMBRIDGE

LONDON   NEW YORK   NEW ROCHELLE

MELBOURNE   SYDNEY

Published by the Press Syndicate of the University of Cambridge
The Pitt Building, Trumpington Street, Cambridge CB2 1RP
32 East 57th Street, New York, NY 10022, USA
10 Stamford Road, Oakleigh, Melbourne 3166, Australia

First published 1984

Printed in the United States of America

Library of Congress Cataloging in Publication Data

Cooter, Roger.
  The cultural meaning of popular science.
  (Cambridge history of medicine)
  Bibliography: p.
  Includes index.
    1. Science – Great Britain – History.   2. Science –
Social aspects – Great Britain – History.   3. Great
Britain – Intellectual life – 19th century.   4. Phrenology.
I. Title.   II. Series.
Q127.G4C66   1984   509.41   84–12078
ISBN 0 521 22743 7

For Margaret and Sebastian
and for my teacher
Robert M. Young

To be sure, the history of science is no more the true center of British history in the 19th century than is the history of Parliament. But it is no less so. And historians of Parliament, or of politics, have amply had their chance, from Halevy on, to produce full and convincing history. And they have failed. So have "social" historians. And attempts to construct "cultural" history on the basis of literary culture alone are not very promising. The leadership in the re-writing of history will have to be assumed by historians for whom the totality of the past is an omnipresent pressure, limiting and defining the heroes at the same time that it gives a stage for their personal existence and gives a rationale for their all-too-human actions, just as it does for all humans.

Susan Cannon, *Science in Culture* (N.Y., 1978), p. 257

Many forces make history. But none makes more history than that which underlies and energizes all other human motivations – the hunger for meaning. For that, people will kill and die, build and destroy. They will even face their own bad dreams and brave the terrors of rebirth.

Theodore Roszak, *Person/Planet: the creative disintegration of industrial society* (St. Albans, Herts., 1981), p. 53

CONTENTS

ILLUSTRATIONS

PREFACE

This book explores a body of knowledge that was the product of one of the most important intersections in modern history. But like the history it explores, this book is itself the product of an intersection. The period over which it was researched and written as a Cambridge doctoral thesis, between 1974 and 1978, was that in which enthusiasm began to mount for the work of Mary Douglas relating patterns of belief to salient characteristics in social structures. At the same time, in the wake of the transatlantic influence of Thomas Kuhn's *The Structure of of Scientific Revolutions,* there reemerged a sociology of knowledge with an emphasis on scientific knowledge. From across the Channel came the *histoire des mentalités,* structuralism, and the daunting genius of Michel Foucault. With the help of Frankfurt scholars, there blossomed an antidogmatic Marxist tradition willing to look hard at science and culture, while within the latter orbit came the stirrings of a vigorous community of social historians, a part of whose reaching beyond empiricism involved the rediscovery of the insights on ideology and culture of the Italian theorist Antonio Gramsci. All of these events bore upon the creation of this study and upon the way it would treat the problem that lies at its heart – the problem of the relations between knowledge and power.

In converting the thesis to a book, I have eliminated some material and added other, especially in Chapter 2 and in the Conclusion (which now brings the history of the subject matter up to the end of the nineteenth century). Notes have been revised, economized, and brought up to date. But mostly, I have sought only to refine the material and its organization with a view to rendering some of the historical complexities clearer and some of the nuances more apparent. Opportunities to publish papers have helped in this, although the only publication in which the reader will find any direct borrowing from some of the material presented here (in Chapters 1 and 3) is that on "Deploying 'Pseudoscience': then and now" (in M. P. Hanen *et al.*, eds., *Science, Pseudo-Science, and Society* [1980], abridged in Patrick Grim, ed., *Philosophy of Science and the Occult* [1982]. Important in enabling me to clarify various interpretive issues was the writing of "The Power of the Body" (in Barry Barnes and Steven Shapin, eds., *Natural Order: historical studies of scientific culture* [1979]. "Phrenology and British Alienists, c. 1825–45" (now reprinted in Andrew Scull, ed., *Madhouses, Mad-Doctors, and Madmen: the social history of psychiatry in the Victorian era* [1981]) deals with an area of phrenology's history that is possible to refer to only in passing in this study; while "Phrenology: the provocation of progress" (*History of Science*, 1976) critically reviews some of the secondary literature on phrenology that reappears in the Introduction and Chapter 1.

I am lastingly obliged to the Canadian Branch of the Imperial Order of the Daughters of the Empire for providing the initial funding for my research; thereafter, generously, the Social Sciences and Humanities Research Council of Canada (SSHRCC) made the completion of the study possible. A Fellowship in 1979 with the Calgary Institute for the Humanities, University of Calgary, and a Killam Fellowship at Dalhousie University in 1980 allowed the rewriting to be undertaken in highly congenial atmospheres. The final drafts of this book were written while I was based at the Wellcome Unit for the History of Medicine, University of Oxford, engaged in new research funded by the SSHRCC and the Wellcome Trust and made all the more pleasant by being a Fellow of St. Antony's College. For so much sustenance mere words of gratitude must always be insufficient. Nor can words alone convey the pleasure I derive from acknowledging the small travel grant I received from the William Ramsay Henderson Trust of Edinburgh, for this trust was established at Henderson's death in 1832 for the popular promotion of phrenology (see Chapter 5).

Many librarians and archivists have had to put up with my endless requests and queries. For being so tolerant, I am especially grateful to the staffs of the University Library, Cambridge, the Bodleian Library, Oxford, the National Library of Scotland, and the Wellcome and British Libraries in London. For their help in providing photographs and granting permission to reproduce them, I would like to thank the following: the Trustees of the National

Library of Scotland (Figure 5); the Guildhall Library, City of London (Figure 2); the Trustees of the John Johnson Collection, Bodleian Library, Oxford (Figures 6, 7); the Wellcome Institute Library, London (Figures 1, 3, 4); the British Library (Figure 8).

Those who gave me encouragement, advice, and support during my research and writing know how much I owe them; but I would particularly like to thank Karl Figlio, Bill Luckin, Keith McClelland, Terry Parssinen, Roy Porter, Tina Posner, and Steven Shapin, who always gave more than was called for. I was fortunate in being able to draw endlessly on the historical acumen and good sense of my colleagues at the Wellcome Unit – more than they realize, Joan Austoker, Penelope Goak, Irving Loudon, Margaret Pelling, and Paul Weindling helped me to avoid many embarrassing mistakes, as did Jean Loudon in pouring over the Appendix; while Charles Webster, who read the entire manuscript and offered an abundance of helpful criticisms, did as much again for my sometimes flagging spirit.

To those to whom this book is dedicated I owe the most. At Bob Young's suggestion the project was begun, and throughout its long gestation he has remained a patient and inspiring counsel for its interpretation. Margaret Cooter – helpmate, friend, and surefooted critic – provided continuous and unstinting support, while my son Sebastian effectively spurred the book to its completion through the potent mixture of his love and my guilt. The finished product inadequately indicates my debt.

The shortcomings are all my own.

R.J.C.

NOTE ON SOURCES AND
ABBREVIATIONS

Over four thousand printed phrenological sources have been consulted in the writing of this book. To list them all, along with the equivalent number of other sources consulted, proves impractical, and a bibliography of works cited would be redundant. An index to the primary and secondary sources has therefore been included to permit the reader to locate readily the full reference in the Notes of any work cited. Provided also at the end of the book is a list of manuscript sources along with a chronological list of British phrenological journals. The place of publication for books is London unless stated otherwise. Throughout the text and notes, "Combe" refers to George Combe.

ABBREVIATIONS

BAAS   British Association for the Advancement of Science
DNB   *Dictionary of National Biography*
DSB   *Dictionary of Scientific Biography*
EPS   Edinburgh Phrenological Society
LPS   London Phrenological Society
NLS   National Library of Scotland
NMW   *New Moral World*
PA   Phrenological Association
‡   denotes entry in Appendix of Public Lecturers on Phrenology (pp. 272–300 of this volume)

INTRODUCTION

Science, medicine, and technology stand routinely before us, yet curiously little is known historically of their social and cultural as opposed to merely their practical effects. There are indeed social histories of scientific institutions, societies, and professional groups, as there are social studies of the relations between science and technology and the interactions between science and philosophy. There is a critical literature on the scientific "age" seen as a conceptual and social *Weltanschauung*, and there is a burgeoning sociology of scientific knowledge that, extending to the social construction of rejected scientific and medical ideas, undermines conventional views of science as "neutral" and/or "responsible, moderate, unsentimental, and otherwise good." Now, even in the biographies of great scientists, and in otherwise parochial studies of the rise of particular scientific disciplines, one is likely to find at least token recognition of science as the historically contingent product of men (mostly men) in specific social and political contexts.[1]

But if science has been profaned as merely another social product, has had some of its ethnocentric biases exposed, and has come to be seen as indivisible from the power relations of its producers through these very acts science has been kept separate from the rest of history and science itself exalted. As a result, scant attention has been paid to the role and the ramifications of science in common cultu_e among common people (in spite of all the works whose titles explicitly link science with culture and society).[2] As yet, we have hardly passed beyond the recognition that "the little men and women in the French and Industrial Revolution who are so convincingly and sympathetically treated by Albert Soboul, George Rudé, Louis Chevalier, and E. P. Thompson, have not yet found a counterpart in the history of science."[3] How science actually functioned in society, at what levels, when, and by what means, and with what force, we have scarely begun to consider. What people really thought of science and how they used it are questions that have been raised and recognized as "every bit as historically important as science as scientists conceive of it," but the answers to these questions have not been forthcoming.[4] For all the professed concern with science as "the dominant force in designing the psychological and metaphysical basis of our politics,"[5] it is surprising, too, how little interest has been shown in the design process itself – least of all for the early nineteenth century when science began to outstrip religion as the major cultural force. The current literature rarely passes beyond the assumption that science and technology rendered people's thought secular and scientistic. Where it has not been boldly reasserted that the mass of mankind were simply the dupes of a stern training by rationalist intellectuals,[6] this presumption for the most part has remained unquestioned. Thus to those outside the subdiscipline of the history of science, it often appears that between the sociology of collective behavior and the history of scientific ideas there exists a veritable wasteland.[7]

This study endeavors to reclaim a part of that wasteland through the examination of phrenology, the nineteenth century's most popular and popularized "science" and one of its most fecund in the period preceding Darwin. But this study does not attempt the impossible – directly to measure the impact of this knowledge on consciousness and behavior. No less than politics, economics, or religion, science has never existed in a vacuum as a separate force. Like other ideas, the impact of scientific ones can only be quantified at the expense of reducing them and their holders to the status of passive things. Partly this is the reason why "cultural" figures in our title: as Theodor Adorno suggested, "culture ... might be precisely that condition that excludes a mentality capable of measuring it" – a sentiment perhaps to be read into Mary Douglas's definition of culture as "a blank space, a highly respected, empty pigeonhole."[8]

More specifically, "cultural" is used here to denote concern with the normative assumptions contained within and conveyed through scientific knowledge. Since our interest in this aspect of science is closely bound to the way in which phrenological knowledge is perceived in this study, it is appropriate to begin with some description of the subject matter itself.

In outline this is easily accomplished. As developed at the end of the eighteenth century by Franz Joseph Gall,‡ a successful Viennese physician, phrenology (or "craniology," as he preferred to call it) was a combined theory of brain and a science of character based on the following tenets: (i) the brain is the organ of the mind; (ii) the brain is not a homogeneous unity but an aggregate of mental organs; (iii) these mental organs or physical faculties are topographically localized into specific functions; (iv) other factors being equal, the relative size of any one of the mental organs can be taken as an index to that organ's power of manifestation; and (v) since the skull ossifies over the brain during infant development, external craniological means can be used to diagnose the internal state of the mental faculties.[9]

Though only the last aspect of Gall's doctrine is popularly recalled today, in its context two centuries ago all of the parts of the doctrine and the system as a whole excited serious attention. As historians of medicine have pointed out, Gall's doctrine represented a significant departure from earlier writings on the brain and its functions since, for the first time, questions on mind and brain were reduced to the single domain of dynamic physiology and biology. Although, as Gall himself was aware, both the notion of the brain as the organ of the mind and the idea of cerebral localization could be found in antiquity,[10] Gall was the first to treat mental phenomena as well as the human passions (previously located in the heart and elsewhere) as purely organic problems of neuroanatomy and neurophysiology. And he was the first to insist that the localization of brain functions needed to be determined by empirical, naturalistic studies of humans in society and of species in nature. If one traces the concept of "function" as applied to psychological and social phenomena back from its late-nineteenth-century and twentieth-century uses, one finds its source in the writings of Gall and his followers.[11] Further assuring Gall's place in the history of medicine was his pioneering work in neuroanatomy. Not until the publication of his *Atlas* in 1810 was it clearly established that "the cerebral convolutions were not haphazard coils, like so much bowel or marcaroni, but structures with an establishing patterning."[12]

A part of what renders Gall's achievement historically complex, however, is that his doctrine did not depend upon his anatomical and physiological researches. As a behaviorist psychology premised on innate mental faculties, phrenology drew credibility merely from the association with anatomy and physiology, as it did from Gall's extensive neuropathological and physiognomical correlations. Gall's own description of his experimental method makes this clear:

I assembled a number of persons at my house, drawn from the lowest classes and engaged in various occupations, such as fiacre driver, street porter and so on. I gained their confidence and induced them to speak frankly by giving them money and having wine and beer distributed to them. When I saw that they were favourably disposed, I urged them to tell me everything they knew about one another, both their good and their bad qualities, and I carefully examined their heads. This was the origin of the craniological chart which was seized upon so avidly by the public; even artists took it over and distributed a large number among the public in the form of masks of all kinds.[13]

Thus, although phrenology's anatomical and physiological premises gave it a more scientific profile than either of those other Viennese products, mesmerism and psychoanalysis, it would be quite mistaken to infer from the fact that modern physiological psychology can be traced back to Gall, that Gall's craniology and its renown had any strict dependence on his medical achievements.

Nor was Gall original in attempting to relate character to physiognomical signs or "signatures." Aristotelian links were in fact explicit in the docrine's retention of the four descriptive classical humors as a starting point for human classifications. Though Gall's hagiographers made much of the fact that at the tender age of nine, Gall had made the observation that his schoolmates with good memories were those who also had large and protruding eyes, they overlooked that straightforward physiognomical correlations with character were common in the folk culture of Gall's time. Within that tradition were physiognomical writings of Gall's contemporary, the Swiss priest Johann Caspar Lavater (1741–1801), which became popular toward the end of the century. Lavater, though an Evangelical and a firm believer in miracles, was also a student of medicine, and it is worth noting that among the ideas he maintained was that of the cavity of the skull being

visibly fitted to the mass of substances it contains and follow[ing] their growth at every age of human life. Thus, the exterior form of the brain, which imprints itself perfectly on the internal surface of the skull, is, at the same time, the model of the contours of the exterior surface.[14]

Lavater, too, based his theory on extensive empirical observations, though, unlike Gall (whose doctrine was independent of Lavater's), he neither attempted, nor was popularly regarded as having attempted, to *account for* the aspects of human nature that he correlated with facial signs. As an early nineteenth-century commentator remarked, physiognomy never pretended "to tell what were the original propensities of man, much less to indicate the simple fundamental faculties of our nature."[15]

Gall's concern with accounting for human nature rendered phrenology not just another doctrine of character, nor even merely a theory of brain but, ultimately, a secular means for assessing and deliberating on man's place in society and nature. Whether or not one took the short step from the idea of the brain as the organ of the mind to the idea of mind as material brain, Gall's reduction of mental phenomena to functions of organized matter could be seen to undermine the Cartesian rationale for the existence of God by undermining the dichotomy between mind and matter or body and mind. According to the mechanical philosophy of Decartes, mind was sentient, as proven through the act of thinking and consciousness; unlike dead matter animated by the mere collision of particles, sentient life necessitated an immaterialist principle, which the mechanists attributed to God.[16] Indirectly, mind proved God. Conversely, to render mind merely a part of the body or merely the function of organized matter was to eliminate the need for the immaterialist principle, hence to spurn God's unique gift to man and, by extension, to spurn God Himself. Gall tried to cover himself on this point (see: Chapter 1) but his doctrine was widely perceived by others as entirely materialist and God-denying.

Which is not to say that in these matters Gall was entirely on his own, no more than he was on his own in seeking to formulate a science of physiognomy.[17] Materialistic approaches to nature were common in the eighteenth century, and even approaches to the brain in these terms were not unknown. Indeed, at the same time as Gall was conducting his researches, the French *idéologues* were also endeavoring to treat mental phenomena in purely physiological terms. Cabanis was among those at the time intent on finding a science relating outward appearances to inward natures.[18] Gall differed from the *idéologues* in that he held to an innatist psychology that was directed against sensationalist or Lockean–environmentalist psychology, and he differed further in that he drew upon and elaborated a neurology that conflicted with that relied upon by the *idéologues*. But in terms of the underlying objectives of his naturalistic researches into brain, Gall and his theory were as much the products of their time as the works of the *idéologues*, the intellectual climate of the late eighteenth century being one in which there was a flourishing interest in the relations between brain and behavior, especially social behavior.[19]

What made Gall's doctrine outstanding was thus neither its approach to the brain nor its underlying motives; rather, it was the fact that it rendered both approach and motive impossible to overlook. Like Galileo's outspoken shattering of the already-cracked Aristotelian cosmology of the early seventeenth century, Gall's doctrine forced unequivocal enagement with materialistic and naturalistic approaches and intuitions by fastening attention to them. Under any circumstances his was the kind of doctrine to excite popular interest on the one hand and to bring down the weight of conventional authority on the other, and in the late eighteenth century and early nineteenth century this response was virtually guaranteed. By its aspiration comprehensively to explain human nature on the basis of a mapped-out hierarchical division of mental labor; by its promise to provide at a stroke practical solutions to the mysteries of character, personality, talent or its lack, crime and madness (hence, potentially, directly to manipulate and control behavior); and by its ready comprehension to even the meanest intellect, Gall's doctrine beckoned into its orbit every one of the social, psychological, intellectual, political and religious concerns that had been aggravated and heightened by the conditions of rapid and pervasive social and economic change. To those open to its possibilities it seemed to offer a revolutionary new basis for conceiving and hence organizing social life. Resembling popular versions of ethology and psychoanalysis and even some forms of Marxism in our own time (though far more popular and available than any of these), phrenology became for some a dogma of enlightenment and promise as well as a refreshing river in which to wash away or drown confusions and disorientations. However, in large part because of this popularity and dogmatism, Gall's ideas appeared to others as the greatest charlatanry of the age, deluding the public and leading them to vain and dangerous expectations. But whether accepted or rejected, totally or in part, and whether on specific social, political, scientific, medical, philosophical, religious, or psychological grounds, phrenology raised the abstraction of "the mind of man" to new heights. In the period between the Age of Reason and the Age of Capital it was this abstraction, whether as object or target, that became the focus for struggles of power.

Although Gall's own writings were hardly consulted in Britain – his *Anatomie et Physiologie* (1810–19) not being translated into English until 1835[20] – his ideas were known in Britain at least since 1800 when the *Medical and Physical Journal* described them as "deserving the attention of the curious." Thereafter, in a context of acute postrevolutionary shock and urban–industrial future shock, his ideas became widely diffused and vigorously debated in nearly every medical, literary, and popular journal.[21] From the mid-1810s impetus was given to the spread of his ideas in Britain through the popularization carried out by J. G. Spurzheim‡ and, subsequently, by George Combe.‡ Spurzheim, a former student and collaborator with Gall who parted company with him before coming to Britain in 1813, and Combe, an upwardly mobile Edinburgh lawyer, were primarily interested in the applications of phrenology to the reform of society and morals. Without substantially altering the doctrine in any of its essentials, they elaborated it differently from Gall in order to have it appeal to an expanding population of practical-minded improvers. Thus, as dozens of scholarly publications testify, phrenology was to become in the English-speaking world an important vehicle of liberal ideology, helping to effect major reforms in penology, education, and the treatment of the insane.[22] Luminaries of early Victorian culture, such as Samuel Coleridge, John Stuart Mill, Harriet Martineau, Samuel Smiles, George Henry Lewes, Auguste Comte, and Henri de Saint Simon, became in some respects phrenology's intellectual guardians. To the sociology and psychology of Herbert Spencer, the evolutionary biology of Robert Chambers and Alfred Russel Wallace, and the physical anthropology of James Hunt and Pierre Paul Broca, phrenology was to be fundamental. In English literature, too, phrenology was to leave its mark, especially in the writing of Charlotte Brontë, Edward Bulwer-Lytton, George Eliot, Edgar Allan Poe, Walt Whitman, Nathaniel Hawthorne, and Herman Melville – many of whom have been studied (if somewhat apologetically) specifically from the viewpoint of their interest in phrenology.[23]

By any standards, phrenology's contribution to the various intellectual and social facets of early Victorian culture must be considered impressive. But like tracing contemporary aspects of neurology and psychology back to Gall, there are hazards in pursuing phrenology in terms simply of its contributions to the fragmented priorities of modern academics. On the one hand, this pursuit burdens the subject anachronistically, while on the other, it obfuscates phrenology's enduring and less obvious political significance as a body of knowledge standing at the apex of the search for the truth about man's place in nature during the period of the most dramatic changes in social relations and values since the seventeenth century. Social histories of nineteenth-century phrenology that conceive of the subject only in terms of a reform movement likewise do little to recover the wider temporal and political significance of the knowledge. To be sure, there was an important phrenology "movement" in the nineteenth century that had its own journals, societies, following, and areas of "influence"; but when studied discretely as such, phrenology as a science of human nature remains essentially epiphenomenal to society, or as something foreign to it and merely affecting it.[24]

Although this study is designed to provide a comprehensive history of phrenology, it is motivated and informed by a different conception of phrenology's historical value – one in which the knowledge and the society it inhabited are seen as part and parcel of each other. Accordingly, with an emphasis on phrenology as a body of natural knowledge, this study looks up through the phrenological conceptions of man, mind, and nature to draw out the nature of their relation to interconnected economic, political, and religious realms.

Uniquely, phrenology invites this approach, and for the same reasons that once made it seem either an antiquarian topic beneath serious historical consideration or suited only for fragmented insights into modernity. Because phrenology is poised between the intellectual boundaries that have come to be erected between science and pseudoscience, nature and culture, science and society, it provides the incentive to expose and evaluate those boundaries. Phrenology is doubly illuminating in this respect because phrenologists themselves actually popularized these demarcations, responding to contemporary opposition to the knowledge as socially "invented." Hence through the history of this discarded scientific knowledge of human nature we can hold a mirror not only to our present image of science, but also to the making of its boundaries.

Because phrenology now appears in many respects as a Dickensian caricature of science, its study can also magnify both the way in which social and ideological meanings are implicit in science and the way in which these meanings are redefined according to social contexts. Received in Britain as a scientific system of exaggerated symbols, phrenology demonstrates how these symbols may serve as alternative codified renderings of social structures and relations (i.e., as "mediations"). As will be seen in Chapter 4, of the many ways in which phrenology helps reveal the expression of social interests through science, none is so clear as the symbol of the head and its internal mapping.

It has not passed unnoticed that phrenology is a useful illustration for the social reinterpretation of the history of science. In a series of essays, Steven Shapin has made brilliant use of phrenology's career in Edinburgh to demonstrate the way in which the social context governs not only the deployment of science but also the perception of specific natural phenomena.[25] Shapin's is all the more convincing a demonstraton for being staged specifically for an audience of historians who conceive of "the social" as merely an additional factor to be inserted into any historical explanation or evaluation of scientific knowledge.

Here, Chapters 1 through 3 are intended partly as an amplification of the kind of interest in and approach to phrenology outlined by Shapin. Throughout, however, the underlying priority is the reverse of Shapin's and, in Chapters 4 through 8, the historical objectives are quite different. Primarily, this book is written for those who have tended to conceive of "the scientific" as merely an additional "factor" to be inserted into social accounts of historical reality and who, moreover, have tended to regard the pre-Darwinian period as one in which these scientific factors figured only incidentally in popular thought and culture. Phrenology's extensive popularization and popularity among common people in the nineteenth century (including popularity among not-so-common artisan radicals) allows the condescensions wrought by the entrepreneurs of the "Darwin industry" to be undermined. The thousands of phrenological publications of the early nineteenth century and the existence of hundreds of phrenological lecturers make clear the naïvity of considering "Darwin" the magic password to Victorian science. These sources reveal that long before "Darwinism" the sluicegates had been opened for the lay application of scientific naturalism to all manner of social, moral, political, and evolutionary thought. While Darwin, just back from his voyage on the *Beagle* in 1838, was starting his first notebook on the "Transformation of Species," the public and theological–philosophical state of mind for the eventual reception of his ideas had already been well prepared by phrenological rationalists and was continuing to be groomed by them. The leading social and moral elaboration of phrenology, Combe's *Constitution of Man* (discussed in Chapter 4), had been in print for over a decade and had already sold over forty thousand copies in a cheap edition available since 1835. Historical fuss over Thomas Huxley's confrontation with Bishop Wilberforce in Oxford in 1860 has obscured that, overall, the amount of intellectual and emotional heat generated by Combe's book far surpassed that raised by the publication in 1859 of Darwin's *Origin of Species*; it has also obscured that the anonymous publication in 1844 of the *Vestiges of the Natural History of Creation* (by Combe's friend and fellow phrenologist Robert Chambers) raised more discussion than the *Origin*. Yet the *Vestiges* was less controversial and less read than the *Constitution of Man*.[26] Turning the historical telescope around, Darwin thus appears less a starting point than a further manifestation and source of final adjustment to public controversy over scientific naturalism. His work becomes, as Owen Chadwick among others has suggested, not a "cause" but a further "occasion" of Enlightenment rationalism.[27]

Not that phrenology was the only purveyor of naturalism and rationalism in Britain prior to Darwin (nor that that was all that phrenology purveyed). Contemporary students and popularizers of geology, botany, and physiology and, more generally, Benthamism assisted in the cause. Phrenologists were merely some of the most visible and vociferous agents for this kind of thinking in the early nineteenth century. To them can be attributed much of the reversal of the earlier reaction (by Malthus and others) to the French prerevolutionary faith in the inevitability of science and progress. Yet popular phrenology did more than help reopen the moderate and decidedly unromantic rationalist–humanist faith in science and progress that had existed in eighteenth-century Britain: Its particular accomplishment was to open and accelerate that faith among persons whose rank and station in life, or whose political outlook, had hitherto sheltered them from it. To this public, which was generally less aware of and less concerned than were their elders with the theological niceties of natural philosophical discussion, the phrenological rendering of mental action into the category of a natural *thing* governed over by *natural laws* was the chief means to the perception of science as a universal deterministic, or natural causative, cosmology.

It is with this perception, rather than with the defense of the claim for phrenology's role in the making of that perception, that this study is concerned. The claim for phrenology's historical role will, hopefully, justify itself in the course of exploring the ideological nature of the perception. Which brings us back to the title of this book, for to address the problem of people's entry through popular science into a particular set of perceptions of reality is to deal with more than merely the social deployment of science and with more than merely the characterizing of and accounting for its popularization. In league with a definition of culture as that which informs "the good and bad, the permissible and forbidden, the beautiful and ugly, the sacred and profane,"[28] it is, at root, to probe into people's renegotiation of reality and into the effects of that reshaping upon social and personal consciousness. To focus on that for the socially diffuse and ideologically complex events of the Industrial Revolution, the historical pursuit of phrenology provides us with a wide and versatile lens.

PART I

Historiography

What hand can grasp that which dwells in the *head*, beneath the skull of man! what finger of flesh and blood, reach from the outward shell, the abyss of powers that repose or ferment within? The deity itself has covered this sacred mount, the Olympus or Lebanon of men with a grove, the usual shade of its mysteries, to be the abode, the laboratory of its most recluse energies. We tremble to think that orb circumscribed, in which a creation dwells, whence one flash that emerges from the chaos may adorn and irradiate, or desolate and crush a world.

Johann Gottfried Herder, "Testimonials in Favour of Physiognomy," in J. C. Lavater, *Physiognomical Fragments* (Leipzig, 1775–8), as trans. in *Analytical Review*, 5 (1789), 457

1

From out the cerebral well

Gall came out of the cerebral well, and looking upon the surface found that it was a landscape, inhabited by human natures in a thousand tents, all dwelling according to passions, faculties and powers. So much was gained by the first man who came to the surface, where nature speaks by representations; but it is lost again at the point where cerebral anatomy begins.

James John Garth Wilkinson, *The Human Body and Its Connexion with Man* (1851), p. 22

Truth is undoubtedly the sort of error that cannot be refuted because it was hardened into an unalterable form in the long baking process of history. Moreover, the question of truth, the right it appropriates to refute error and oppose itself to appearance, the manner in which it developed ... does this not form a history, the history of an error we call truth?

Michael Foucault, "Nietzsche, Genealogy, History," in *Language, Counter-Memory, Practice* (Oxford, 1977), p. 144

Historical interest in phrenology is almost as old as phrenology itself, and in many ways its study is as revealing. Pursued as a topic in its own right through its own textual sources, the history of this historical interest is nearly as complex as phrenology's actual history. Not surprisingly, this history (of the historical interest) also bears a diversity of orientations similar to the diverse uses of phrenology in its day. At one extreme are serious philosophical ruminations on the origins of physiological psychology, such as those by J. D. Morell (1840), George Henry Lewes (1857), and Frederick Lange (1881), which were written when the dust had hardly settled on the initial disputes over the scientific claims of phrenology;[1] at the other extreme are trivial and anecdotal pieces on craniology canvased by popular commercial magazines as well as by antiquarian journals of science and medicine; while in between these two extremes are the various informative and mostly recent social histories of phrenology and phrenologists.

But if the secondary literature on phrenology is disparate in its orientation, it shares, from the reader's point of view, a common interpretative problem, namely, that of deciding where social and ideological interests end, and where, if at all, detached historical analysis and reflection begin. Before we enter into the examination of phrenology as a social and ideological knowledge resource in the early nineteenth century, it is as well to examine the way in which these histories of phrenology have themselves served implicitly and explicitly as knowledge resources for social and ideological interests. Since our ulterior motive in this chapter is to establish the need for a sociological approach to past belief and disbelief in the truth of phrenology, the consideration of other treatments of phrenology's history can usefully serve not only to beckon and set our own approach into relief, but also, to a degree, to presage the argument for the social and ideological relativity of the veracity of phrenology in the early nineteenth century. The consideration of previous historical treatments can also provide us with a means of presenting historical and biographical information essential to our subsequent discussion.

WHIGS AND REVISIONISTS

Until very recently, phrenology was approached historically in either one of two ways. Though not mutually exclusive, these approaches can in most cases be distinguished. For the sake of convenience we can refer to them as "Whig" and "Revisionist."

The Whig interpretation of phrenology holds true to the criterion for which Herbert Butterfield initially assigned the label in *The Whig Interpretation of History* (1931). To a degree difficult to exaggerate, its reading of the past backward from the present, and its maintenance of the view that nothing can be true in the past that conflicts with what is known in the present, makes it abound with condescension, oversimplification, and overt moral intonation. Although ever since Butterfield wrote his pamphlet Whig accounts of phrenology have been receding, they have by no means ceased to exist. Most frequently they are found in the "after-hours" writing of persons whose expertise lies in science and medicine but whose authority is felt (or hoped) on that account to extend to history. Hence an emeritus professor of medicine, writing in 1977 in the *Journal of the Royal College of Physicians* on two distinguished nineteenth-century physicians who happened also to be leading advocates of phrenology, submits: "Regarding phrenology, it is indeed remarkable that men of such high intelligence should have given such nonsense any credence, but, for a time, it ensnared the nation, particularly its upper classes, and is by no means the only instance of the gullibility of the public and the medical profession."[2] That the emeritus professor has his facts wrong with respect to the popularity of phrenology only serves to highlight the smug arrogance and presumption to judge the past that characterizes Whig writing.

But this is the lesser of its shortcomings. More serious is its implicit legitimation of the view of modern science and medicine as objective and neutral. Since most Whig accounts of phrenology have been written by persons with unequivocal stakes in modern scientific knowledge, it is not surprising that their accounts lead in this direction. Indeed, many involved in modern science and medicine have written on phrenology specifically in order to defend the neutrality of science, (just as others of a similar ilk have taken to Lysenkoism and social Darwinism for this purpose). Phrenology, it has seemed to these persons, is a readily accessible example of knowledge patently "flawed" by extrascientific factors and, therefore, able effectively to be contrasted with "real" science. Circularly, by referring to "correct" science, an explanation is thought to be had for "incorrect" science. But in fact, dogmatically explaining phrenology as incorrect science or "pseudoscience" renders not an explanation of past belief in it, but rather an accumulation of scientistic capital to be expended in furthering the image of modern science and its practitioners as divested of social and ideological interests.[3]

Very often such phrenologically derived capital has been deployed rhetorically in attacking other perceived scientific bogies. The psychologist Karl Dallenbach, for instance, in an article in the *American Journal of Psychology* in 1955 sought to deride what he took to be the scientific pretentions of psychoanalysis by simply likening psychoanalysis to phrenology. More recently, a similar attempt to deploy phrenology against the "olympian glibness" of psychoanalysis as a part of a broader project to carve a sharp distinction between science and myth has been made by the Nobel

Prize–winning scientist turned literateur Sir Peter Medawar. The critic and biologist Steven Rose, too, in an effort to undermine the scientific validity of intelligence testing, has twice in a recent essay singled out the protagonist Hans Eysenck as operating in "the manner of a nineteenth century phrenologist," as if by this comparison Eysenck's credibility would be demolished. Apparently forgotten by Rose is that his opponent has already played this card: In his popular works on the facts and fictions in psychology Eysenck praised Dallenbach's article and justified his own scientificity against the likes of Rose by drawing the exact same contrast with phrenology.[4]

Important to note about these uses and counteruses of phrenology is not the obvious points their deployers have wished to score. Rather, it is the way these deployments have covertly served to legitimate the framework in which the scoring has been conducted – the dichotomized framework of fact–value, science–myth, science–society, nature–culture, science–scientism, and science-ideology. These demarcations have become so ingrained in modern thought that it is seldom recognized by general historians (let alone by those whose expertise lies in science) how they constitute a central part of a historically contingent, humanly created metaphysic – a metaphysic that ever since the early ninteenth-century writing of Comte has tended to go by the name of "positivism."[5] While it is interesting that Comte himself drew heavily on Gall's phrenology in sharpening his distinction between the "metaphysical" and the "scientific" stages of a discipline's development (see: Chapter 4), the origins of the dichotomy extend much further back in history. As Everett Mendelsohn among others has tried to make clear, the process of identifying certain bodies of knowledge as "incorrect" (because of their having unquantitative human, social, or metaphysical dimensions) in order to establish the impression of *other* bodies of knowledge as value-transcendent touchstones of truth was "socially imposed and self-consciously accepted" during the emergence of the capitalist order in the seventeenth century.[6] It was then, amid the expansion of the new quantifiable system of knowing external nature and, some would argue, simultaneously the "emergence into a position of dominance of a class defined by its role as controllers of the labour process," that hermeticism, alchemy, and magic (the internal forms of knowing) were driven underground as deviant and countercultural.[7] The origins of the metaphysic of separating science or the new knowledge of external nature from everything that might transcend the political authority being based upon it was thus part and parcel of the process of rationalizing and legitimizing the newly altered social order and its intellectual controls. As George Lukács pointed out as long ago as 1923, modern science and its methodology were the chief instruments in reifying and making to appear as natural and objective or nonmetaphysical the social relations upon which modern science was reared.[8] Through the development of modern science the power relationships of capitalist society were concealed. Thus, as abbreviated forcefully in the dictum of R. M. Young: Modern science "*is* social relations," or *is* the social relations embedded in its historical origins.[9]

Considered from this perspective, those seeking directly or indirectly to legitimate the value-free wisdom of modern science by drawing upon phrenology as an instance of socially infiltrated knowledge must be seen as engaged in nothing less than an ideological campaign. In forgetting that the science–pseudoscience split was the active creation of intellectuals in a specific socioeconomic context, evaluations of phrenological knowledge, or evaluative deployments of it, only further conceal the subjectively "objectified" terrain of capitalist social relations. As we will see, this ideological campaign is a part of the same one that in the nineteenth century was waged by the bourgeois phrenologists themselves when they attempted to separate out a "pure" version of their science from an ostensibly "corrupt" version and when they militantly attacked their opponents in the establishment as mere "metaphysicians." If anyone is to be reckoned as "acting in the manner of a nineteenth-century phrenologist," therefore it is not he or she whose work happens (or is hoped) to be ethically out of fashion, but rather all those who aspire to capitalize on the beleagured doctrine of skulls by flogging positivist interpretations of it.

On the face of it, the whole basis of the Whig account of phrenology has been undermined by Revisionist accounts written by professional historians of society and medicine.[10] Reacting to the avoidance of serious historical discussion of the subject, these historians have performed a good service by showing that in its context phrenology had considerable depth and far-reaching sig-

nificance at intellectual and popular levels. Yet it cannot be said
that in challenging the obvious ethnocentricism of Whig accounts
Revisionists have succeeded in undermining the less obvious positivist terrain of phrenology's study. On the contrary: Far more
concerned with the writing of accurately contextualized history
for its own sake, than with considering the social–metaphysical
implications of the Whigs' approach to science, Revisionists too
have inadvertently validated that terrain and its constitutive social
relations. By focusing on phrenology's role as a sociomedical
"movement" and leaving unquestioned and unexamined the nature of the knowledge itself, Revisionists for the most part have
produced only partial studies of phrenology as a "scientism."[11]
That is, mainly by offering insights into only the social uses and
functions supposedly extrapolated from the science, they (like those
who have written on the nature of social Darwinism without at
the same time discussing the social nature of Darwin's thought)
have left intact and thereby helped to sustain the metaphysics of
distinguishing between "pure" and "socially abused" knowledge.

The implicit positivism of Revisionist accounts becomes explicit
where they attempt to explain the rise and decline of the phrenology "movement" in the 1820s and 1830s. For this they accept
in part what Whigs have always taken as self-explanatory: that
phrenology was a "fad." Hence to varying degrees Revisionists
too have evaded social explanation through social description.
However, by focusing especially on the more serious-minded advocates of the science, Revisionists reject the Whigs' overtly condescending view that *all* believers in phrenology were naïve and
gullible followers of fashion. As they see it, the rise of the phrenology movement is in large measure to be explained by the fact
that in its context phrenology was at least a quasi-legitimate science. After all, many contemporary critics of phrenology in science
and medicine accepted *some* parts of Gall's doctrine. Revisionists
then go on to explain the decline of the phrenology movement in
its elitist intellectual form (in the late 1830s and 1840s) partly in
terms of an exhausted fad, and partly in terms of a growth of
knowledge that ultimately pushed phrenology from the scientific
stage. Thus Revisionist accounts of phrenology, insofar as they
touch on "scientific truth," are really only slightly more sophisticated versions of the Whig's "propaganda of the victors." Like
Whigs, Revisionists believe that one-time proponents of phren-

ology eventually "came to their senses" through the inevitable progress of science.[12]

Actually, it was only through the advance of neurophysiological research in the second half of the nineteenth century that some aspects of phrenology became scientifically credible for the first time. It was in 1861, in a famous session of the Anthropological Society of Paris, that Pierre Broca (1824–80) displayed his discovery of the *circonvolution de language*. After this, through subsequent observations, Broca was to prove that the posterior part of the third frontal convolution of the brain was indispensable to articulate speech. Considering that he had set out to disprove the phrenologists, it is a striking irony that "Broca's convolution," as it is known today, was located where Gall had placed the seat of the faculty of language. This coincidence aside, Broca's discovery confirmed the general validity of the phrenological concept of localized brain function and greatly accelerated further research into it.[13] The work of J. Hughlings Jackson, John Bucknill, James Crichton-Browne, David Ferrier, and Charles Sherrington at the end of the nineteenth century in effect confirmed basic phrenological principles. Crichton-Browne could write in 1924 that "the phrenologists were right, ... we are all phrenologists today ... for we have come to accept all the cardinal principles upon which the phrenologists insisted. Why, even their weakest point – their skull doctrine ... has been made good."[14] As contemporary neurophysiologists are well aware, when it comes to discussing the structure of the cerebral cortex the influence of Gall and the phrenologists still persists.[15]

Far, then, from being pushed off the scientific stage in the late nineteenth century, phrenology was actually pushed onto it. But what challenges the Revisionist historical schema of phrenology's rise and decline is that in being thus "scientifically" advanced, phrenology was not in any way advanced socially or scientistically. Though some late Victorians heralded the new scientific findings as the basis for a new phrenological movement, their efforts went almost entirely unrewarded.[16] The only popular phrenology that survived with any strength into the twentieth century was that still to be found on the piers of Blackpool, Brighton, and Morecambe until the Second World War: character-reading and fortune-telling from bumps on the head.

The career of phrenology in the latter part of the nineteenth century thus highlights an incongruity between phrenology as a science and phrenology as a subject of social relevance that is left unexplained by both Whigs and Revisionists. But it is not just the career of phrenology in the latter part of the century that posits this incongruity requiring explanation. For the earlier part of the century, too, a discrepancy can be seen to exist – a discrepancy based on the inverse of the above relation between phrenology's attributed veracity and its scientistic inutility. It is appropriate to spell this out at this point in order both to meet the needs of chronology and to establish the need for seeking (in the following two chapters) historical understanding based other than on the truth–utility schema adhered to by Whig historians and reproduced in part by Revisionists.

PHRENOLOGY'S BRITISH RECEPTION

Far from being regarded as a wholly credible science earlier in the nineteenth century, phrenology from the commencement of its career in Britain was often seen as pseudoscientific and pseudo-philosophical. In one of the earliest notices of the science, that by John Yelloly, M.D., in the *Monthly Review* in 1802, a lasting precedent was set with the dismissal of the science as "visionary."[17] In a reaction not unlike that to Methodism in the eighteenth century, other journals concurred with the view that phrenology was spread by harebrained enthusiasts and crafty imposters who naturally appealed to the simple, the eccentric, the curious, and the gullible. It was the latter, according to the *Literary Journal* in 1805, who flocked to Dr. Gall's lectures on the Continent, fondly imagining that they had "found a key to very great discoveries with respect to the abilities of mankind."[18] Although the view of Gall's doctrine as whimsical and wild temporarily underwent change among some medical men in 1808 when Gall and Spurzheim presented their *Memoir* on the brain and nervous system to the National Institute of France,[19] the general impression of Gall as a "philosophical charlatan" was not readily altered in the newspapers and periodical press. Before 1820 phrenology was regarded with disdain in the *Edinburgh Medical and Surgical Journal*; *London Medical Respository*; *British Critic*; *Monthly Critical Gazette*; *Critical Journal*; *Literary Journal*; the *Monthly, Quarterly, Augustan, Eclectic,* and

Edinburgh reviews; the *Gentleman's, New Monthly,* and *Blackwood's* magazines; and the *Literary Gazette,* to mention only the most widely circulated. In their collective wisdom the science was everything from crude, shallow, puerile, dull, dogmatic, absurd, foolish, and extravagant to a scientific farce and the most frontless piece of charlatanry that the age had produced, while the "cunning craniologers" who were beginning to roam the country were seen as quacks, empirics, manipulating imposters, and itinerant mountebanks to be looked upon "as rather knaves than fools."[20] This same impression of the science as "a sick man's dream" (as Bentham once dismissed it) could be had through the visual puns in George Cruikshank's *Phrenological Illustrations* (1826) or the grotesque caricatures in the style of Hogarth's "Physiognomists" drawn by E. F. Lambert and R. Cocking, among others.[21] For those with a liking for satiric rhymes and doggerel there was "Craniology" by Thomas Hood and "Phrenology" by Charles Tennyson (both published in 1827)[22] or *The Craniad: A Serio-Comic Poem* (1816) and the ninety-page *Craniad; or, Spurzheim Illustrated* (1817) assumed to be written by the editor of the *Edinburgh Review,* Francis Jeffrey, with the assistance of John Gordon. A member of the City Philosophical Society produced *Craniology Burlesqued in Three Comic Lectures by a Friend to Common Sense* (1816). In the same vein, as early as 1805, there appeared Isaac D'Israeli's "A Dissertation on Skulls: Lavater, Camper, Blumenbach, and Gall";[23] later delights including *Encephalology* (1824),[24] John Trotter's pseudonymous *Travels in Phrenologasto* (1825), the *Metropolitan Quarterly Magazine's* "A Phrenopatetic History" (1826), and the Wesleyan preacher James Everett's pseudonymous *The Head-piece; or, Phrenology Opposed to Divine Revelation by James the Less* (1828) with its sequel *A Helmet for the Head-Piece; or, Phrenology Incompatible with Reason, by Daniel the Seer* (1828). As late as 1830, shortly after Richard Cobden (later a patron of phrenology) had had his dramatic spoof, *The Phrenologist,* rejected by Covent Garden Theatre,[25] the *Edinburgh Literary Journal* commented on that theater's production of Thomas Wade's *The Phrenologists: A Farce in Two Acts:* "Though phrenology be an excellent farce in itself . . . it is not the cause of excellent farces in others."[26] In short, as the *Gentleman's Magazine* prefaced its comments on the subject in 1806, there was considerable agreement that

The very top
And dignity of Folly we attain
By studious search and labour of the brain.[27]

Whig historians might well have justified attaching the label "pseudoscience" to phrenology on the basis of these satires and lampoons. But there has been no need. For reaffirming the uniform wisdom of modern science a far more compelling, seemingly authoritative, body of literature exists: the extensive scientific and medically based writings that coexisted with and fed the lampoons. In these were incorporated the appropriately phrased negative statements on the science by some of the most eminent scientists and philosophers of the time.

One of the first of such statements was that which appeared in the *Edinburgh Review* in April 1803.[28] Occasioned by Charles Villers's published letter to George Cuvier on Gall's doctrine, it was written by Thomas Brown, subsequently the holder of the chair of moral philosophy in Edinburgh. Although in 1803 Brown (1778–1820) was just completing the requirements for the Edinburgh M.D., he had already distinguished himself as a serious critic of the philosophy of mind of Erasmus Darwin.[29] Like most of the articles in the *Edinburgh Review*, Brown's was dispassionate in tone, giving it the impression of being written with no other purpose than that of furthering the intellectual integrity of a journal fast becoming the Koran of the educated public. This impression was supported by Brown's dismissal of the charge of materialism that had been brought against the doctrine. Referring to materialism as the doctrine relating mental states to bodily organs, Brown saw no reason why Gall's dividing up of the mental faculties should make him more of a materialist than anyone else who believed in the mind–body dualism. Though Gall in fact endeavored to be agnostic on the question of materialism, this was not known by Brown, nor acknowledged by any of his contemporaries.[30] Moreover, Brown himself, unlike most subsequent antiphrenologists, had a strong attachment to the ideas of certain French materialists.[31] It was thus in his interest to suggest that the accusation against Gall's doctrine of implicit materialism or denial of the soul was based primarily on a religious emotionalism that should have no place in serious rational discourse.[32] A truly intellectual critique of the doctrine, he claimed, must be grounded entirely upon an examination of its actual philosophical and scientific pretentions, and it was to these that he duely turned.

Philosophically, he criticized Gall for having, through anatomy, physiology, and pathology, reified or lent a misplaced concreteness to the faculties of mind that in the metaphysics of Reid and Stewart were really only reflective concepts. Although 70 percent of the names Gall attached to his physiological faculties were similar to those that the Scottish Common Sense philosophers attached to their psychological concepts, Brown, unlike some modern scholars, did not accuse Gall of having stolen his nomenclature.[33] Rather, he charged him with having unwittingly denied the reflective categories of mental philosophy their rightful meaning and of having transformed those categories into discrete operational vectors located physically on the surface of the brain.[34] Of Gall's craniological speculations, Brown perceived that these were really a "species of physiognomy" stemming not from the anatomical principles that Gall – to his credit – had brought forward, but merely from "inference from the inspection of the skull." The physiological premises, too, and all the evidence brought forward in support of them left Brown with the impression that while there was much that was sound in principle in Gall's theory, far more was deeply flawed. After examining it all, he concluded that the doctrine was simply "not very convincing."

Also arriving at the pseudoscientificity of phrenology on the basis of similar seemingly commonsensical and universal logic and reasoning was the article on Gall and Spurzheim's doctrine in the *Edinburgh Review* twelve years later. Occasioned chiefly by the much-discussed publication of Spurzheim's *The Physiognomical System of Drs Gall and Spurzheim* (1815), this article was written by John Gordon, M.D. (1786–1818), a fellow of both the Edinburgh Royal Society and the College of Surgeons who was well on his way to becoming John Barclay's equal as a medical lecturer in Edinburgh.[35] Gordon wrote in the immediate wake of the Napoleonic Wars when Anglomania was running strong and when "materialism," as a result of the reaction to the "sensual excesses" of the French Revolution, had lost much of its acceptable association with orthodox Newtonianism and Cartesianism and had come to bear far more of an antitheistic connotation with overtones of social and political subversion.[36] Nevertheless, just as Brown's article bore no explicit indebtedness to French Enlightenment

thinking, so Gordon's article disclosed few signs of overt exploitation of anti-French, antimaterialist sentiment. His tone was much
less dispassionate than Brown's, however, and he could not resist
from remarking, for example, that Gall and Spurzheim's observations were

a collection of mere absurdities, without truth, connexion, or consistency; an incoherent rhapsody, which nothing could have induced any
man to have presented to the public, under a pretence of instructing
them, but absolute insanity, gross ignorance, or the most matchless
assurance.[37]

But it was primarily with the discrediting of the physiological and,
above all, the anatomical speculations of Gall and Spurzheim that
Gordon was concerned, and in this he serves the Whig historical
purpose well, for his highly detailed and technically involved criticisms remain undeniably persuasive. Although Gordon did not
in fact cite what was to become the most treasured piece of evidence against the craniological part of the doctrine – the existence
of the frontal sinuses that prevent all direct cranial reading in that
region of the head of supposed phrenological organs beneath – he
did raise the general problem of cranial cavities. He also took up,
and soundly refuted, the notion of a correspondence between brain
size and intellectual power; the failure of Gall and Spurzheim to
specify the physical limits of each mental faculty and to specify
the exact nature of the boundaries between them; the inadequacy
of their comparative anatomy as a means of determining their
identification and numbering of the parts of the brain; as well as
more than a dozen other substantive points. Gordon also seriously
questioned Gall and Spurzheim's method of dissection and the
thoroughness of their actual knowledge of the known structures
of the brain and nature of cerebral tissues. Turning, finally, to
their drawings of the brain, Gordon made it clear that not one of
their "views of the parts of the external or internal surface of the
brain . . . is in all respects correct; in several, the omissions are
great; in a considerable number the errors are extravagant." In all,
Gordon concluded, Gall and Spurzheim

have not added one fact to the stock of our knowledge, respecting either
the structure or the function of man . . ., [but present] such a mixture
of gross errors, extravagant absurdities, downright mistatements, and
unnecessary quotations from Scriptures, as can leave no doubt, we ap-

prehend, in the minds of honest and intelligent men, as to the real ignorance, the real hypocrisy, and the real empiricism of the authors.[38]

Gordon took his criticisms of the doctrine still further in *Observations on the Structures of the Brain, Comprising an Estimate of the
Claims of Drs Gall and Spurzheim to Discovery in the Anatomy of that
Organ*, which was published in Edinburgh two year later.[39] Thus
a year after that, in 1818, when the physiologist and savant Peter
Mark Roget came to write his entry on "Cranioscopy" for the
Supplement to the sixth edition of the *Encyclopaedia Britannica*, he
could appear as expressing the intelligent person's view of the
doctrine as "preposterous" on the basis of many of the same kinds
of evidence brought forward by Brown and Gordon. Like Brown,
Roget also wished to appear as wholly free from all "irrational"
religious prejudice. Hence at the outset of his article he asserted
that his interest was only in assessing the physiological claims of
the doctrine. Irrelevant to his purpose, he said, was the "senseless"
religious clamor against the knowledge as materialist and deter-
minist (the latter charge of an innatest psychology denying free
will having by then become common). The particulars of Roget's
article need not detain us here; it only needs to be said that, just
as in Brown's article or in the comments on phrenology in 1824
by the Regius Professor of Medicine at Oxford, John Kidd, Roget
singled out as subjects for praise the physiological premises of
phrenology and the cerebral anatomical methodology of Gall and
Spurzheim, but did so in the midst of a total condemnation of the
theory of cerebral localization and the attendant craniology.[40]
Thereby, Roget conveyed the idea that some parts of Gall and
Spurzheim's doctrine – notably the parts that were least socially
contentious – were more legitimate or more "scientific" than others. Some basically sound physiological principles, Roget's reader
was led to believe, had unfortunately been driven to quite ridiculous lengths.

By 1842, when Roget's article was republished unaltered in the
seventh edition of the *Britannica* under the new title of "Phrenology," the authoritative backing for its opinions had expanded
impressively.[41] To Brown and Gordon's criticisms could be added
the comments on the doctrine's philosophical weaknesses and anatomical fallacies pointed out by Dugald Stewart and John Barclay
in 1821 and 1822.[42] Reference could be made to aspersions on Gall's

neuroanatomy made by Sir Everard Home in his Croonian Lecture before the Royal Society of London in 1821, to those made there by Charles Bell two years later, and to those repeated by John Kidd in his Bridgewater Treatise of 1833.[43] Reference could further be made to yet another article in the *Edinburgh Review* written in 1826 by the editor, Francis Jeffrey, in which were marshaled to great effect all the previously made philosophical, anatomical, and theological criticisms, as well as explicit antiforeign sentiments.[44] For some of the most academically rigorous strictures on phrenology, one could point to the papers by Sir William Hamilton[‡] that were delivered before the Royal Society of Edinburgh between 1825 and 1829.[45] To the same body, and to the Royal Medical Society of Edinburgh, additional criticisms were made in 1828 and 1829 by the medical upstart Thomas Stone, M.D.[46]

Roget's lack of need to alter his 1818 opinions was also reinforced by the research carried out by the French physiologists François Magendie and M. P. J. Flourens, by the Berlin physiologist Karl Rudolphi, and by the American professor of physiology at Columbia University Thomas Sewall. As well, there were the criticisms by Drs. John Bostock, James Copland, and James Cowles Prichard,[‡] and by the leading figure in the Royal Institution of London in the 1830s and 1840s, William Thomas Brande.[47] By the latter date the opposition had gained still further strength from the renunciation of phrenology by various former supporters, on the grounds, they claimed, of its "scientific" inadequacy (see: Chapter 3).

Whig historians, then, however misguided in their motives, were largely correct to call phrenology "pseudoscientific" in the sense of it being discredited knowledge in its own time. Clearly there were, as Hazlitt argued in 1829, "a thousand instances on record in which this science has been contradicted by facts."[48] The Whigs' *only* mistake, it might almost be said, was that they looked at merely one side of the coin and, in avoiding the other, were able to conclude that phrenology lacked serious historical worth. The error in this supposition becomes manifest when we turn the coin over and look to the kind of evidence that Revisionists could point to in documenting the rise of the phrenology movement.

THE MEDICAL PROFESSION AND PHRENOLOGY

For the early decades of the nineteenth century the strongest support for phrenology came from the medical profession. This is well reflected in the membership of the twenty-eight or so phrenological societies in Britain before 1840, some of which were almost wholly composed of medical men and in few of which did the medical profession represent less than one-third of the registered members. As late as 1838, after medical recruitment had fallen off, the phrenological statistician Hewett Watson[‡] could still claim with some accuracy that at least one-third of the one hundred writers on phrenology in Britain who could be identified at that time, and one-sixth of the thousand members of phrenological societies, were physicians or surgeons.[49] Support, though not always unequivocal, came from such leading medical authorities as John Abernethy, Sir Astley Cooper, William Lawrence,[50] and John Elliotson, and by the mid-1820s – after Gall had visited London and had had his lectures reported in full in *The Weekly Medico–Chirurgical & Philosophical Magazine*[51] – the most powerful medical journals of the time all came out in strong support of the science. *The Medico–Chirurgical Review* maintained that phrenology was "the most intelligible and self-consistent system of mental philosophy that has ever been presented to the contemplation of inquisitive men," and its editor, James Johnson, elsewhere publicly endorsed the science; the *British and Foreign Medical Review* gave space to several highly flattering articles on the science, and its editor, John Forbes, was a member of the council of the Phrenological Association; while the *Lancet* from the time of its founding in 1823 to 1851 devoted over six hundred pages to what it regarded as a "beautiful and useful" science, and its editor, Thomas Wakley, was a member of the London Phrenological Society (LPS) from 1824.[52]

One consequence of this coverage in the medical press was that medical students at the time had little chance of escaping the subject; not only were they to find it favorably discussed in leading journals, but also they were to find it recommended in medical texts and in many of the lectures forming a part of their courses. Indeed, by the time the first full course on phrenology in a British medical school was delivered (by the surgeon Henry Holm[‡] in London Hospital in 1832), the science had become a familiar part of medical education and the suggestion had been made to Sir Robert Peel that phrenology become an official part of medical instruction.[53] The cockney hero of medical students, John Elliotson, who founded the LPS in 1823, included discussion of the science in the many editions of his medical texts, as he also did in

THE WEEKLY

MEDICO - CHIRURGICAL & PHILOSOPHICAL
MAGAZINE.

No. III.   SATURDAY, FEBRUARY 22, 1823.   *Price 4d.*

"FLORIFERIS, UT APES, IN SALTIBUS OMNIA LIBANT
OMNIA NOS, ITIDEM, DEPASCIMUR AUREA DICTA."

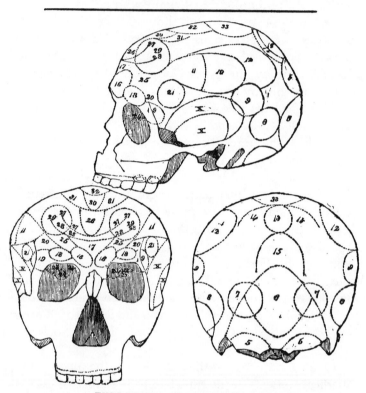

EXPLANATION OF THE PLATE.

1. Organ of the tenacity of life.—2. Of the organ of self preservation.—3. Organ of the choice of nourishment.—4. Cerebral organs of the external senses.—5. Organ of sexual gratification.—6. Organ of the reciprocal love of parents and children.—7. Organ of attachment and friendship.—8. Organ of courage.—9. Organ of the instinct to assassination.—10. Unknown organs.—11. Organ of cunning.—12. Organ of circumspection.—13. Organ of the instinct of rising in rank or estimation.—14. Organ of the love of glory.—15. Organ of the love of truth.—16. Organ of the sense of locality.—17. Organ of the sense for collecting and retaining facts.—18. Organ of painting and the perception of colours.—19. Organ of the arithmetical sense.—20. Of the musical sense.—21. Of the mechanical sense.—22. Organ of verbal memory.—23. Organ of the disposition for learning languages.—24. Organ of the memory for distinguishing and recollecting persons.—25. Organ of liberality.—26. Organ of the genius for comparison.—27. Organ of the metaphysical genius.—28. Organ of the spirit of observation.—29. Organ of wit.—30. Organ of goodness.—31. Organ of music or theatrical talents.—32. Organ of holiness.—33. Organ of perseverance.

VOL. I.   c

Figure 1. Title page of the *Weekly Medico–Chirurgical and Philosophical Magazine*, 22 February 1823.

his teaching at St. Thomas' Hospital and at Grainger's Theatre of Anatomy in Southwark (the proprietor of the latter, Richard Grainger, being a member of the LPS from 1825).[54] W. W. Sleigh and John Epps[‡] probably included discussion of the science in their lectures at Dermott's School of Medicine, as Erasmus Wilson appears to have done at the Middlesex School. Joseph H. Green, a demonstrator on anatomy at St. Thomas' and subsequently professor of anatomy at the College of Surgeons, included the first abstract of Gall and Spurzheim's method of brain dissection in his *The Dissector's Manual* in 1820, and in subsequent editions this was expanded with the help of his friend John Flint South, a member of the council of the LPS and lecturer on anatomy at St. Thomas'.[55] In 1825 Wakley published in the *Lancet* a full course of eighteen lectures on phrenology by Spurzheim, and in 1836 a course of twenty lectures on the subject by the French medical authority François Broussais.[56] By the latter date Elliotson, then professor of practical medicine at the new University of London, had taken the science with him into University College Hospital, where he lectured to some of the largest audiences of medical students ever assembled. Archibald Billing, senior physician and lecturer at London Hospital, who joined the LPS early in 1833 after Holm's lectures at the hospital, likely kept the science before his students, as he did through the later edition of his textbook *First Principles of Medicine.*

Considerable discussion of phrenology also went on at the reform-minded Westminster Medical Society to which Johnson, Epps, and the phrenologists Forbes Winslow, Edward Wright, Robert Dunn,[‡] and John S. Streeter all belonged. It is probable that similar discussion went on in the Royal Medico–Chirurgical Society to which Elliotson, Lawrence, Dunn, and the phrenologists Thomas Forster[‡] and Joseph Moore belonged; in the Physical Society of Guy's Hospital to which Moore and Streeter belonged; and in the London Hospital Medical Society to which the phrenologist Edward Moore belonged. It is probable, too, that phrenology was on the agenda of the reformist Association of Apothecaries and Surgeons' Apothecaries, since its president, Joseph Hayes, was a leading figure in the LPS in the 1820s and had a keen interest in the popularization of science.[57]

Outside the metropolis, too, phrenology was similarly propagated in medical schools by men who were nearly all either heads of phrenological societies or prominent community spokesmen for the science. Among these were physicians and surgeons such as John Fife[‡] and T. M. Greenhow at the Newcastle Medical School, Cordon Thompson at the Sheffield School of Anatomy and Medicine, Charles Cowan[‡] at the Bath School of Medicine, Daniel Noble[‡] at Manchester's Chatham Street School of Medicine, John Mackintosh at Edinburgh's Argyle Square School, and William Macdonald and William Weir[‡] at Glasgow's Andersonian University (Weir also being the coeditor of the *Glasgow Medical Journal*).[58]

Many advocates of phrenology were also among the senior honorary physicians and surgeons of dispensaries and infirmaries. Both founders of the Plymouth Dispensary for Diseases of the Eyes, John Butter and Edward Moore, for instance, were among the corresponding members of the LPS, as was the senior honorary physician to the Chester General Infirmary, Llewelyn Jones, and the surgeon–apothecary at the London Infirmary for Diseases of the Lungs, William Henry. Edward Barlow, one of the founders of the Bath Phrenological Society, was physician to the Bath United Hospital.[59] Striking, too, are the number of advocates of phrenology who were medical superintendents of county and private lunatic asylums. Among these were the leading alienists of the time: Sir William Ellis, John Conolly, and W. A. F. Browne,[‡] all of whom claimed to derive from phrenology essential insights for their reformed, humanitarian treatment of the insane.[60] Also worth noting is the approval and advocation of phrenology that came from court physicians such as Sir James Clark , James Stewart, Andrew Combe, and Sir William Knighton.[61]

It is not difficult to explain in terms specific to medical science why so many in the profession in the early nineteenth century responded favorably to phrenology. The abundant literature that they left behind leaves us in little doubt that they felt that for the first time the mysteries of the mind had been opened to them. To Forbes Winslow, for instance, the future editor of the *Journal of Psychological Medicine*, Gall's physiological psychology, by uniting the mind with neurology on the one hand and the biology of adaptation on the other, seemed a conceptual triumph of the highest order, for it transformed abstract metaphysical conceptions of mind into actual organic entities amenable to the interests and understandings of the practical-minded.[62] The reification of mind that was objected to by Thomas Brown and other students of Scottish faculty psychology was thus by these men taken as a cause for celebration. Woolly metaphysics, they claimed, had produced only heaps of "crude indigestible masses of metaphysical speculation" along with vague, contradictory, and idle theories; but, thanks to phrenology, the brain now became "part and parcel of the human organism, and as subject in common with the liver and lungs etc., [applicable] ... to similar laws and sympathies."[63] "Unless rules of investigation apply to the brain's physiology which differ from those relating to the remaining organization," explained Daniel Noble, the principles of phrenology could not possibly be denied.[64] Hence the conclusion of the *Lancet* in 1825 that "the physiology of the brain, as taught by Gall and Spurzheim is ... the only one having the slightest analogy to truth, or in any way calculated to explain the multifarious mental phenomena."[65] The supposed utility of the science for medical understanding could itself be taken as a measure of the science's truth, for as "Bacon inferred that Aristotle's philosophy was false because it was barren ... it is a legitimate inference from the same principle, that phrenology is true because it is fruitful."[66] This Baconian measure of truth could be further applied to Gall and Spurzheim's empiricist methodology, for they had, it was claimed, worked from no "preconceived view of creating, or supporting, a favoured hypothesis; but were led ... into a train of observations on the functions of the brain; from which they, at length, drew those inferences."[67]

Virtually all the leading supporters of phrenology likewise maintained that they had only been won over to the knowledge by submitting to a similar train of empirical correlations, frequently only after having initially dismissed phrenology as "pseudoscientific." David Uwins, for example, who was held by others in the medical profession to be a man of "vast erudition and experience," claimed to have been "*bitten* by phrenology" after writing a hostile account of it in the *Eclectic Review* in 1815. In much the same manner as Edward Barlow in his address before the newly formed Provincial Medical and Surgical Association in 1834, Uwins related in 1836 how his scepticism had fallen before the invincible march of phrenological "facts." The endorsement of the science that he provided in major articles in the *London Encyclopedia* (1829) and the *New Monthly Magazine* (1832) appeared to rest, as much as his former opposition had, upon impartial medical evidence and not upon the justifications of "particular creeds and professions," to which he now attributed the writings of antiphrenologists.[68]

It would not be amiss to add that elsewhere Uwins candidly remarked that it did not matter to him whether or not the phrenologists were right in their claims. What mattered, he insisted, was that they had endeavored to apply physiology to "morals, and ethics, and medicine" and, in so doing, had uncovered "the proper mode of conducting man's energies and faculties."[69] Much other explicit evidence of the importance of phrenology to medical men in providing insights into the "proper mode" of individual and social conduct could also be brought forward at this point. But it is better saved for later, for while it does not alter the fact that in the context the grounds for supporting phrenology could be seen and felt to be as logical and rational as the reasons put forward against it, such evidence too readily obscures what is equally significant and worthy of emphasis: that the scientific–medical opponents of phrenology often put aside their scientific and medical evidences to complain about how it was "a crime to entertain such a doctrine" and "a consummate folly to boast of it."[70] The latter kind of evidence, in particular, helps make it clear that to characterize the debates over phrenology as an instance of a crude popular scientism intimidating transcendent Truth and Reason is not only to distort historical reality but, as well, to act in a highly subjective and inconsistent manner. Selecting supposedly rational scientific facts and methodologies in the consideration of the claims of antiphrenologists but only "extrarational" social values in the consideration of the claims of phrenologists is clearly wrong-headed. But the Revisionist effort to "correct" the Whig historical record by pointing to the rationalism of the phrenologists is obviously no less wrong-headed. Both historical exercises are in fact amazing reflections of the imperatives of our culture – amazing, because there is probably no better instance than the debates over phrenology where hindsight permits us to see that neither side had, as it were, the "correct" information on the nature of the brain.

In the absence of any absolute truth, the real value of phrenology's historical consideration must be seen to lie not in wittingly or unwittingly enforcing the demarcations between "science" and "nonscience," but rather in persuading us that when it comes to the Truth about nature and human nature, there can be no touchstones other than those that exist in the minds of the participants in history (including those writing its history). If this is indeed the case, as thinkers from Paracelsus to Marcuse have all along suggested, then it follows that the task before the historian of so-called pseudoscience is not to make further privilege for positivist science, but to determine how and why some conceptions of reality acquire the mantle of objective scientific truth and enter into the domain of common sense while others come to be regarded as arrant nonsense.[71]

PART II

Science and social interests

Scientific concepts are not simply asymptotic approaches to underlying truth. They are products of a particular social structure and may in turn either reinforce or challenge the social status quo. Not only the daily practice and social use, but also the content of science would be different in a differently organized society.

Norman Diamond, "Politics of Scientific Conceptualization,"
Science for the People, 8 (1976), p. 14

Men, who produce social relationships in conformity with their material method of production, also produce ideas and categories, that is to say, the abstract, ideal expressions of these same social relationships. Thus the categories are no more eternal than the relationships which they express. They are historic and transitory products.

Karl Marx to P. Annenkov, 28 December 1848, in *The Letters of Karl Marx*, ed. Saul Padover (Englewood Cliffs, N.J., 1979), p. 51

2

The social sense of brain

Were it merely a question among anatomists relative to a particular structure of the brain, or a dispute among medical philosophers respecting some litigated right to a discovery, it would
have little interest for the general reader: but a system of Cranioscopy is something very different, and as it involves in its conclusions, most important moral consequences, it claims from every
one, . . . a serious and patient investigation.

"Observations on the Anatomical Peculiarities of the System of
Gall and Spurzheim," *Glasgow Enquirer*, 1 (November 1820), 33

In fact, with some exceptions, the term "mind" has not functioned as a scientific concept at all but as a rhetorical device, even
when its use has been forbidden. More exactly, it has acted to
communicate – and sometimes exploit – a fear rather than to
define a process, a fear of subjectivism.

Clifford Geertz, "The Growth of Culture and the Evolution of
Mind," in J. M. Scher, ed., *Theories of the Mind* (New York,
1962), p. 714

Of the little we know of Gall's motives for constructing his science,
we know at least this: that his scientific and anecdotal evidence
flowed *from* his philosophical-cum-social interests. Even before
commencing his anatomical investigations he had set down his
views on mind and matter, body, and soul, in his first publication
on the philosophy of medicine in 1791.[1] On the one hand he
rejected theories of mind as independent from brain and, on the
other, rejected that experience was the only source for the contents
of the mind and organization of thought; that is, he was both
antiidealist and antisensationalist. After 1796 Gall developed his
ideas further in public lectures in Vienna, but in focusing too much
attention on socially sensitive areas, they were soon forbidden by

the emperor of Austria on the grounds that they were conducive to materialism, immorality, and atheism. Through this denunciation Gall's reputation was made and his theory put into lively circulation. Born a Catholic, educated by a priest, and originally destined for the priesthood, Gall died with his books on the Index and was buried (apparently by choice) in unconsecrated ground.[2]

Hence, although there was always considerable ignorance in Britain of Gall's actual writings, it was difficult for anyone ever to be unaware of the social unorthodoxy of what Gall himself called his "truth, though opposed to the philosophy of ages."[3] If this nonconformity was not clear from the opponents' casting of the doctrine into the "fungus school of Spinoza, Hartley and Darwin," it was clear from some supporters' claim that their philosophy was "opposed to the principles and practices of all governments and almost all laws and institutions."[4]

Yet if Gall's ideas were virtually synonomous with social unorthodoxy and dissent, and hence implied change, there was nothing in them qualifying any particular form of dissent or specifying any particular kind of change. Unlike many of his detractors and his glorifiers, Gall himself was neither an ideologue nor a social dogmatist. What his ideas stood for was indeterminate since his philosophy, unlike his cerebral theory, was more reactive than constructive. Epistemologically and socially his doctrine could be worked in a number of different ways. Certainly the radical materialism espoused by some supporters of the doctrine was not endorsed by all. Throughout the nineteenth century, in fact, phrenology was to have links with immaterialist traditions – occult, hermetic, Neoplatonic, and romantic. Indeed, Gall himself has sometimes been considered as a representative of the "Romantic school" and of having produced a hybrid "Romantic psychology expressed in positivist language and methodology."[5] It was the romantic Johann Herder, apparently, who convinced Gall that he should study comparative anatomy and, although the significance of this has more to do with the organicist evolutionary framework of the phrenological doctrine than with anything specifically antimaterialist or antirationalist (see Chapter 4), it is true that Gall's ideas were to hold a certain fascination for Goethe and other German *Naturphilosophen*.[6] In Britain, the mystically inclined engraver, sculptor, and friend of William Blake, John Flaxman (1755–1826), readily incorporated phrenology within his anti-Newtonian scheme of things, as did various other Swedenborgians. Coleridge, too, initially expressed considerable interest.[7]

Most of the supporters of phrenology referred to in the preceding chapter might well have appreciated the attraction of young idealistic romantics to the new way of understanding human nature. However, their own motives for expressing opposition to consensual philosophical and intellectual norms through embracing Gall's heterodoxy could hardly be described as romantic. What these motives were can be determined in large part by collectively considering their biographies in relation to the collective biography of their intellectual opponents. To this end we will confine ourselves here to only those supporters and opponents of the knowledge who had claims to scientific or medical expertise. Further, we will include among our sample only those who advocated or contested the knowledge prior to 1835, the date after which phrenology became widely recognized and seized upon as a vehicle for liberal social reform (a recognition largely made through the popularization of Combe's *Constitution of Man*). Thus in the terms of intellectualist historians the following comparison between British phrenologists and antiphrenologists is chronologically situated at the period prior to the knowledge's manifest social and ideological "pollution." Excluding from an assembled list of 133 scientific–medical supporters of phrenology those for whom biographical information is insufficient for comparative purposes, the following analysis is based[8] on 60 proponents and 17 opponents and includes all the major figures referred to in the preceding chapter.*

---

*Opponents (note: for criteria of selection see: Chapter 1): Matthew Baillie (1761–1823), John Barclay (1758–1826), Charles Bell (1774–1842), John Bostock (1773–1836), Thomas Brown (1778–1820), James Copland (1791–1870), John Gordon (1786–1818), Sir William Hamilton (1788–1856), Sir Everard Home (1756–1832), Francis Jeffrey (1773–1850), John Kidd (1775–1851), Edward Milligan (1784–1833), James Cowles Prichard (1786–1848), P. M. Roget (1779–1869), Michael Ryan (1800–41), Thomas Stone (1793–1854), John Yelloly (1774–1842).

Proponents (note: for those not discussed elsewhere in the text [see index] or in the Appendix listing lecturers [‡], criteria for selection here includes membership in a phrenological society and/or phrenological publications and/or evidence from the *Phrenological Journal*): Disney Alexander,‡ Matthew Allen,‡ Edward Barlow (1779–1844), Archibald Billing (1791–1881), W. A. F. Browne,‡ John Butter (1791–1877), G. D. Cameron,‡ Richard Chenevix (1774–1830), James Clark (1788–1870), Andrew Combe (1797–1847), John Conolly (1794–1866), Charles Cowan,‡ Robert Dunn,‡ John Elliotson (1791–1868), William Ellis (1790–1839), W. C. Engledue,‡

PHRENOLOGISTS AND ANTIPHRENOLOGISTS: A
SOCIAL MAP

The first and most noticeable difference between the phrenologists
and the antiphrenologists in our sample is that of their ages. In
1818, the year of John Gordon's death, the average age of the
sixteen antiphrenologists for whom we have dates was forty-one,
while the average age of the fifty-one phrenologists for whom we
have dates was twenty-four. Only eleven of the phrenologists in
1818 were over thirty; only six were over forty. Though in several
cases it was much less than a generation (reckoned at twenty-five
years) that separated the supporters and opponents, overall the
difference in age is wide enough to support the idea of a generational conflict. Indeed, this was clear to many of the supporters,
especially the more evangelical of them. Like the active supporters
of Darwin's theory later in the century or the advocates of reductionism in biology in Berlin in the 1840s, they felt, as one
phrenologist in our sample (aged twenty-four in 1818) put it, that
it was to the "rising generation . . . alone we must look for a belief
in, and earnest cultivation of, any new doctrine in any department
of knowledge."[9] As in all cases of the assertion of new knowledge
by a younger generation, however – be it Puritanism in the seventeenth century, *Romantische Naturphilosophie* in late-eighteenth-
century Germany, or National Socialism in Germany in the 1930s
– age differences between the contestants do not in themselves
command explanatory power.[10] To cite generational conflict is
merely to identify one of the common symptoms and clues to
underlying dissatisfaction with the existing institutionalizations of
power. As Timothy Lenoir has pointed out, it is not age itself that
matters in the consideration of generational factors in relation to

John Epps,[‡] John Fife,[‡] John Forbes (1787–1861), T. M. I. Forster,[‡] Richard Grainger
(1801–65), T. M. Greenhow (1791–1881), William Gregory,[‡] John Harris (1804–48), Joseph
Hayes (1769–1830), G. C. Holland,[‡] H. H. Holm,[‡] Robert Hunter,[‡] James Johnson (1777–
1845), Sir William Knighton (1776–1836), William Lawrence (1783–1867), William
MacDonald (1804–74), Sir George Mackenzie,[‡] William Mackenzie,[†] John Mackintosh (d.
1837), G. Miller,[‡] Edward Moore (1794–1858), Joseph Moore (d. 1855), D. Noble,[‡] H.
Overend,[‡] Richard Poole (1783–1871), John P. Porter (1771–1855), J. Q. Rumball,[‡] T.
Sandwith,[‡] James Scott,[‡] John Robertson Sibbald (1799–1868), John Flint South (1797–
1882), J. G. Spurzheim,[‡] John Soper Streeter (1802–73), E. Sweetlove,[‡] Cordon Thompson
(1793–1876), David Uwins (1780–1837), Thomas Wakley (1795–1862), H. C. Watson,[‡]
W. Weir,[‡] Charles Wheatstone (1802–75), Robert Willis,[‡] W. J. Erasmus Wilson (1809–
84), Forbes Winslow (1810–74), Edward Wright (1791–1859).

social and scientific change so much as the fact that roughly coeval individuals have been exposed to the same kind of social and historical experience.[11]

That that experience was similar among the phrenologists in our sample is reflected in their economic and social status relative to that of the antiphrenologists. Whereas the majority of the antiphrenologists by 1830 were either at or beyond their professional primes with incomes, social power, and prestige secured, most phrenologists were still struggling to establish themselves. Many would never achieve the social distinction that most of the antiphrenologists achieved, and it seems fairly certain that had their lives suddenly been terminated in, say, 1840, almost all of them would have fallen through the specially strung net of the end-of-the-century compilers of the *Dictionary of National Biography*. As it is, the *DNB* misses but 2 of the opponents in our list, yet has entries for only 27 of the 60 proponents (the 27 being selected here from the 133 supporters *because of* their *DNB* entry). Retrospective judgments on phrenology aside, the exclusion of phrenologists from the *DNB* is to be explained in part by the fact that the social experience of those who decided who was to qualify for entry in the *DNB* was much closer to that of the opponents than to the proponents.[12] By the criterion of education, for instance, of the 60 supporters, none had ever studied in Oxford; only Elliotson and T. M. I. Forster (both of whom the *DNB* include) and John Harris studied at Cambridge, while Richard Chenevix and Archibald Billing (both also included in the *DNB*) studied at Trinity College, Dublin.[13] Most of the others, coming from relatively deprived social backgrounds, had to struggle to pay for their medical education, were early apprenticed in apothecaries' shops and to surgeons, or, like Johnson and Clark (who struck it rich by chance encounters with royalty), took or bought university medical degrees after working in the lowest ranks of the medical profession, as naval surgeons.[14] Conolly, Johnson, and Uwins took to writing for pecuniary reasons in periods of unemployment; Matthew Allen[‡] for a time found subsistence through lecturing on phrenology, and W. A. F. Browne[‡] assisted himself in the same way; while Forbes Winslow (who was certainly one of the most impecunious of the supporters) wrote his 1832 essay *The Principles of Phrenology* while a student in order to help pay for his courses.

For almost all the antiphrenologists, on the other hand, the experience of social and economic insecurity was far removed. Most of them had sheltered upbringings and gentlemanly educations befitting the sons of titled and wealthy families – families whose connections could greatly ease the opportunities for the qualifications sought by the compilers of the *DNB*. While none of them were educated at Cambridge, and only four at Oxford, the University of Edinburgh served most of the others in similarly privileged ways. Indeed, the University of Edinburgh was something of a closed shop for them: All three holders of the chair of moral philosophy, Stewart, Brown, and John Wilson (the coeditor of *Blackwood's Magazine* who also opposed phrenology), had previously attended the university; moreover, Brown, Gordon, and Jeffrey were all students of Stewart, while Gordon was also a student of Barclay. As George Combe[‡] understood when he entered the "open" competition for the university chair of logic in 1836, his outsider status gave him no real chance; and no one was surprised that the chair went to the leading exponent at the time of Reid and Stewart's Common Sense philosophy, the outspoken antiphrenologist Sir William Hamilton.[‡15]

As pointed out in the preceding chapter, there were university professors and hospital lecturers among the phrenologists. But as opposed to nine professors and lecturers among the antiphrenologists in our sample who were in status institutions, there were among the phrenologists only Billing at London Hospital, Charles Wheatstone at King's College, London, and Elliotson and Conolly at the new "godless institution in Gower Street," University College. Neither Lawrence at St. Bartholomew's Hospital, nor Richard Grainger by the time he came to be lecturer on anatomy at St. Thomas', nor John South by the time he became professor of surgery at the Royal College of Surgeons was an open supporter of phrenology, while Wheatstone appears to have kept his advocacy of the science separate from his professional duties.[16] The Andersonian University, where William Weir,[‡] Robert Hunter,[‡] and William Mackenzie[‡] taught medicine and where William Gregory[‡] became a lecturer in chemistry in 1837, was primarily a place of popular and practical instruction with low academic status.

This same picture of the phrenologists' lower social and intellectual status relative to that of the antiphrenologists is reinforced by noting who among the sample were fellows of the Royal Societies of London and Edinburgh. Among the supporters before 1835, nine of the sixty had this honor (three of them being fellows before being introduced to phrenology), while no fewer than twelve of the seventeen opponents had this distinction, receiving it either before or during the period of their active opposition to the knowledge. If only because election into these societies depended upon inside sponsorship and support as well as financial standing, the greater preponderance of fellows among the opponents reflects, as the *DNB* entries do, the opponents' greater conformity with dominant interests and social norms as reflected in scientific organizations. Though Elliotson, Wheatstone, and Clark were able to become fellows of the Royal Society of London, and Gregory of the Royal Society of Edinburgh, while supporting phrenology, only Elliotson was well known at the time as an advocate.[17] It is noticeable that all of the phrenologists who were elected fellows after 1835 (Billing, W. A. F. Browne, Grainger, and W. J. Erasmus Wilson) were elected only after they had shed or disguised their interest in phrenology. In this they were like Sir Astley Cooper, who suppressed his radicalism before being elected a fellow of the Royal Society in 1802, and like Lawrence, who kept his radical materialism to himself once he was elected president of the Royal College of Surgeons in 1846.[18]

Religious beliefs similarly divided the two parties, though comparative data on this for the period with which we are concerned is difficult to come by. Of the six supporters of phrenology known with certainty to have belonged to the Established Church, four (H. C. Watson,[‡] Conolly, Cordon Thompson, and William Ellis) are notable for their apostacy and, in the case of Conolly and Thompson, for their conversions to Unitarianism, or, in the case of Ellis, to Wesleyan Methodism. Calvert Holland,[‡] the son of a Sheffield artisan, had his education supported by Unitarians. What is known of the other supporters (excepting Charles Cowan,[‡] who was the son of a clergyman and was active in Low Church politics, J. Q. Rumball,[‡] who was an arch antimaterialist, and J. F. South, who became an enthusiastic Anglican later in life) points to healthy strains of antireligious materialism (such as was voiced by Elliotson and William Engledue[‡]), outspoken rationalism (as witnessed in Browne's observations *On Religious Fanaticism* [1835] or in Hall Overend's[‡] announcement of conversion from Quakerism to "free thought"), or vocal nonconformity (as expressed in Epps's[‡] *Some Fallacies Put Forth by the Church of England, and the Duty of Dissenters* [1834] and in Disney Alexander's[‡] lay preaching for the Methodists).

Among the opponents of phrenology, excepting the Unitarian John Bostock, there was a much firmer outward commitment to established faith and to socially undisturbing natural theology. Barclay was the son of a Perthshire minister and was himself a minister in the Church of Scotland before taking up medicine; Matthew Baillie, fellow opponent of phrenology with Everard Home in the Royal Society in the 1810s, was the son of a Presbyterian minister who became a professor of divinity at Glasgow University; and Charles Bell was the son of a prominent Episcopalian clergyman. Unlike many phrenologists, none of these men rebelled from the faith of their fathers. The only Quaker among the opponents, James Prichard,[‡] is noteworthy for his conversion to Anglicanism (apparently not just to meet Oxford degree requirements), while John Kidd and Bell were the authors of Bridgewater Treatises, undertaken to illustrate "the Power, Wisdom and Goodness of God, as manifested in the Creation" (the intentions of Bridgewater's will for the writing of these treatises being entrusted to the president of the Royal Society). Bell also coedited with Henry Brougham an edition of Paley's *Natural Theology* (1835). Though none of these opponents wanted to be thought of as opposing phrenology purely on religious grounds, they all probably shared Hamilton's view of the science as being "implicit atheism" and had few objections to its being attacked on those grounds.[19] While not all phrenologists sided wholeheartedly with Lawrence in his celebrated controversy with Abernethy in the late 1810s and early 1820s over theories of life (to which Gall's ideas contributed by being both French and linked to antivitalism), none of the opponents of phrenology wished to have any association with materialism.[20]

Inextricably connected to the religious dissent among the phrenologists was their political liberalism, epitomized in Wakley's defense of the Tolpuddle Martyrs and the Chartists, but more representatively witnessed in John Fife's[‡] campaign for the Reform Bill and his support of the Anti–Corn Law League. Admittedly, political boundaries between phrenologists and antiphrenologists are not easily drawn, and the terms *Whig, radical,* and *liberal* are hardly more than crude distinctions that harbor a wide variety of

political and social choices.[21] To some extent the difficulty in drawing clear political boundaries between phrenologists and antiphrenologists is a consequence of certain shared elements in their
thought, a subject that will be taken up in the following chapter.
For the moment it will do to say that for the most part phrenologists were radicals in the 1820s, usually becoming liberals later,
while most antiphrenologists supported the Whig (usually reformist) status quo as qualified by Francis Jeffrey in the *Edinburgh
Review*.

In summary, what was ostensibly an intellectual debate about
scientific truth by politically disinterested spokesmen of science
and medicine reveals itself, through the collective biographical
consideration of those involved in the debate, as closely correlated
with the disputants' socioeconomic experiences and sociopolitical
interests. What *by and large* distinguishes those attracted to phrenology was their recently heightened sense of social worth being
incommensurate with their place and power in the social process.
This was particularly so among those who can be seen as constituting the phrenological "hard core." By fully or partially attaching themselves to a body of knowledge that rejected the reigning
philosophical bases to social power and authority and that (by
purporting to maximize peoples' competence to predict and control behavior) bore an immediate challenge to dominant forms of
the manipulation and organization of social life, the supporters of
phrenology signified in a form of knowledge appropriate to their
professional calling a demand for total integration into a reformed
society – a society in which would predominate what they believed
to be their more meritocratic values. Antiphrenologists, on the
other hand, can be seen as having been anxious to preserve institutionalized social and ideological interests. Their attempts to prove
phrenology "false" or to show that phrenologists were "third-rate
intellectuals" may be seen as the "scientific" mode through which
they hoped to legitimate restraint on the incorporation of emergent
values. The fact that these antiphrenologists were well aware of
the strong tide of utilitarian social and political reform and, at the
same time, relatedly, of the evident decline in the attraction of the
metaphysics of Reid and Stewart in the face of scientific empiricism
goes far to explain the lengths to which they were willing to go
in order to prove phrenology false. In Edinburgh, especially, as
Shapin has shown, it was no idle curiousity, but rather a desperate

need to defend vested values and interests, that, for example, drove Sir William Hamilton to devote himself to the study of anatomy solely in order to prove that phrenology was "idiotcy grafted upon empiricism."[22]

THE LIMITATIONS OF COLLECTIVE BIOGRAPHY

Exposing the relative sociopolitical and socioeconomic differences between phrenologists and antiphrenologists undermines claims that might be made for the intellectual autonomy of the disputants and, given the type of knowledge at issue, makes it extremely difficult to consider any aspect of the dispute as outside a framework of social interests. Yet in the final analyses the value of the technique of contrasting the collective social biographies of intellectual disputants ("prosopography" in the widest sense) is mostly only heuristic. It forces us to think about knowledge and knowledge claims in terms wider than those permitted either by intellectualist history, with its stress on autonomous cognitive events, or by the psychologistic history of great figures, which holds that the fountainhead of all thought is the personality of the individual. Methodologically, therefore, the prosopographical means of aligning certain abstract ideas to networks of social interests answers to the lament of Mannheim that, while the philosophers, in conceiving of ideas as heavenly descended entities, made the history of thought appear artificially homogeneous and indiscriminate, the literary and "great men" historians atomized it.[23] Transcending both, prosopography goes some way to meeting the need of the social historian of ideas to establish the connections between knowledge and power.

However, as a passive methodological device, prosopography is also limited and can be potentially misleading. On the one hand, Arnold Momigliano, although thinking of prosopography in the more restricted family-connection sense, has criticized it for being insufficiently appreciative of concrete situations and of presupposing rather than really explaining the material and spiritual needs of groups of individuals.[24] On the other hand, more conventionally, Charles Rosenberg has asserted that

one must distrust any approach which fails to recognize that human beings, in any culture, come in assorted psychological shapes and sizes. No analytical strategy which assumes that the behavior of groups can be explained by considering them as undifferentiated individuals writ large can prove intellectually satisfactory.[25]

Although one might be just as distrustful of any claim to know what is or what is not "intellectually satisfactory," and although the identification of mutual social interests among the respective proponents and opponents of certain ideas in no way implies their psychological homogenity, it is true that on both sides of a dispute there are nearly always seemingly exceptional individuals whose social interests do not align with the majority and whose support or opposition may be unique in terms of its concrete circumstances.

Among our antiphrenologists, for instance, special accounting could be said to be necessary for the presence of James Copland who, as a younger and self-made man, had far more in common with many phrenologists than with most antiphrenologists.[26] Neither can the Unitarian John Bostock or his friend P. M. Roget be easily bounded within the same upper class, Church-connected social orbit as the major Edinburgh antiphrenologists. Though Roget was the nephew of Sir Samuel Romilly, was an Anglican, and was a power within the Royal Society, he was by association and marriage more closely allied to bourgeois mercantile sources of wealth, status, and power and had (like Bostock) an ideological affinity with philosophical radicalism.[27] Antiphrenologists like this, who moved within the provincial literary and philosophical societies and the Royal Institutions, who were leading figures within the new London and provincial medical schools, societies, and hospitals, and who fraternized on the senate of London University and in the councils of Henry Brougham's Society for the Diffusion of Useful Knowledge, inhabited a world that, while on the one hand was familiar to many phrenologists, was on the other hand quite differently nuanced from the world inhabited by the Hamiltons and Jeffreys of Edinburgh (in which a horror of both popular and philosophical radicalism figured prominently).[28] Different again, was the antiphrenologist John Kidd. By his family background, his studies under Sir Astley Cooper at Guy's Hospital, his High Church anti-Calvinism, and his opposition to Dugald Stewart's philosophy, he can be seen as having characteristics in common with both parties, yet as having close sociopolitical rapport with neither.[29]

Exceptions such as these do not invalidate sociological methods of approach to scientific knowledge and debate. On the contrary, beyond reminding us of the historical truism that one cannot always make a general finding fit with all the particulars out of which the generality was drawn, the exceptions might be said only to highlight certain crudities in our application of the methodology. Clearly unrefined is, first, the attempt to cover thirty-five years of uneven debate over phrenology (the last at least twenty of which coincided with the most intense economic and ideological disruption of society since the seventeenth century) and, second, the attempt to take Britain as a whole as the context of analysis. The fact that social differentiations between phrenologists and antiphrenologists can be qualified at all over that stretch of time and across that broad context must be seen as lending considerable weight to a social interpretation of the debates and as amply justifying the interpretative procedure. But completely overlooked thereby is how different perceptions of the knowledge could relate to differences in the structures of local economies and class relations, to differences in inherited local political, religious, intellectual, and cultural traditions and institutions, to differences in the custodial care of those traditions and institutions, and, above all, to differences in the degree to which all of these might have been felt to have been undergoing change. As several regional studies of phrenology have shown, these variations were substantial in the period prior to 1835, the arbitrary cutoff date of our sample of contestants.[30]

There is not the space here to enter into or to try to add to local studies of early-nineteenth-century phrenology. However, the points that a comparison of these regional studies could be said to establish – namely (i) that science is never directly reflective of ideology and is therefore always open to a range of epistemological and political positions; (ii) relatedly, that the use of science is never contained within a single discourse or a single sociopolitical tradition; and (iii) that imperatives change as circumstances change – can be illustrated as well by focusing on a few of the early and (by our sociological criteria) "exceptional" supporters of phrenology. In so doing we will be keeping with our brief in this chapter of accounting for why individuals sought to place themselves in opposition to consensual norms by embracing phrenology, or why they sought by those means to make their opposition manifest.

EARLY VARIETIES OF BELIEF

But at the outset it has to be confessed that very often there *is* no way of knowing why an individual choses to engage or not to engage in a particular intellectual activity. Not only are the wider historical determinates for accepting or rejecting certain ideas at certain times unapparent to most people, but also, the rationalizations that people have for taking up certain bodies of knowledge are frequently left unstated. Sheer lack of biographical contextualizing information often precludes speculation on motives. Such limitations are apparent even with respect to J. G. Spurzheim,‡ Gall's collaborator between 1800 and 1813. We know hardly more than that he was raised a Lutheran and that prior to studying medicine in Vienna at the turn of the century he was a student of divinity and philosophy at the University of Treves. Once charitably referred to as having "perhaps too great a faith in his own opinions," he was undoubtedly egotistical, was obsequious among what he called "good families," was indifferent to the sufferings of the poor, and was as firm a believer in law and order as he was in "liberal principles." But why exactly he disliked the "mechanical direction which [Gall's] anatomical investigations had taken," why he loathed Saint-Simon yet admired Robert Owen as an educationalist, or why he desired to point out a "standard of natural morality" that Gall had never hoped for – all these are questions difficult to answer satisfactorily due to the paucity of the right sort of biographical material.[31] Interestingly, Coleridge referred to Spurzheim in 1817 as "beyond all comparison the greatest Physiognomist that has ever appeared," but by 1830 had decided that while likeable, " he is dense, and the most ignorant German I ever knew."[32] Like other comments on Spurzheim, these by Coleridge tend to tell us less about Spurzheim than about the commenter and his changing attitude to the science. It may be a sufficient explanation that Spurzheim needed to establish his independence from Gall; but his deeper motives for advocating phrenology remain opaque relative to the clearly socioreligious and ideological ones of Combe and his followers.[33] That Spurzheim was more the bearer than the inventor of phrenological notions, that he was transculturally mobile, and that he was as adept at accommodating himself and the ideas he bore to different contexts as he was at changing his middle name (from Christoph to Gaspar, and sometimes to Kaspar) all contribute to the difficulty of making any real social and political sense of his motives for advocating phrenology.

Equally opaque in many respects is John Elliotson, who, next to Spurzheim and Combe, was the person most responsible for proselytizing phrenology in Britain. Elliotson turned to phrenology around 1822 when he joined the Edinburgh Phrenological Society (EPS) (a year after his brother Thomas had joined) and organized the LPS in 1823 after having experienced no difficulties in entering the upper echelons of the medical profession while still a young man. All that can be seen to have prompted his celebration of the knowledge was an impish compulsion continually to shock respectable society and continually to test the threshold of toleration of his peers in the medical profession. He was among the first in the profession to discard stockings and wear trousers, to advocate the clinical methods of Laennec and the use of the stethescope, to recommend acupuncture, to deny the contagiousness of typhus, and to administer to his patients heroic doses of creosote. It is difficult to see his overtly materialist advocacy of Gall's doctrine, and his consequent denunciation of Spurzheim as one who had bowdlerized Gall's doctrine for the flattery of the conventional and fashionable, as other than one more egotistically satisfying means of affronting the conventional. (This does not mean, however, that he did not at the same time sincerely believe in the truth of Gall's doctrine.) Only in the 1840s, when his advocacy of mesmerism and phreno-mesmerism cost him his job at University College, do we see Elliotson beginning, belatedly, to share some of the social insecurity of many of those previously attracted to the knowledge he championed. But prior to then, it is difficult to account for his compulsive turning to unorthodox knowledge and behavior in any satisfying political or psychosocial way. Perhaps only in the fact that his father was a prosperous London apothecary might there be a clue. It may be, more than we suppose, that Elliotson shared the characteristic ambivalence of the socially and intellectually upwardly mobile: on the one hand, seeking through the mantle of learning to bury a past connected with crass petty commercialism, while on the other hand endeavoring to defy the smug superiority of those born into traditional power and privilege and to challenge those seeking to reproduce traditional modes of professional conduct. Doubtless, too, the fact that Elliotson was scarcely over five feet in height also accounts for some of his manner. But, as with Spurzheim, in the absence of essential autobiographical information, it is only possible to speculate on the problem of motives.[34]

That locating the relevant biographical fragments *can* enable us to make social and political sense of seemingly socially "exceptional" early supporters of phrenology is a reason for turning to a figure who occupies no place of significance in the history of phrenology, Rear Admiral John Ross (1777–1856), the Arctic and Antarctic navigator. In the absence of further information it would have to be concluded that Ross's joining the EPS in January 1823 relates only to an asocial interest in the practical applications of the science to naval discipline, a subject upon which he wrote a pamphlet in 1825.[35] In Ross's case links between support for phrenology and forms of opposition to orthodoxy seem remote, and, superficially at least, he seems to have had much more in common with antiphrenologists than phrenologists. He was older than most supporters and, as a commander in the Royal Navy, he obviously had power and status within the traditional establishment.[36] He also had good connections with the scientific elite of his time, numbering among his friends Sir Joseph Banks, the president of the Royal Society, and various others within what Susan Cannon styled the "Cambridge Network."[37] It was through those connections that Ross was appointed to lead the 1818 expedition to search for the North West Passage.

Quite unlike Elliotson, Ross was not in the least inclined to deviant behavior. Appended to his pamphlet of 1825 was an unflattering phrenological delineation of the political radical Joseph Hume, while the contents of the pamphlet reveal none of the humanitarian "progressive" rhetoric of later phrenological writers on the related subject of prison discipline.[38] Ross's pamphlet supports and rationalizes the necessity of the prevailing methods of naval discipline and expresses the desire to see phrenology employed in order to maximize the effectiveness of those methods: Through phrenological analysis, he believed, the psychological sources of a sailor's disobedience could be located and hence the most appropriate conventional punishments applied. The son of a minister, Ross was also orthodox in religion, and there is no reason to doubt his claim that he at first rejected Gall and Spurzheim's teachings because of their association with fatalism and materialism. Apparently it was only after reading Spurzheim's works, the *Transactions of the Edinburgh Phrenological Society*, and Combe's early essays that Ross came to the conclusion that phrenology, by revealing human imperfections, actually exposed one's "dire need for the Saviour Jesus."[39] In this and other respects his path to phrenology was not unlike that of certain members of the Church of Scotland who, as Ross believed

under information, and the ideas that [phrenology] was a dangerous doctrine, studied it as a duty, that they might the better be enabled to "crush it in the bud," [but in the process] became proselytes to the science, and some of them, who have become the greatest proficients, have not hesitated to declare its doctrines not only conformable and congruous to those of Christianity, but (next to the scriptures) to be its most rational and natural support.[40]

By pointing this out and by insisting that phrenology vindicated a truth "founded on facts, ascertained by consciousness and observation," Ross was quite consciously attempting to forestall the casting onto himself of the animadversions "lavished on those who expouse the cause of phrenology."

But if Ross recognized phrenology as socially deviant, why would he bother to join a phrenological society? It could be argued that having to his satisfaction rationalized a faith in the science as nondeviant socially and religiously, he saw no contradiction in supporting what could be shown to reinforce orthodox practices and beliefs. However, were this representation of his chain of reasoning correct, it would still not quite answer why he chose to join phrenological ranks when he might as well have held privately to his belief in the practical value of phrenology. A better explanation for his open support (and one that reveals this representation of his reasoning as incorrect) emerges when we recall the particular circumstances in which he found himself in the early 1820s.

In his 1818 expedition to the Arctic, Ross blundered by claiming that access to the Pacific through Arctic waters was blocked by the existence of what he indicated were the "Crocker Mountains." The explorer William Parry and the astronomer Sir Edward Sabine, both of whom accompanied Ross on his expedition, doubted the existence of the Crocker Mountains and were able to confirm their doubts in the expedition commanded by Parry in 1819–20. Sabine meanwhile published a highly polemical attack on Ross, and, upon Parry's return, Ross's credibility as an explorer and geographer was shattered.[41] The government and scientific elite no longer sought his counsel on matters of Navy exploration nor sponsored any further voyages by him. Ross's status and place within the scientific community were thus rendered ambiguous: If he was not quite an "outsider," he certainly no longer commanded "insider" status and power.

In making his faith in phrenology public, Ross can be seen as acting in ways analogous to many of the young professionals who joined phrenological societies whose experiences of social and economic insecurity were predetermined by background. Ross, too, it would seem, was both gesturing resentment and seeking to challenge the monopolizers of power who had shut him out. Seeming to underline this point is the fact that once Ross had restored his reputation and had worked his way back into the corridors of power (in 1829, through the private financial backing of the distiller Felix Booth), he no longer maintained any public connection with phrenology and phrenologists, though he continued to pursue the science privately.[42] Ross only differed from the majority of those in the phrenological societies in that he did not seek to combine his use of the phrenological resource to challenge authority with any politically linked ambition to fundamentally alter social structures and relations. For Ross, as for many others involved with phrenology prior to its full Combean elaboration, association with the knowledge was more personally than socially opportunistic. But it was no less "political" for that.[43]

Had Ross been unable to restore his reputation and self-esteem, it is conceivable that he would have retained association with phrenologists and possibly have taken up the social and ideological attitudes of the majority of those in the phrenological societies. Some such process of adopting attitudes that eventually came to rival those belonging to social background occurred in the case of Sir George MacKenzie,[‡] the squire of Coul. A gentleman–amateur in science, MacKenzie was a friend and pupil of the founder of the Wernerian Natural History Society, the geologist Robert Jameson. On the basis of his work in mineralogy and for his part in a valuable geological survey of Iceland, he had been elected a fellow of the Royal Society of Edinburgh in 1799 and the Royal Society of London in 1815.

MacKenzie became interested in phrenology in 1816 during the debates in Edinburgh between Gordon and Spurzheim. He was then delivering in parts to the Royal Society of Edinburgh what in 1817 was to be published as *An Essay on Some Subjects Connected with Taste*, an essay in which he not only dared to question some of the opinions of Dugald Stewart, but to account for why Stewart's metaphysics had fallen out of fashion. Arriving at the conclusion that metaphysics were useless because they offered nothing tangible that could be practically applied, it was almost inevitable that MacKenzie should have been led to an interest in the radical phrenological alternative to metaphysics. Indeed, by the conclusion of his delivery in the Royal Society, he was opting enthusiastically for Spurzheim's doctrine as "the only true explanation of the differences of taste and of taste itself." The basis for friendship with phrenologists established, MacKenzie became an intimate of Combe in 1817. Shortly thereafter his faith in phrenology was cemented when he experienced a convincing delineation of his head (an experience common among phrenological zealots, though, as MacKenzie's intellectual movement indicates, not essential to the desire to pursue phrenology).[44] In 1820 he published a volume of *Illustrations of Phrenology* and joined the EPS.

Unlike Ross's public commitment to phrenology, MacKenzie's obviously cannot be related to a single or sudden experience of alienation from his scientific and social peers. Nevertheless, once committed to the doctrine, he was to undergo experiences that could only help to channel his antimetaphysical interest in the knowledge into explicit antielitism and so strengthen the ideological rapport with Combe and other bourgeois social reformers.[45] In 1825 the Royal Society of Edinburgh denied MacKenzie the privilege of responding to the antiphrenology papers delivered in the society by Hamilton. The frosty reception that he received from that body in December 1829 when he was finally permitted to respond (after Hamilton had had further occasion to deliver antiphrenological papers), the society's refusal to print his reply in their official proceedings, and their subsequent spurning of his deliberately provocative presentation of the volumes of the *Phrenological Journal* further contributed to his movement toward and

self-identification with the nonaristocratic, overtly entrepreneurial–utilitarian bourgeois–liberal ideology of the Combean phrenologists. The point is underlined both in the fact that it was in
March 1832, the very month of the third reading of the Reform
Bill, that MacKenzie made his presentation of the volumes of the
Phrenological Journal to the Royal Society and that it was in the
liberal *Scotsman*, the voice of the new middle class in Edinburgh,
that he published his reply to Hamilton.[46] MacKenzie was thus
not unlike certain of the improvement-orientated landowners involved with the Royal Institution of London who, as a result of
much less acute political experiences in science activity, similarly
took up ideological positions that did not objectively "belong" to
them.[47] MacKenzie's "false consciousness" was exceptional only
to the extent that phrenology itself was exceptional in making the
links with social and ideological deviance highly visible.

Though MacKenzie was the only aristocrat to both articulate
and fully embrace a Combean style of phrenological thinking, he
was not alone in combining an interest in the knowledge with an
interest in conventional science and in having the social signifi-
cations of the latter modified by the reactions to the former. The
chemist and mineralogist Richard Chenevix is another who appears to have traced a similar-looking trajectory, though he was
far less a science dilettante than MacKenzie. He had studied chemistry at the University of Glasgow, won the Royal Society's Gold
Medal in 1801, and been offered a fellowship by the society upon
his first scientific communication. He had also been invited by the
Royal Institution to serve on their Committee for Chemical Investigation and in every other way was destined for a high reputation in scientific circles.[48]

According to the *Phrenological Journal*, Chenevix first became
interested in Gall's ideas around 1802 when he was twenty-eight,
making him the second British subject to "embrace" the science.
According to his own testimony, it was in Paris in November
1807 that he listened to Gall's lectures with "intense interest."[49]
Although there is no evidence either for or against the supposition
that his interest in the knowledge was heightened (in the manner
of Ross's) as a result of the faux pas he committed in the Royal
Society in 1803 over the discovery of palladium, there is clear
evidence that his belief in mesmerism (dating from 1816) hardened
his opposition to the scientific establishment who were as close-

minded on that subject as they were on phrenology.[50] Significantly, the year in which Chenevix began to practice mesmerism and to appeal for impartial inquiry into it (1828) was the same year in which he came forward in the *Foreign Quarterly Review* with an impressive article on phrenology that strongly endorsed its claims.[51] The following May he communicated to the Royal Society (while Roget was the editor of its *Transactions*) Spurzheim's paper on the anatomy of the brain. Given his conversance with the whole phrenology controversy up to that time and, in particular with Roget's and the Royal Society's part in it, Chenevix could hardly have missed the significance of or have been surprised at the statement of the secretary who read Spurzheim's paper – that it could not be printed in the official proceedings because "it did not contain any new matter." As bluntly stated by Davies Gilbert, the president of the Royal Society at the time of Chenevix's death in 1830, the speculations into which Chenevix had fallen were *"wholly unworthy of being noticed in this place!"*[52]

Chenevix's background was that of a wealthy Huguenot family exiled in Ireland – a background that goes far to explain why he should have given backing to knowledge persecuted by authority, why he should have been friendly with the Edgeworths and other reformers, and why he delighted in opposing German chemistry, which he saw as linked through *Naturphilosophie* to counterrevolutionary politics.[53] That same background, however, that extends to his marriage to a countess and to his spending the largest part of his adult life on the Continent also inhibits consigning Chenevix's support for phrenology to any narrowly conceived sociopolitical school. His example also highlights the problem inherent to and effaced by the rigidity and passivity of sociological maps of supporters and opponents of particular sets of ideas – the problem of degrees of commitment. Chenevix clearly sympathized with phrenologists and gave them his support, but he can hardly be called a "strong" supporter of the knowledge. There is no evidence that he ever belonged to a phrenological society, and although his posthumously published *Essay on National Character* (1832) was held by phrenologists to be an elaboration of their principles, the book's actual reliance on phrenology is minimal.[54] Thus although Chenevix's example supports the correspondence between ruptured relations with the orthodox scientific community and socially meaningful interest in bodies of dissenting knowledge, it also points to the importance of heeding the additional complicating factors in that relationship, factors emotional, temporal, and spatial.

Many of these same considerations apply to the involvement with phrenology of the final figure we have space to consider here, Thomas Ignatius Maria Forster.[‡] He merits our attention as the person who not only added the organ of "mystery" to the phrenological chart (subsequently labeled "supernatural") and as the first person to lecture on the subject in Edinburgh, but also as the person who, in 1815, coined the word *phrenology*. Forster's background, like Chenevix's, was one of independent wealth, valuable family connections with many of the leading scientific, medical, and literary figures of the day, and dissent. His ancestor was Benjamin Furly (1636–1714), the Quaker merchant and friend of Locke, whose exile in Rotterdam provided a haven for radical republican intellectuals and freethinkers. Forster's father, grandfather, and uncles, all of whom had a hand in Forster's Rousseau-inspired upbringing at the family estate near Epping Forest, carried on the family tradition of merchant banking, the pursuit of science (especially botany), commitment to English and French Enlightenment principles, and devotion to humanitarian causes (many of them Quaker-associated, though the family seems to have become nondenominational).[55] Forster, by the time he was in his midtwenties and before he had begun his medical studies at Cambridge, was already being regarded as one of Britain's "most indefatigible and successful cultivator[s] of the natural sciences."[56] He had written on meteorology, ornithology, insanity, and botany (the last resulting in a fellowship in the Linnean Society) and had begun to cultivate his other life-long interests in medicine, astronomy, aeronautics, vegetarianism, and temperance. In 1817 he married the daughter of an amateur physicist and fellow of the Royal Society, Henry Beaufoy.

Unlike Chenevix, however, Forster's commitment to phrenology was highly public and unequivocal. In his autobiography he claimed to have first been attracted to Gall's doctrine in 1806 (possibly, therefore, after having read the favorable account of it published in the *Medical and Physical Journal* in that year) and to have faithfully followed the progress of the science thereafter. But it was not until 1814, when, through Lawrence, he met Spurzheim in London and had his head read phrenologically, that he became an enthusiastic convert. Befriended by Spurzheim, he studied brain physiology under him, introduced him to Sir Joseph Banks and other savants who were family friends, and traveled with him on parts of his British tour. In Cambridge in 1815 Forster apparently tutored John Herschel, Babbage, and Whewell on the science, and it was his paper on phrenology to the Wernerian Society of Edinburgh in June 1816 that set the stage for the intellectual drama in that town a month later when, in Barclay's lecture theater, with the *Edinburgh Review* in one hand and a skull in the other, Spurzheim delivered his famous point-by-point refutation of John Gordon's critique of the doctrine. In March 1825 Forster was elected an honorary member of the LPS.[57]

Since many of Forster's scientific communications as well as his writings on phrenology were made in the same journal in which he coined the word *phrenology* – the *Philosophical Magazine* – it is not unreasonable to associate him with the professed objects of that journal: to open out science by "diffus[ing] Philosophical Knowledge among every Class of Society" and making it more "useful ... especially to the Arts and Manufactures of Great Britain."[58] More particularly, we might align Forster with the members of the London Askesian Society and the London Philosophical Society, the chief ideological organ of which was the *Philosophical Magazine*. The Askesians, who established their society in 1796, were mostly "new men," largely self-made, intellectually active, socially mobile, and deliberately practical rather than contemplative. Although the society was weighted with nonconformist medical men (primarily Quakers and Unitarians), the newspaper entrepreneur who was the editor of the *Philosophical Magazine*, Alexander Tilloch, was a typical early member.[59] The son of a Glasgow tobacco merchant, Tilloch (1759–1825) was educated at the University of Glasgow before emigrating to London in 1787, where he purchased the *Star* newspaper and joined the Sandemanians. By the end of the century he had established himself economically and, like other Askesians, was concerned not simply with status, but with expressing through the mode of science activity the desire for accommodation within a slightly more democratic social and cultural power structure than that then existing. After the Askesian Society merged with the Geological Society in 1807, Tilloch moved into the slightly more radical, but still wholly bourgeois, London Philosophical Society, established in 1811. Its pledge, as printed in the *Philosophical Magazine*, was to "eradicate unphilosophical prejudices . . . but above all, to remove that barrier erected by pedantry against universal knowledge, which has introduced an *esprit de corps* into philosophy, and rendered it the territory of a sect rather than the promise of the world."[60] Unlike the Askesian Society, the London Philosophical Society gave backing to phrenology, and although the *Philosophical Magazine* had given impartial reports on Gall and Spurzheim's doctrine since 1802, it is not until the 1810s that they can be read as counterculturally significant.[61] The appearance after 1815 of Forster's many articles on the doctrine can be taken as confirming Tilloch's appreciation of the science as such, for these were not just accounts of the science, but fulsome tributes to it that left no doubt about the extent of the knowledge's challenge to accepted thought. As Forster humbly submitted in one of his phrenological articles in 1815: "I only wish to excite others to lay aside, as I have done, the notions of the old philosophers, to discard all previous opinions and to reason by facts which can be demonstrated."[62]

Yet by no means does it necessarily follow merely from the fact that Forster made statements such as these in the *Philosophical Magazine* that the significance he himself attached to the science was the same as that of those who seized upon the knowledge he labeled. Forster was neither an Askesian nor a member of the Philosophical Society, and although he is known to have corresponded with the radical publisher Richard Carlile, he seems to have been generally happier in the company of the more retiring John Abernethy than the radical William Lawrence.[63] Unlike Mackenzie, Forster had little interest in utilizing phrenology to advance a utilitarian–meritocratic social philosophy, and unlike Elliotson he had virtually no interest in mounting, through phrenology's materialist study of mind, an attack on the major ideological edifice of traditional landed society: established religion. In some respects, as Spurzheim perceived, Forster was more like Gall, for he was both a child of the Enlightenment and a romantic dissident from some of the Enlightenment's basic philosophical assumptions.[64] Moreover, like Gall, he never really lost his political innocence or ever consciously attempted to deploy what was philosophically deviant to an ideology of social change. Being relatively secure socially and economically, he had no need to. Nor was he forced to do so out of any experience of alienation from his peers: Well within an ostensibly liberal-minded – Banksean – intellectual elite, he could decline the Royal Society's offer of a fellowship in 1816 on the grounds of certain of its rules while continuing to attend Bank's Sunday morning private assemblies in Soho.[65]

It would be mistaken, therefore, to attempt to read Forster's dismissal of the "absurdities" of Berkleyian philosophy, "the studied sophistry of Hume and the verbiage of Dugald Stuart [*sic*]," as an expression of the desire to alter social relations by attacking their philosophical foundations as impractically idealist and elitist.[66] Far from subscribing to the practical-minded and empiricist rhetoric of those within the Askesian mold, Forster was always as proud of his contributions to metaphysics as he was of his contributions to the practical sciences and arts.[67] Indeed, therein lies the clue to his dismissal of previous philosophies and the clue to the difference between his interest in phrenology and that of others referred to in this chapter: For Forster, although he was reform-minded, the attack on reigning philosophical notions was not a part of a negative reaction to existing social relations, but rather a part of a purposeful quest (entirely metaphysical as far as he was concerned) for a nonmaterialist and holistic understanding of man and mind in relation to nature. Like Coleridge, the basis of whose anti-Cartesian and anti-Newtonian *Naturphilosophie* Forster may have acquired from his idealist colleagues in Cambridge (especially Whewell), Forster was searching for what have been called "the laws of interconnections between diverse phenomena" or for the spiritual reality beyond the material world.[68] His insatiable encyclopedic appetite for knowledge reflects that search, and it is in the terms of it that his celebration of phrenology is to be understood, for to him the merit of Gall's doctrine was its transcendence of the Cartesian dichotomy between mind and body through its revelation of mind and material brain as indivisible. To Forster, Gall was to be lauded for having provided within the mind of man a microcosm of the organic unity between developing interactive parts.

Although there are points of similarity between this interest in phrenology and that exemplified by Combe and Elliotson, for the most part they diverge and reflect very different philosophical premises and imperatives. They also reflect different degrees of political awareness: Although the whole of the search in which

Forster was engaged can be seen as mutually constitutive with the economically rooted and politically manifested contemporary ruptures in the connective tissues of society, Forster remained unaware of the wider sociopolitical significances of his intellectual activity. Only in the early 1820s when, in the wake of the Lawrence–Abernethy dispute, charges of political sedition came to be leveled against physiological and psychology materialism, and as phrenology pari passu began to be mobilized for radical social dissent, did Forster become cognizant of the political resonances and social implications of his advocacy of phrenology. Significantly, as he gained this awareness, he began to retreat from the science. Though, like Ross, he never repudiated the scientific basis, nor the practical value of phrenology, he no longer devoted the same amount of attention to it that he had in the past, while the attention that he did devote to it was largely given to distinguishing his interest from that of those beginning to take it up. To argue against what he called the "bad interpretation" of phrenology as pure materialism and to vindicate an apolitical nonmaterialist reason for his having taken an interest in it were the prime motives for writing his autobiography in 1835. In it he took to particular task those "Scottish anatomists" who, in his opinion, had been seduced by their trade into thinking that through the phrenological depiction of the physical parts of the brain they could understand mind. Such persons, Forster wrote, echoing Thomas Brown, were reifying humanness by pushing physics beyond its proper limits; they were revealing reasons for being interested in phrenology that, at a philosophical level, were entirely contrary to those that had led him to his advocacy.[69]

In thus coming to defend an antimaterialist philosophy, Forster was thrust unwittingly into a conservative position relative to the supporters of Elliotson or Lawrence. Moreover, he was forced to become sociopolitically aware of this. In the manner of Godwin and Wordsworth before him, he now began actively to defend conservative political interests. In 1827 he wrote appreciatively of Prime Minister Canning, and in 1830 he wrote of England's liberty and prosperity under Wellington.[70] Yet just as it is mistaken to see the growth of Forster's interest in Gall's ideas as directly related to concern with changes in social relations and structures, so it is an oversimplification to interpret his "retreat" from phrenology as immediately linked either to preserving the political status quo or to a heightened concern with social respectability. In fact, it could be argued that he did not retreat from phrenology because of its radical materialist associations so much as he outgrew any need for it upon finding in the Catholicism to which he converted in 1824 the "centre of unity" for which he had always been searching.[71] This interpretation is attractive since on the one hand it is only with difficulty that Forster's ongoing scientific activities in the 1820s can be seen as relating (at any level) to a heightened concern with social unorthodoxy, while on the other hand an espousal of Catholicism in Britain in the early 1820s can hardly be regarded as any less unorthodox than an advocacy of phrenology.

In reality, Forster's turning to Catholicism and his disassociation from radical phrenological materialism were the connected parts of a single process. Both aspects may be traced to the year 1823 when he visited his "friend" Gall in Paris and expressed his disagreement with the idea that the "spirit" was merely a function of the organization of brain matter.[72] In the same year he published his *Somatopsychonoologia* in which, while defending Lawrence's antivitalist theory of life against Abernethy, he at the same time argued the irrelevance of science itself for understanding the truth about human existence.[73] Instead, in the manner of sixteenth-century humanists, he argued the need to return to a pure Catholicism in which Reason and Faith would be entwined. Upon his conversion to Catholicism the following year and through its religious obligations he claimed to have found access to "a new order of things."[74] In his own terms he had succeeded in his ambition to make his world whole. It is pointless therefore to debate whether Forster's retreat from phrenology was determined by his personal "spiritual" growth or whether the spiritual development was determined by his reaction to the emergent sociopolitical meaning of psychological materialism. It would seem more important to recognize from his example, as indeed from the others considered in this chapter, that human reality is "total" and that any attempt to carve out a separation between material sociopolitical concerns and spiritual or intellectual ones can only be productive of misleading historical abstraction.[75]

More generally, the consideration of these examples of early supporters of phrenology makes it clear that there could be as many individual motives for turning to and deploying Gall's unorthodox ideas as there could be particular dissatisfying circumstances seeming to require confrontation. Nothing in the knowledge itself determined the kind of opposition to be expressed through the knowledge (though there was, as we will come to see, a particular kind of *order* mediated through the knowledge). So far as biographical information permits us listening in on these early advocacies, what is heard is discordant: In taking the same protest song, each sang it according to a melody determined by his own immediate needs and interests. To acknowledge these individual variations in motive and expression, however, is not to invalidate claims for the social nature of the production and use of the knowledge, nor to suggest that "personal" factors can therefore be *juxtaposed to* "social" factors in explaining people's interest in the knowledge. Even though it might be said of some of these early supporters that they were more interested in expressing and, through expressing, coping with, their personal miseries, frustrations, and longings than they were interested in society and social facts,[76] this does not necessitate that, even in those cases, we forfeit social considerations for entirely psychological ones. Indeed, it is impossible to see how we can, since in all cases the knowledge was pursued not apolitically for its own sake (or, at least, not only for its own sake), but always as an expression of dissent from the existing intellectual order of things and, hence, from the existing rationales for the social order.

What cannot be said of these early supporters of phrenology is that they foresaw or necessarily predicated the future social and ideological meaning and use of the knowledge. Even Elliotson, in aligning Gall's antiidealism with radical materialism, could not have understood the full social implications of his action, since no more than anyone else in the 1810s and 1820s had he the power to visualize the social, economic, and cultural shape of things to come. His particular kind of expropriation of the knowledge was important to emergent social groupings because the kind of opposition it aroused clearly revealed the appropriateness of applying phrenology to an antitraditional, antiauthoritarian ideology of change. But in the first instance, Elliotson's deployment of the knowledge was prompted more by self-interest than social consciousness. Likewise we could say of the other early propagators of Gall's ideas that they fertilized the imported seed and made its agitational function manifest, but it was not their efforts so much as the changing composition of the soil itself that determined the way the plant was to grow as well as the kind, quality, and marketability of the fruit it was to bear.

3

The rites of passage

Thus there are historically formed specialised categories for the
exercise of the intellectual function. They are formed in connection with all social groups, but especially in connection with the
more important, and they undergo more extensive and complex
elaboration in connection with the dominant social group. One
of the most important characteristics of any group that is developing towards dominance is its struggle to assimilate and to con-
quer "ideologically" the traditional intellectuals.

Selections from the Prison Notebooks of Antonio Gramsci,
ed. Q. Hoare and G. Nowell Smith (1971), p. 10

A new science proves its efficacy and vitality when it demonstrates
that it is capable of confronting the great champions of the tendencies opposed to it and when it either resolves by its own means
the vital questions which they have posed or demonstrated, in
preemptory fashion, that these questions are false problems.

Ibid., p. 433

It will now be seen whether Phrenology is a "fraud," a piece of
"specious quackery," a system of "bumps and lumps," and its
"pretended discovers philosophical imposters," or a system
founded in nature, and having truth for its basis.

Lancet, 16 April 1825, p. 41 (on Spurzheim's lectures)

"Who would have supposed," remarked Richard Chenevix in his
article in the *Foreign Quarterly Review* of 1828,

that from the perceptions of a mere brat of nine years old, a system could
have ensued, which, in the hands of Dr. Spurzheim, would in the year
1826, have filled not only the large lecture-room of the London Institution, but all the staircases, corridors, and passages leading to it, with
hearers?[1]

The question was rhetorical, but the fact was, that from the early
1820s many Britons had arrived at the "painful conviction, that

this delusive doctrine is widely spreading, in circles where scientific information is but sparingly distributed, and where specious pretension is admitted as an equivalent for solid learning."[2] Moreover, it was clear to most contemporaries that the growth of this interest in phrenology among predominantly middle-class groups could not be attributed simply to a fascination with skulls, craniology, and cerebral physiology. Though curiosity and novelty doubtless played a part in drawing to Spurzheim's lectures in the London Institution the largest audience in that institution's history,[3] the fact that it was in that kind of forum, and at that particular moment in history that interest in phrenology was awakened, deprives curiosity and novelty, or mere fashion alone, of explanatory power in and of themselves. Nor can we attribute the phenomenon solely to the force of personality, since Spurzheim was not the only person to experience such lecturing successes – successes that often occurred in the very places where the knowledge had previously been spurned.[4] Finally, while we can indeed relate the growth of interest to the growth of belief in phrenology's scientific veracity, it should be obvious that only the most causally specious a posteriori logic would permit the latter to explain the former. That the members of the London Philomathic Institution spent four nights in 1825 debating the question "Is there reason to believe that the doctrines of Phrenology are founded in Truth?" before devoting a large part of their journal to extolling phrenology's practical benefits, confirms, as much other evidence does, that the image of scientificity and truth were considered as vital.[5] But if only because such discussions were conducted in full awareness of the prohibitions on the subject in the more established scientific institutions and were, therefore, social discussions a priori, the matter of phrenology's truth must be seen only to beg the question of *how* and under *what* conditions that truth came to be constituted in those quarters.

Such is the brief for this chapter. Since it is a part of our contention, however, that the answers to historical questions about social phenomena are not to be found wholly in the phenomena themselves, nor only in the power of ideas behind them, we begin by turning to the general social and institutional contexts in which phrenological knowledge came to be elaborated and deployed.

SCIENCE ACTIVITY'S SOCIAL LANDSCAPE

Although no society is ever out of the processes of "destructuration" and "restructuration," British society in the period between the 1790s and the 1840s was in many respects in the almost formless conjunction in between. In the 1820s especially, virtually every cultural tissue that in one way or another had bonded preindustrial society was in a state of dissolution, while the new cultural tissues that would bind industrial society were only at the point of their formation. Antonio Gramsci's term *organic crisis* characterizes the situation well (if unintentionally), for although the social transformations centered in this period were radical and systemic, they involved no moment of revolutionary break with the past.[6] The hallmark of this period was more one of experience and feeling than of spectacle and direct observation. All the changes in manners, habits, and outlooks, like all the overt and covert political activity generated directly and indirectly from the shift in the economic mode of production (itself a gradual shift), were class-orientated, yet were manifested in the absence of discretely perceived class structures and relations. Like the organism unwittingly liberated from the usual restrictions imposed upon it by inheritance and design as a result of a new external force, social class structures were at a moment of release at the same time as they were assuming their new dialectically bound internal and external forms.

That the rapid growth of science activity during the Industrial Revolution was a part of this process of "the making" of class is no more in doubt than the observation of E. P. Thompson, that "the bourgeois revolution and the scientific revolution in [seventeenth century] England...were clearly a good deal more than just good friends."[7] Although historians have largely shied away from the task of analyzing in class terms the relationship between economic and scientific activity during the so-called second scientific revolution, they have made it clear nevertheless that while interest in science in places such as the London Institution or the provincial literary and philosophical societies – "Lit & Phils" – was integral to the Industrial Revolution, there was no essential connection between that interest and the scientific–technical necessities of industrial production. To the new generation of professional men who mostly inhabited these institutions, the links between science and economy were social, political, and cultural.[8] Though the London Institution was formed in 1805 by a group of commercially minded dissidents from the Royal Institution who were seeking to provide the City's answer to the science of landed society offered in Mayfair, in it, no less than in the Lit & Phils, the pursuit of the knowledge proclaimed as "practical" was independent of the knowledge's technical utility or validity.[9] Primarily, scientific knowledge functioned in these forums to provide a cultural space for indirectly expressing and rationalizing distance from the priorities, underlying values, and implicit assumptions and legitimations of the preindustrial agrarian-based social order and power structure. Through the pursuit of knowledge that was ostensibly practical and rational, a challenge was made, explicitly or implicitly, to the contemplative and introspective means, whether intellectualist–metaphysical or spiritual–religious, whereby the traditionally constituted power structure was seen as sanctioned. As this "natural knowledge" was used to delegitimate what by implication were the "unnatural" bases of the traditional social structure, so it was also used to legitimate the transformation to, if not actual existence of, a social world in which urban utilitarian and meritocratic values would predominate.

That the need for this social world was expressed intensely within these particular forums cannot be separated from the fact that many of their members were outside or only on the edges of existing social elites. To a certain extent they were like the institutions themselves at certain moments in their histories, in that they were seeking incorporation within higher-status groups. Characteristically, this upward mobility was often accompanied by simultaneous denunciation of those same higher-status groups. But the fact that not all members can be characterized as social "outsiders" or "marginal men" or culturally "liminal" persons, while those who might be thus categorized were often ambivalent about the social center to which they were aspiring, suggests that the raison d'être of these institutions in the period prior to the 1840s was not simply that of facilitating upward mobility.[10] (There were, after all, more effective ways of seeking gentlemanly status and power than joining a Lit & Phil.) Rather, as Ian Inkster has recently suggested in a revision of his previous view, one must understand these institutions more in terms of their providing *identities* for those whose "marginality" was less crucially determined by their economic and social standing than by the fact that they were "neither overtly of the capitalists and often decidedly not of the working masses."[11] For young medical men, above all, the sense of ambiguous social place could be intense. Often it was heightened by experience in infirmaries and dispensaries where lay governors regarded them as "comparable to factory managers or engineers – men with skills but employees or tradesmen rather than capitalists."[12] Unlike their eighteenth-century predecessors in medicine, law, and the Church, whose status as "gentlemen" of learning, leisure, and culture had been conferred on them by the landowning class, the new generations of professionals (of whom there were simply many more per capita than ever before) had to rely far more upon occupational qualifications and merit in order to acquire status.[13] By the standards of preindustrial Britain they were not even "professionals," for in ungentlemanly fashion they had to seek fees for specialized services and had to do so in highly competitive and almost entirely urban markets. Moreover, like other entrepreneurs, they frequently had to sell their products as "safe and rational" to a public that was often highly sceptical. It is not surprising, therefore, that it was the medical profession in particular that was most intellectually active in the new science institutions of the early nineteenth century,[14] nor surprising that they tended to exaggerate bourgeois aspirations and competitive individualist values and to be outspoken in their commitment to social change.[15]

By thus locating themselves in Lit & Phils and similar places, the new professionals confirmed through the use of natural knowledge and the rhetoric of utility the legitimacy of bourgeois dominance. Thereby, reciprocally, over time, these "new men" – the self-styled "thinking class" – also confirmed their own elitist identity and integration into the ruling class that was being remade. Thus from behind value-neutral façades, through knowledge associated with radical social dissent but rendered "polite" (by, among other means, the adoption of Royal Society rules prohibiting overt discussion of politics and religion), the members of these institutions engaged in a struggle of class making that was allied to and inseparable from the political, economic, and social fortunes of bourgeois industrial capitalism.

BACONIAN APOTHEOSIS

If "science and active benevolence" in general provided these men with the "power of speech" (as was said of the phrenologist Dr. Charles Cowan), phrenology in particular gave unmistakable expression to their purpose.[16] As specially "revived" by and for the new urban professionals in the 1820s, phrenology metaphorically and literally drove their social aspirations to a head.[17] As a body of natural knowledge that not only celebrated intellect, but celebrated it through a physiological interpretation of cerebral reality that located intellectual and moral faculties physically at the top of a value-laden hierarchy of mental organs, phrenology indeed was almost a caricature of the aspirations of the "thinking class." Its naïvely empiricist methodology – the purported observation of mental functions through craniological formations – highlighted the differences with, at the same time that it challenged the introspective intellectual processes and productions of, the metaphysicians. By comparison, phrenology's methodology made the latter's productions appear deliberately obfuscatory – as "scholastical *double* dutch," "a labyrinth of obscurities and absurdities."[18] Typically, Robert Chambers wrote: "To me, Phrenology appears to bear the same relation to the doctrines of even the most recent metaphysicians [as] Copernican astronomy bears to the system of Ptolemy."[19] Unlike the mysterious, excluding methods of the elitist mental philosophers (which phrenologists likened to alchemy), phrenology was democratically open to the observations and common sense of all.[20] As its findings were visible, so its theory and practice were easy to grasp. Thus the defense of phrenology was always inseparably a defense of the rights of "the people" against the rule of privileged groups.[21] By the same antioccult token, phrenology championed a material–practical world in which there was little room for the spiritual. Though, in truth, phrenology's revivalists (no less than spiritual revivalists) were seeking to perceive reality through a glass clearly, the reality they sought to grasp immediately and directly, and the means by which they pursued it, were wholly different. As opposed to the pursuit of inner truth through emotional or sensual–spiritual experience and/ or blind faith, phrenology's mainstream apologists in the 1820s (unlike some earlier romantics and later socialists) sought a wholly quantifiable external truth by means intellectual and "rational."[22] In the words of a religious-orientated educational magazine in 1835, "phrenology is to the science of mind, what astrology was to astronomy or alchemy to chemistry; with this difference, that it seeks to mystify by assumed facts, instead of occult mystery."[23] The celebration of the physiological "facts" of mental organization for the amelioration of man's social condition never held phrenologists back from likening the spread of their message to that of

Christ, however.[24] Indirectly, too, they drew upon and gained rhetorical strength from traditional spiritually inspired antischolasticism. But it was hardly in the tradition of Calvin, Luther, Wesley, or the cobbler and mystic Jacob Boehme that these phrenologists regarded themselves when they scorned the dead languages, the classics, and other symbols of elitist obscurantism.[25] Nor was it in the more naturalistic, antiauthoritarian, and antiintellectualist tradition of Paracelsus and Van Helmont that they saw their pursuit of plain and puritanical understanding. Rather, and almost exclusively, they considered themselves as following in the footsteps of Francis Bacon. Emphasizing observation, absolutizing "objective facts," and stressing accessibility, practicality, and progress, they enlarged the Baconian image of science in order to reiterate Bacon's rejection of all arguments based on mere political and religious authority. More than others, phrenologists were responsible for both the making and the spreading of the notion of Bacon's method as "the one God had approved for Englishmen" (as Charles Kingsley put it).[26]

It was characteristic of this Baconianism that it paid scant attention to those aspects of Bacon's writings that supported careful analysis and inductive logic – to those aspects, that is, that made Bacon intellectually attractive to natural philosophers such as John Herschel and William Whewell. In fact, it was precisely because phrenology ignored academic niceties, or dismissed them as academic pedantry, that it appealed the more strongly to those who were mostly engaged in practical affairs and who had little or no desire to critically reflect. Phrenology's reification of mind and wholly empiricist comprehension of mental function legitimated the abdication of reflection by denying an active principle in cognition.[27] Which is to say, more generally, that phrenology appealed because it always oversimplified: As it was the ultimate form of psychological reductionism, so it inspired a wholly simplified grasp of all intellectual and social reality. Though hardly unique in this respect, insofar as this simplification of reality permitted coping with uncertainty and ambiguity in a social situation conducive to their intensification, we might assign to phrenology, at the level of the individual, much the same function that Malinowski assigned to magic and that Parsons extended to "pseudoscience" at the level of society as a whole.[28] We will elaborate on this psychosocial function of phrenology in our discussion of the attraction to the knowledge of George Combe; at this juncture it is only necessary to point out that it is precisely the positivist distinction between "scientific" and "irrational" systems of thought that Malinowski and Parson's functionalist explanation of the "irrational" was intended a priori to reinforce, that the history of phrenology's popularization undermines. Here, after all, was a body of knowledge that was anything but "magical" or "irrational," however much it may have been derided as nonsense by some contemporaries. If phrenology was extraordinary, it was not as "pseudoscience" in the Parsonian sense, but rather as "suprascience," for what distinguishes its appeal was its ultrarationalism and ultraantisupernaturalism, or, as we would say today, its ultrapositivism. It cannot be stressed enough that in investigating phrenology's construction and appeal in these terms we are exposing not an exceptional body of knowledge, but one that is ultrarepresentational.

MAKING SUPRASCIENCE

In the Lit & Phils, as in the societies exclusively devoted to phrenology, it was primarily the evidence of medical spokesmen that gave the greatest legitimacy to the other members' belief in phrenology's scientific integrity. It needs recalling that to the majority of lay persons the antiphrenological literature written by the scientific elite was not readily available nor all that interesting. Far more available and stimulating were the bigoted religiously motivated attacks. Hence to those seeking to establish society on a more "rational" footing, the very presence of numerous medical supporters of phrenology could enhance conviction as well as allow for the dismissal of accusations that the supporters of the knowledge were persons ignorant of anatomy and physiology – "lawyers, divines, and merchants, who know nothing about the brain."[29] But it was the supposed value-neutrality of medical knowledge that mattered most. Since the leading opponents had also to rely on medical knowledge, it was not in the capacity of the opposition to reveal medical knowledge as socially constructed. The sanctity of medical science remained inviolate (as indeed it does in much medical history) since it was in everyone's interest that it should appear so. Hence journals such as the *Gentleman's Magazine*, which began in the early 1820s to cater to the new breed of men in the Lit & Phils, could simply draw on the expertise of the medical profession to justify their new phrenological recommendations.[30]

In the lecture halls the scientific expertise and supposed objectivity of phrenology was visibly reinforced by the very artifacts of medical science – the skulls, busts, casts, and charts of brains with which lecturers surrounded themselves. Spurzheim, who did more than any other itinerant to disseminate phrenology in the Lit & Phils in the 1820s, was particularly fond of thus equipping himself, and, as critics pointed out, "few were prepared, by previous knowledge, to estimate the real merits of his demonstrations."[31] As indicated by the outline of Spurzheim's lecture course to the London Institution (Figure 2), the case for phrenology appeared to be argued by facts alone, to which were added sensible-sounding practical conclusions.

Significantly, the central factual illustration in phrenology, the phrenology head, had itself become scientized by the mid-1820s. Whereas in Gall and Spurzheim's early diagrams the head was portrayed in a natural lumpy manner and the countenance was of a real person, by the 1820s the head had become a stylized sphere (cf. Figures 3 and 4) The image of scientific precision, authority, and definitiveness that this allowed was further enhanced by the redrawing of the lines demarcating the mental faculties. The cranial topography that had appeared to John Gordon in 1815 "like the maps of revolutionized France" or "like the scales of a salmon magnified" was thereby rendered into something far more reminiscent of an illustration from physics or mechanics.[32] Whether or not this gave to phrenology an unexpected and becoming simplicity (such as Barthes attributes to $E = mc^2$), there can be no doubt that imagistically it was a part of a submission of human quality to mathematical quantification or a severing of those links to art, religion, sense, and spirit that had been integral to Lavater's physiognomy.[33] Hence, to some extent, the scientized visage of phrenology might be regarded as the iconographical response to the charge that Spurzheim laid himself open to in his lectures in the London Institution in 1825 when he carelessly referred to the "invention of phrenology." "Surely," retorted the *Monthly Magazine*, "whatever is *invented* cannot be *science*. Invention belongs to *art*, and to the creation of *genius*. Science analyses facts, and develops principles. It discovers, but it does not *invent*."[34] By

London Institution.

1827.

PROSPECTUS

OF

Dr. SPURZHEIM's

LECTURES ON PHRENOLOGY.

LECTURE I. *Wednesday April 4th.*
Introduction—The Brain is the organ of the Mind—
Plurality of the mental powers and their respective organs—
Division of the head into various regions.

LECTURE II. *Wednesday April 11th.*
Means of specifying the powers of the mind, and of
pointing out their cerebral organs.—Orders in which the
organs of the mind may be treated.—Nomenclature.

LECTURE III. *Wednesday April 18th.*
Organs in the occipital region—Amativeness—Philopro-
genitiveness—Inhabitiveness—Adhesiveness—Self Esteem.
Love of Approbation.

LECTURE IV. *Wednesday April 25th.*
Organs in the lateral regions — Combativeness — Destructiveness—Secretiveness—Cautiousness.

LECTURE V. *Wednesday May 2d.*
Organs in the Sincipital region, comprising those of the
moral and religious sentiments—Benevolence—Veneration.
Firmness—Conscientiousness—Hope—Marvellousness.

LECTURE VI. *Wednesday May 9th.*
Ideality—Mirthfulness, Imitation—Intellectual Faculties.
External Senses—Forehead or frontal region.

LECTURE VII. *Wednesday May 16th.*
Perceptive Faculties — Individuality — Form — Size—
Weight—Coloring—Eventuality—Locality.

LECTURE VIII. *Wednesday May 23d.*
Perceptive Faculties continued — Number—Order—
Time—Melody—Language—Reflective Faculties: Com-
parison—Causality.

LECTURE IX. *Wednesday May 30th.*
Philosophical — Moral and religious considerations in
connexion of Phrenology.

LECTURE X. *Wednesday June 6th.*
Phrenology in connexion with Physiognomy and the
arts of Imitation—Natural Language.

LECTURE XI. *Wednesday June 13th.*
Phrenology is the foundation of a sound doctrine of
Insanity—Points necessary to be known to Jurymen and
the Public at large.

LECTURE XII. *Wednesday June 20th.*
Phrenology is the basis of Education and Legislation.

The Lectures commence at Seven o'Clock in the Evening.

Figure 2. Prospectus of Dr. Spurzheim's lectures on Phrenology at the
London Institution, April 1827. (*Source:* London Institution, Syllabuses
of Lecture Courses 1819–1874)

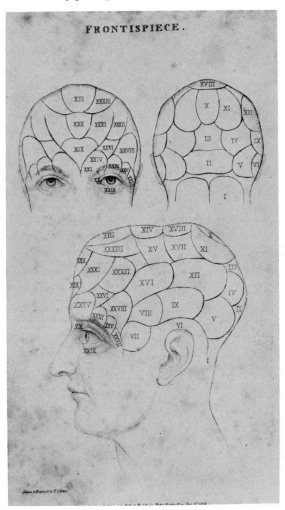

FRONTISPIECE.

Figure 3. Frontispiece phrenological head from J. G. Spurzheim's *Physiognomical System*, 1815. (Courtesy of Wellcome Institute Library, London)

literally plastering smooth the physiognomical realism of the original phrenology head, phrenologists in the 1820s symbolically disguised the human origins of their knowledge, rendering it sacred as "science." Paradoxically, the act of crafting this image of science was, simultaneously, the act of effacing phrenology's creation.

Phrenology's human origins were also disguised and its scien-

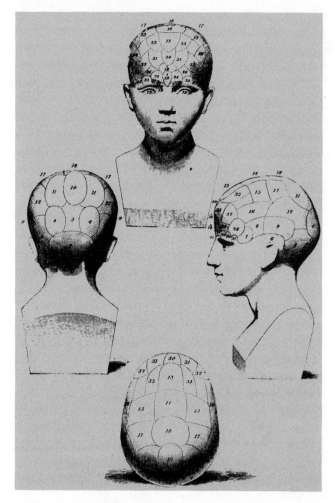

Figure 4. Frontispiece views of a phrenology head from George Combe's *Elements of Phrenology*, 1824.

tificity further enhanced by the revisions made to the original nomenclature. Whereas Gall had provided simply a list of twenty-seven mental organs, Spurzheim organized these, plus additions, into a botanical arrangement of orders and genera. Moreover, he also "botanized" the names of the organs to meet the needs of polite society: hence Gall's *Zeugungstrieb*, for the organ of sexual gratification, was rendered into "Amativeness"; *Jugenliebe, Kinderliebe*, for the love of offspring, became "Philoprogenitiveness";

Würgsinn, for the organ of the propensity to murder, was atten-
uated to "Destructiveness"; and so on.[35] Not only were these terms
as legitimate as any "in mineralogy, and still more in botany,"
phrenologists insisted, but, with the Greek exception of "Philoprogenitiveness" they were "compounded of English words, either
in Johnson's Dictionary, or in very current usage."[36] As always,
phrenologists sought to emulate what they scorned and have it
both ways at the same time – not unlike others with new bodies
of knowledge.

A different but no less deliberate move toward scientificity was
the commencement in 1821 of the "official" *Transactions of the
Edinburgh Phrenological Society*. Consciously modeled on the published proceedings of other elitist scientific assemblies, the *Transactions* conjured all the gloss of socially respectable science. Likewise
the *Phrenological Journal*, the four-shilling quarterly that superceded
the too restrictive *Transactions*, was in its layout an imitative cross
between the prestigious *Edinburgh Review* and the *Edinburgh Philosophical Journal*. Always run at a loss, the *Phrenological Journal*
(1823–47) in the eyes of phrenologists more than paid for itself as
an emblem of scientific status in a context in which that kind of
emblem was coming to matter most.[37]

But perhaps most important for the creation of phrenology's
scientific image was the identification and isolation of persons held
to be advocating a "corrupt" version of the knowledge – in particular, mammonistic lower-class practical "professors" of phrenology and working-class militants exploiting the knowledge in the
interests of atheism and socialism.[38] Although the attack on these
persons was more of a response to a situation that had developed
than a calculated strategy on the part of middle-class phrenologists,
through the act of drawing attention to the "misappliers," and
through deriding "bumpology" and "phrenological palmistry" as
vulgarizations, those seeking to monopolize the social resource of
phrenology were able subtly to elevate the idea that there actually
was, at root, a "pure" phrenology and that they, the respectable
phrenologists, were its proper guardians. By holding up to the
audience from whom they sought recognition a species of scientific
pornography or "scientism," phrenologists from the rising professional class flattered and reinforced their audiences' and their own
integrity, objectivity, and elitism in much the same way that real
pornography served Victorian moralists as a self-justifying "neg-

ative analogue."[39] Even though elitist phrenologists practiced little else at their meetings than craniology, based all of their practical remarks on the reading of heads, legitimated all that was unique in their social reform program on cranioscopic diagnosis, prided themselves on the "astonishing accuracy" with which they could read heads, and told their audiences to look to their own heads for the real proofs of the science (and of course gained their most zealous converts in this way); and even though – indeed because – it was in the name of "the people" and from the perspective of phrenology's easy access to reality that these phrenologists mounted their attack on the arcane, introspective, and mysterious methodology and productions of the old elite, they were able, through the isolation of a "false," "pseudoscientific" phrenology in the hands of charlatans and demagogues to enhance the impression that phrenology was not a superficial means of character reading, but rather a sophisticated branch of human physiology requiring deep and intelligent study.[40] Richard Beamish, for example, while elaborating the profundities of phrenology to his audience in the Cheltenham Literary and Philosophical Society in 1841, made it clear that *he*, a fellow of the Royal Society, did not feel bumps, but he invited those seeking the personal revelations of the science's truth to consult the dependable practical phrenologist, Mr. Wilson, who lived nearby.[41]

Thus "respectable" and respectability-seeking phrenologists in their effort to protect themselves and their knowledge against the charge of being "superficial and declamatory" not only popularized and reinforced a positivist notion of science as objective, value-free knowledge that could be readily distinguished from "ideology," "scientism," or "pseudoscience," but also firmly established that the demarcation was a part of the protection of class interests. Little wonder, then, that the campaign for the purity of phrenology spearheaded the campaign for the sanctity of "science" itself.

Even so, it would be anachronistic to suppose that the image of scientificity would have been enough to ensure phrenology's social success in a culture in which religion was still far more important than science. Without deference to the conventions of orthodox religion, phrenologists realized, they could not hope for a hearing from respectable society. Thus the *Phrenological Journal* in its "Introductory Statement" in November 1823 was at pains to assure its readers, "We will omit no opportunity of removing those grounds of unjust dislike to our science, arising from an erroneous belief that it leads to materialism, fatalism, immorality, or irreligion."[42] Nor did it omit such opportunity. Endlessly it reiterated, on the one hand, that phrenology leaves these questions alone (which, strictly speaking, was true insofar as a materialistic and mechanistic understanding of the brain and its functions did not necessitate a denial of the immaterialist principle of mind); while on the other hand, it insisted that the science was "perfectly consistent with, and most favourable to the doctrine of the *immortality* of the soul, . . . and that it is beautifully in harmony with the precepts of our Holy Faith."[43] Not untypically, Edward Turley,‡ in his phrenology lecture to the Worcester Literary and Scientific Institution in 1834, declared:

> If I thought its study could shake one link in that chain of belief which the creature has in the bounty, and wisdom, and power of his Maker, – or, if I thought it would loosen the ties of morality and religion, I would, had I the power, hurl the demon of Phrenology, and scatter its fragments, to the extremity of space. But no, there is no more danger to be apprehended to Christianity from an examination of the curious and beautiful structure of the brain. . .than there is in examining the structure and properties of a blade of grass.[44]

By the 1840s almost wholly reversed was the widespread opinion of the 1810s that phrenology was "implicit atheism"; from the archbishop of Dublin down to the scurrilous editors of the ultraranting *Protestant Magazine*, and among dissenters of every sort, doubts about phrenology's harmony with religion were nearly everywhere dispelled.[45] Although it is clear that this shift in opinion could not have occurred had not the social center of gravity itself been shifting in the first quarter of the nineteenth century, there can be no doubt that the revised opinion of phrenology also depended upon the deliberate effort of phrenologists to divorce their knowledge (and themselves) from its previous countercultural materialist moorings. In effect, as the majority of phrenologists moved away from being merely the opponents of the old order to being the apologists for and protectors of the reformed order, they endeavored to erase their tracks. For this purpose it was insufficient (and for some phrenologists uncongenial) merely to align phrenology with orthodox natural theology.[46] More effective and more purposeful was a reliance on the same technique that had gone into the building up of phrenology's image of scientificity, namely, the identification and rhetorical exploitation of phrenological "deviants" abusing the science by twisting it to their own infidel ends. Indeed, the campaign for phrenology's religious conformity and that for its scientific purity were part of the same simultaneously occurring process. "Our readers may rest assured," the "Introductory Statement" in the *Phrenological Journal* continued,

that they will not only never find this Journal inculcating or countenancing principles at variance with sound morality and pure religion, but, on the contrary, they they will find it bringing to speedy justice any pseudo-phrenological writers, who may attempt to pervert the science by a contrary course.[47]

Not the least of the reasons why the religious and the scientific purity campaigns were linked was that those who could most easily be picked out and taken to task as the "defilers" were phrenology's supporters among the working class. As we shall see below, when this class-directed campaign was undermined in the early 1840s by certain middle-class phrenologists breaking rank and too openly aligning the knowledge with materialism, phrenology was seriously impaired as an elitist bourgeois movement. Through this act the sought-after contrast between the pure and the defiled was itself defiled.

Quintessential to the technique of drawing sharp contrasts in order rhetorically to exploit them was the phrenologists' emphasis on their persecution. Like the identification of deviants within the movement, the persecutors from without permitted a backhanded skirting of certain issues and a focusing of attention elsewhere. But whereas the identification of the "pseudophrenologists" within the movement served a secondary consolidating purpose, the focus on the persecutors from without was fundamental to the rise of the movement itself. In particular, the rhetoric of persecution was deployed to withdraw attention from the explicit demands of the antiphrenologists for the phrenologists to "prove" their theory in the terms of the antiphrenologists. Like most intellectual insurgents, most phrenologists were well aware of the subjective nature of their opponents' mode of cognition and terms of reference, and they recognized that to respond directly to the demand for "proof" would mean lending tacit approval to that subjectivism. To dwell on the persecution of phrenology was to avoid that pitfall while at the same time to distinguish and legitimate differences in social and ideological outlook.[48]

Typically, phrenologists flattered their audiences' rationalism, nationalism, and liberalism by pointing out how Gall had been forbidden to lecture in autocratic Austria and how, as recently as 1824, the unenlightened Roman Catholic authorities in France had revealed their fear of scientific truth by prohibiting lectures on phrenology without special licence. Effective comparisons with the fate of Galileo were too easy to make and too tempting to resist – all the more so after phrenology was denounced as "contrary to morality and the Catholic Religion" and phrenological works were placed on the Index.[49] What a contrast with the state of affairs in the "freeest of nations," remarked Chenevix, where

the study of man will excite the greatest interest. Without such knowledge, indeed, liberty cannot exist. Such is a cause of the warm reception which phrenology has met with among its partisans in England, and of the no less warm opposition of its adversaries. The reverse, too, has procured it a tepid attention in France; for, whatever be the forms of liberty there, its spirit is yet to be born. It is, then, easy to conjecture what may be the mind of the United States of America toward this doctrine.[50]

Only in the most backward recesses, it was implied, did opposition to phrenology prevail – in places such as the Royal Societies, where the prejudices of "the great" held sway; or in Oxford where, as late as 1830, Spurzheim was refused permission to lecture; or in that bastion of Anglican priestcraft, King's College, London, where the "fettered state of mind" of certain physiologists would permit phrenology no hearing.[51] It was precisely in these places, it was further suggested, that pragmatism and humanitarianism were least cultivated: Not only did their inhabitants oppose the phrenological knowledge that could effect the best management and cure of the insane, the most efficient transportation and reform of criminals, and the surest foundation for education, but in their effort to disprove the phrenological theory of brain they had had to resort to the cruel methods of vivisection.[52] Hence the fact that phrenology had not been endorsed by the scientific establishment and had found its "chief supporters...among the lower ranks of the learned" was readily turned round as a rationale for its support

among those outside the old establishment. That neither did effete
"gentlemen of science" much approve of this most practical body
of knowledge only strengthened the rationale. As Chenevix put
it, nicely capturing the double-edge,

We do not really understand what fashion is in science; neither do we
conceive how truth is to be chosen as a *petite-maitresse* chooses her gown,
or a dandy his mustachios. If persons of fashion will not believe in
phrenology, so much the worse for them; phrenology can do without
them. If fashion and respectability be the same thing, however, the University of Cambridge [where Spurzheim lectured to a large audience in
1826] may count for something, and save the blushes of many who now
fear to be called quizzes by avowing their conviction.[53]

Socially, the importance of the rhetoric of persecution and "rational dissent" for those who had come to realize and resent their
"marginality" was that it clarified reality by artificially polarizing
it. Whereas in fact antiphrenologists for the most part shared with
phrenologists an optimistic uniformitarian faith in gradual progress, in social homogeneity, stability, and hierarchical order, and
shared with phrenologists a nonliteralism in biblical matters and
a view of a lawful rational universe presided over by a benign
Diety; as a result of the collision with and rebound from phrenological rhetoric, antiphrenologists appeared wholly as the retainers of a static and privileged aristocratic society allied to inherited
agrarian wealth, while phrenologists appeared wholly as progres-
sives for an open society allied to the mobile fortunes of commerce.
What in most cases were differences between different factions of
the same class over *degrees* of social reordering and the *pace* of social
change (phrenologists seeking a more collapsed social hierarchy
more speedily introduced) became construed over the course of
the controversy, in relation to the further emergence of urban
industrial society, as competing class views over entirely different
kinds of social orders. The more the debates over phrenology spi-
raled, the more was politicized every aspect and everyone who
claimed to speak with authority on man, mind, and society. The
more, therefore, did the *appearance* of discrete world views in
collision take on a reality of its own, with phrenology coming
both to stand as a symbol of what was new and progressive and
to serve as a wedge between the new and the old that exacerbated
the difference. Actively to support phrenology in the 1820s and

1830s was thus to engage not merely in a modernized Baconian version of the seventeenth-century debate between "the moderns" and "the ancients," but to engage in a debate so sharply focused as to appear no less socially consequential than the struggle between the Newtonian–Cartesian academicians and Jacobin natural philosophers in late-eighteenth-century France.[54] In other words, in a social situation most remarkable for its rapid transformations in the absence of revolutionary class conflict, or in the absence of fundamental and visible ruptures in political structures and social relations, the debate between phrenologists and antiphrenologists (or rather the exploitation of that debate by bourgeois ideologues of change) facilitated a caricaturized or epitomized understanding of social reality that was comparable to that afforded to individual psychology through the knowledge itself. Thus the revived phrenology of the 1820s was "crisis knowledge" not only in that it was the product of the organic crisis of the times, but also in that it eliminated ambiguity by disclosing in black and white what in reality was gray.[55]

Historically, however, what this level of phrenology's appreciation reflects is a reality wholly the opposite to that dramatized for these persons through the rhetorical elaboration of the debates over phrenological knowledge. The simple clash of discrete metaphysical polar opposites presented through the phrenologists' caricature of the battle over their knowledge (and unwittingly reproduced through narrow intellectualist accounts of that controversy)[56] belies the far from discrete and far from mechanically causal interactive historical process behind the growth of the subjective appreciation of phrenology. Historically, that growth bears witness, rather, to the dialectical movement whereby, in a context of pervasive socioeconomic change and rising social aspirations among certain social groups, a new body of "natural knowledge," resisted by hitherto dominant social and intellectual groups, interacted reciprocally with emergent subdominant meritocratic interests to sharpen and strengthen the aspiring group's social significance and articulation.[57] Thereby increasingly defined through phrenological knowledge and its interactions was a new "style of thought" or new way of conceiving, perceiving, and presenting reality. Naturally, as in the emergence of a new and eventually distinctive style of painting (to borrow Mannheim's analogy), the new bourgeois–liberal style of thought that came to be elaborated through phrenology's revival in the 1820s was only gradually perceived and appreciated as mutual socioeconomic interests, aspirations, and perceptions coalesced – the new style and its recognition feeding one off the other.[58] (Naturally, too, once this new style of thought had been nurtured out of infancy, direct phrenological rationalizations of the social interests upon which it was based became superfluous.) But it should be understood, also, that the new approach to thinking and to the perception of reality that was quickened into life and crystallized for many of the new urban professionals through the insurgent phrenologists' active manipulation and polarization of reality never necessitated that all who gradually came to assume this new style should have acted alike at conscious political levels of existence. Certainly there was understatement in the comment of a phrenologist, writing in 1825 on phrenology's relation to political liberty, that "phrenologists themselves have not yet arrived at...unanimity."[59] Nor would they ever achieve coherence in party political affairs. Nevertheless, the presentiment of unanimity registers, even at this level, the increasing sense among phrenologists of a collective and distinctive sociocultural attitude and outlook.

By the 1830s there were few who had not come to appreciate that phrenologists were major representatives of and functionaries for the bourgeois reformist meritocratic style of thought. "Inasmuch, as at this moment, the phrenologists appear to be the most strenuous advocates for putting society on an improved footing," the Benthamite *Examiner* stated in October 1831,

we must say that all haters of the present unequal and unnatural distribution of power and knowledge must feel indebted to them for their exertion....if phrenology conduces to the formation or spread of such opinions as it maintains, that phrenology strictly cannot be a bad thing.[60]

Over the next decade the opinion that phrenology, socially speaking, was a "good thing" was to be taken from innumerable journals, many of whom were the same who had earlier expressed contempt. With increasing frequency appeared the Chenevix-like rationale for this shift, that though the doctrine had "met with words enough to have overthrown the argumentative powers of any Irish barrister," yet it had not sunk into oblivion like the doctrines of Johanna Southcott and Thomas Spence with which it had been compared.[61] (Like most commercial products, phrenology's endurance was to be taken as a measure of worth.) With greater frequency, too, came the argument that

many persons who have been accustomed to regard [phrenological] authors as visionary enthusiasts or artful imposters, have been in a manner compelled to make it the object of a more serious examination, by finding it zealously espoused by men of talents and acuteness, who may be in error but are certainly far above contempt.[62]

Once support for the social worth of phrenology had been rationalized in ways such as these, it was an easy step to open praise – praise that might even run, as in 1841 in the *British and Foreign Review*'s revision of its earlier hostility, not only to acquiesing to "what we [now] conceive to be the more rational and moderate phrenological views," but also to admitting "to a certain extent...cranial characteristics."[63] Thus truthfully it could be said, as the *Hampshire Telegraph* put it after the lectures on phrenology by the president of the Emsworth Literary Society in 1842:

Popular prejudice is vanishing fast before free enquiry.... Men begin to discover, that if Phrenology be consistent with fact, it must, in spite of all appearances, possess the advantage which characterizes all that is real, of being ultimately beneficial to man.[64]

Or, as Edgar Allan Poe stated some six years before,

Phrenology is no longer to be laughed at. It is no longer laughed at by men of common understanding. It has assumed the majesty of a science, and, as a science ranks among the most important which can engage the attention of thinking beings.[65]

Such appraisals "among candid and enlightened men" were rightly interpreted by phrenologists as evidence that their knowledge had come to be properly appreciated. Significantly, however, it was just at this period, when, as Charles Bray put it in 1842, the "reference to the truth or falsehood of phrenology" had ceased much to matter among the "well-informed public," that phrenology itself ceased much to matter among those who were primarily interested only in their own social aggrandizement.[66] Insofar as phrenology was only an intellectual midwife to the emergence of the bourgeois–liberal style of thought, interest in it diminished in proportion as that style of thought and the social relations that went with it were felt to have become dominant. But since this recognition depended upon socially governed individual perceptions of the knowledge and on previous degrees of commitment to it, there was to be no single moment for the withdrawal of support. In 1836, at the same time that Poe was eulogizing the knowledge and five years before the dawn of phrenological enlightenment in Emsworth, it was possible for a reviewer in one of the Unitarian journals to reflect: "Phrenology fairly ran away with us in our youth; but she carried us over ground so rugged and into mists so thick that as we grew stronger we grew desirous of emancipation, and at last burst away out of her labyrinthine recesses."[67]

For those who had been deeply involved in phrenology's propagation, though, it was less easy to "burst away" and still keep face (as we will see, there were also other reasons for them not to). Far more characteristic was the gradual withdrawal of acknowledged interest, such as can be witnessed in the *Lancet* in the late 1830s when, it is also significant, new forms of dissenting knowledge, such as homeopathy and mesmerism, began to come under attack as socially infiltrated "pseudosciences."[68]

A convenient and socially illuminating benchmark for the withdrawal of the initial bourgeois–liberal interest in phrenology is the important article on "True and False Phrenology" that appeared in the *British and Foreign Medical Review* in July 1842. Before we turn to that, however, it is worth referring briefly to the phrenological societies, for in many ways their history, at the narrow institutional level, prefigures that witnessed in the wider social sphere. Moreover, there are direct and noteworthy historical connections between the occurrences at the micro and the macro levels.

PHRENOLOGICAL SOCIETIES

Composed for the most part of a vanguard of the "thinking class" and, in particular, of young physicians and surgeons anxious to display their liberal principles, phrenological societies were often subgroupings of Lit & Phil members. In some cases, such as in Liverpool and Newcastle, they were housed in the same building as the Lit & Phil. Members paid the gentleman's token of a guinea per annum and endeavored to abide by the "no politics, no religion" ruling of the elite scientific institutions.[69] Like the Lit & Phils, furthermore, the phrenological societies reached their numerical apogee between the mid-1820s and the early 1830s. In

1826, the same year in which the charter Edinburgh Phrenological Society (established by George and Andrew Combe and three others in February 1820) reached a membership of 120, it was being remarked that "scarcely have we a city, containing an university, or a town boasting a lunatic asylum, but it has added the beneficial institution of a Phrenological Society!"[70] A decade later twenty-nine such societies had come into being, and by then one did not have to search hard in any major urban center to locate places such as the Liverpool Literary, Scientific, and Commercial Institution (established in 1835) advertising an "excellent and extensive PHRENOLOGICAL MUSEUM open to the use of Members."[71]

For all these societies what mattered most was the fact of formation. So long as there were those, such as the editors of the Anglican *Christian Observer*, who were prepared to rail against the spread of "craniological schools! craniological pulpits! and craniological nurseries!" the formation of phrenological societies seemed worthwhile to those interested in provocation and change.[72] But since "the great object of their exertion[s]" was not the refinement of cerebral physiology, but merely "a triumph over their opponents," once they were in existence their reason for being was more or less fulfilled.[73] Thereafter they had little function other than the reaffirmation of the faith of the members. Though a few of the societies endeavored to exercise some control over the propagation of phrenology when they were under pressure to do so, it was beneath the dignity of most to turn evangelist. Consequently, most of them languished soon after they were founded. "We are," wrote the secretary of the society in Dublin, "all satisfied of the truth of Phrenology, and unless something new were to be discussed few of the members would assemble."[74] By 1830 weekly meetings of the society in Edinburgh were attracting less than a dozen persons; and a decade later it was scoffed that the society in London had "dwindled into a little Tea-and-coffee coterie, meeting at the house of Dr Elliotson."[75] Elsewhere the same apathy to repetitive discussions of skulls of criminals and famous persons soon set in and meetings ground to a halt (though it is worth bearing in mind that geological and similar societies established around this time often suffered a similar fate once initial enthusiasm had worn off).[76] A few phrenological societies managed to keep going, but most of these were not established (or *re*established, as was the case in Sheffield, Glasgow, and Liverpool) until the late 1830s and 1840s, and then on rather different grounds and with members drawn from lower social strata. In Warwick, Warrington, Blackburn, and Belfast, the original societies were able to continue by forming themselves into, or merging with, local geological, archaeological, or natural history societies, and other provincial phrenological societies were encouraged similarly to broaden their scope. In all such reconstituted societies, however, discussion on phrenology per se became less and less.[77] In short, the institutionalization of phrenology was found to be self-defeating, for it turned the key on the exploitation of its persecution, shackling the hidden agenda behind its social success among the reform-minded.

But it would also be true to say that the phrenological societies floundered because members soon came to realize that membership operated against identification with and integration into more socially elitist scientific associations. As the *Phrenological Journal* reflected in 1840 on the problem of the "non-endurance" of phrenological societies,

[it] seems to us to arise chiefly from the absence of sufficient personal advantages to the members individually. . . . the mere fact of membership of a phrenological society at present gives no stamp or credit to the individual member, such as our metropolitan chartered societies for science puposes do give to some extent.[78]

Although entry into phrenological societies was made more for the purpose of countercultural flag waving and mutual support than directly for the seeking of social status, most members were upwardly mobile and, increasingly, were concerned with establishing elitist identities where they could. The best supporting evidence for the view that the phrenological societies failed in part because they could not fulfill this function rests with the history of the last and the largest of the institutionalizations of phrenology, the Phrenological Association.

Projected in March 1835, the PA was the tactical response to the exclusion of phrenology from the British Association for the Advancement of Science. Unlike the relationship between phrenology and the Royal Societies, however, the relationship between phrenology and the BAAS was more complex, since, superficially at least, the BAAS symbolized the same enshrining through science activity of the social and ideological interests purveyed by phrenologists. Although in reality (as phrenologists soon discovered) the BAAS remained in the tight control of a small clique of well-connected intellectuals, it was born (in 1831) out of the same dissenting matrix as the Lit & Phils and the provincial phrenological societies. Like them, it articulated science both as a social anodyne and as an agent for the social accommodation of urban professionals within the reforming bourgeois industrial order.[79] Ideologically, therefore, it was not unreasonable for phrenologists to hope that their subject might be incorporated as an official "section" of the BAAS. Practically, however, this was impossible. Out of its own need to disguise the social interests behind its origins, the BAAS endeavored in its sphere to do exactly as the phrenologists did in theirs: on the one hand, to sharply demarcate science from social interests in order to enhance the value-neutral image of science and, on the other, to bend over backwards to stuff their committees with the titled and lettered in order to enhance the legitimacy and social respectability of their activity. Whewell's threat to resign if "notorious men" such as Robert Owen and Dr. Chalmers were allowed in exemplifies the self-consciousness with which the BAAS tried to build up its image and fully suggests the reason why Whewell and the other ideologues of the association tried to keep out such a socially and scientifically controversial topic as phrenology.[80] Although the BAAS did not exploit phrenology as its own "negative analogue" (in part because there were too many supporters of phrenology among its members), it was obvious to phrenologists that their knowledge, and hence their status, was as much under threat in the BAAS as in any of the unreformed scientific institutions.[81] Discussions of phrenology nevertheless went on at BAAS meetings, initiated by the phrenologists within; but as in the transactions of the Royal Societies, these were suppressed in the official proceedings.[82] Moreover, when, in 1834, the BAAS met in Edinburgh, the provincial Athens of phrenology, it was made explicit by the president, Adam Sedgwick, that members were "to confine their researches to dead matter, without entering into any speculations on the relations of intellectual beings." As if addressing Combe himself, who had just been admitted a member, Sedgwick added that "he would brand as a traitor that person who would dare to overstep the prescribed boundaries of the institution."[83]

Phrenologists dared not. Instead, on the initiative of Sir George

MacKenzie (after he had laid the interests of phrenologists before Sedgwick and been rebuffed), the idea was floated of an independent Phrenological Association to hold its meetings concurrently with those of the BAAS.[84] Membership was to be restricted to members of either phrenological societies or the BAAS, at a fee of 10 shillings per annum. The object was less one of retaliation against the BAAS, therefore, than the emulation of it, and through emulation and proof of mettle the hope of eventual incorporation. Of course, by mimicking the BAAS the PA also mocked it, and while retaining its independence the PA could also signify criticism of those same elitist pretentions to which many of its members aspired.

In large part it was because of the ambiguities in its place and function that the PA received considerable backing, even though by the time of its first meeting in Newcastle in 1838 most of the original phrenological societies were moribund. Between the first meeting and the fourth, in London in 1841, 300 names appear on the membership list, including those of the publisher Robert Chambers, the alienist John Conolly, the statistician William Farr, the educationalists Thomas Bastard and Thomas Coates, the writer and reformer and M.P. for Sheffield from 1832 to 1837 John Silk Buckingham, and the M.P.'s Francis Beamish and Lord Douglas G. Hallyburton.[85] Though drawn from all corners of Britain, members came principally from London, Glasgow, Edinburgh, Manchester, and Liverpool (proportionately in that order), and, as the accompanying table reveals of the 219 members for whom information is available, the occupational breakdown was typical of that to be found in phrenological societies generally. That less than 20 of the members could place prestigious letters behind their names also confirms the phrenologists' relatively low social status.

Although the PA's second meeting at Birmingham in 1839 was a disaster due to the lack of phrenological infrastructure in the town, poor organization, and a relatively low BAAS turnout (as a result of recent Chartist activity), on the basis of both the first meeting in Newcastle and the third meeting in Glasgow, phrenologists had reason to be gratified. Not only were their proceedings reported in the press as if they constituted an official section of the BAAS, but also, because the public tended to be far more interested in the "science of human nature" than in the drier stuff of the BAAS, they tended to receive a disproportionate amount

Occupations of Phrenological Association members, 1839–41

Medical	74	Tradesmen and artisans	7
Manufacturers and merchants	47	Civil engineers	6
Legal	20	Ministers	6
Writers, journalists,		Public lecturers	5
publishers, and printers	12	Architects	3
Clerks (in law and		Army and Navy	3
commerce)	8	Dentists	3
Independently wealthy	8	M.P.s	2
Schoolteachers	7	Accountants	1
Artists	7	Total:	219
		Total membership:	300

of press coverage. At Glasgow, Combe completely upstaged the BAAS, and had his revenge on it, when he lectured publicly to an audience of over six hundred on the subject of national crania – a lecture that he had offered and had had turned down by the BAAS in 1834.[86]

But the success, such as it was, was short-lived and, in itself, was a contributing factor to the demise of the PA as originally conceived. With a strong membership, the greater proportion of which came from London, it was decided after the Glasgow meeting to part company with the BAAS and meet at a different time in London. To Combe this was the realization of his worse fears and the main reason why his support for the PA had never been more than lukewarm: Metropolitan phrenology under Elliotson's aegis had always been different in character and aspiration than that defined by Edinburgh, in part because the size of London imposed fewer social constraints on phrenologists but, more so, because Elliotson's own relatively autonomous social position encouraged a following that tended to despise the socioreligious pretentions of Spurzheim and Combe and to openly endorse a wholly materialist conception of man and nature.[87] The strong presence of London phrenologists within the PA meant that internally there was a replication of many of the same tensions over image building and social status that existed between the BAAS and the PA as a whole. With the PA based in London, it was almost inevitable that these tensions would be brought to the surface.

Though Elliotson's diplomatic skills permitted the meeting of

1841 to pass off without incident, all phrenologists agreeing on
the greater necessity of publicly vindicating phrenology as a rep-
utable science, at the meeting the following year the fragile coherence among phrenologists was shattered when Elliotson's
colleague, William Engledue, a twenty-eight-year-old Portsmouth
physician, delivered an opening address in which not only was
the materialism of "cerebral physiology" asserted uncompromisingly, but the latest social heterodoxy of mesmerism was also
strongly endorsed.[88] Well calculated to win the sympathies of infidel artisans (see Chapter 8) Engledue's address predictably con-
vulsed   the   Edinburgh-orientated   respectability-seeking
phrenologists who saw undermined, at a single stroke, two decades of carefully rehearsed, endlessly reiterated, and successfully
sown rhetoric on phrenology's harmony with socioreligious views.
Not even the latinate pretention of the word *phrenology* was left
them. Not surprisingly, therefore, a desperate attempt was made
by some phrenologists to save the situation. The Scottish advocate
James Simpson and the city editor of the *Times*, Marmaduke Sampson (another close friend of Combe), whipped up a "Declaration
of Expediency" that, while denying that materialism was the only
basis of phrenology, argued that Engledue's charge ought not to
be the cause for "an inconsiderate alarm." Seventy-one members
of the PA signed the declaration and, though it was ridiculed by
Engledue and Elliotson in their new materialist journal *The Zoist*,
it did in fact assist in the holding of a sixth meeting of the PA in
London in July 1843.[89] To this meeting, however, the turnout was
meager and any lingering hopes of phrenology being recognized
by and phrenologists being integrated into more elitist scientific
groupings through the institutional route were quashed by the
reassertion of dissident materialism and mesmerism.

THE FIRST END OF "THE SICK-MAN'S DREAM"

It was two months after the disruptive fifth meeting of the PA
that the article on "True and False Phrenology" appeared in the
British and Foreign Medical Review. The article made explicit that
a watershed had been reached between a popular "phrenologism"
and a socially respectable "scientific" phrenology, and that the
time had come either to purge the science of its "half-proved truth
and empty conjecture" and the unbecoming popular trappings that

arrested its scientific progress or to abandon it altogether.[90] Assumed by many to have been written by the editor of the journal, John Forbes, who had been a leading member of the PA before resigning after Engledue's address, the article was in fact written by Forbes's colleague and alter ego, Daniel Noble.[‡] Noble, too, up to this time had been a leading promoter of phrenology; he had been president of the Manchester Phrenological Society between 1835 and 1838 and, while deeply involved in various local and national social and medical reform movements, had written dozens of papers supporting phrenology as well as lecturing on it in the Manchester Literary and Philosophical Society.[91] Like Forbes, and along with Andrew Combe, Samuel Solly, and Sir George MacKenzie, among others, Noble, too, had resigned from the PA upon hearing Engledue's address.

But it would be wrong to suggest that the medically couched sentiments expressed in Noble's article and the disassociation from phrenology that they justified were historically dependent upon or directly attributable to Engledue's address. After all, the majority of medical men had left the phrenological societies by the mid-1830s, while two years *before* Engledue's address the botanist Hewett Watson had resigned as editor of the *Phrenological Journal*, suddenly convinced that "much is stated in the writings of phrenologists which is doubtful, if not erroneous."[92] Watson, like most other renegades from phrenology, gave no explanation for why it had taken him until 1840 to recognize phrenology as "pseudoscience," after having led the attack on the antiphrenology of Roget and Sir William Hamilton in the 1830s.[93] But while his rebellion from his father's Toryism and his dissent from the Anglican Church in which he was raised are suggestive of the reasons why he had located himself among the van of phrenological counterculturalists in the 1820s and 1830s, so his application for the chair of botany in Ireland in 1846 provides an inkling of the changing imperatives behind his withdrawal.[94]

Engledue's address, then, might be likened to the phrenologists' caricaturing of the debate with antiphrenologists in the 1820s and 1830s, in that it did not *cause* opinions to shift, so much as it heightened awareness of the way in which personal and social circumstances had changed and, through that heightening of awareness, helped to force choice. However embarrassing at the time, Engledue's address offered what must, in retrospect, have

appeared to former supporters of phrenology as a well-timed ex-
cuse for severing their connections with a social resource that had
effectively served its purpose and was now felt only to be compromising. Forbes doubtless realized this in 1841 when he was
appointed physician to Prince Albert and the queen's household.
Its a safe assumption, too, that Noble, having been offered a county
magistracy and become one of Manchester's leading physicians
and consultants by the 1840s, no longer wished to be reminded
that he had once played the Leveller's part in securing for the
Manchester Phrenological Society a cast of the head of William
Cobbett.[95] Aware that the cohering ideological function of phrenology was blighted (along with professional prestige) if phrenology was rendered too obviously the tool of devisive political creeds,
Noble, in his article in Forbes's journal, offered his colleagues a
face-saving alibi for the abandonment of their former faith: It was
not that they had ever been misled in endorsing phrenology, he
suggested, but rather that this "true theory of brain" had become
degraded by falling into the hands of the "facile" and "superficial."
In the face of this scientistic overkill, it was only proper that those
who were, as it were, "free from ideology" and interested only
in "neutral knowledge" should disassociate themselves. A few
years later Noble followed his own counsel and opted for the
respectable brain physiology of his major critic, William
Carpenter.[96]

A similar story can be told through the biographies of many
former phrenologists (just as it can through the histories of many
former advocates of orthodox "natural knowledge").[97] In a slightly
different way, the story is repeated through the lectureship on
phrenology that was established at the Andersonian University in
December 1845. Behind this (made possible through the funds
provided in the will of one of the earlier wealthy patrons of phrenology) was the anticipation that medical practitioners then "between the ages of forty and fifty" who had sought the advantages
of phrenology in the 1820s and 1830s would be anxious to send
their sons through a course of phrenological instruction. When
only twelve students enrolled, however, it was strikingly evident
that the lectureship was to be almost wholly a tribute to phrenology's *past* relevance.[98] Standing socially on much firmer ground
than that once stood upon by many of their fathers, the sons (now
along with their fathers) could by 1845 nod sagely in agreement

with the much-quoted statement of Benjamin Travers, surgeon extraordinary to Victoria and Albert, that phrenology owed its existence "to the countenance which it derives from a twilight of truth, though only sufficient to serve as a beacon to the absurdities with which it is enveloped."[99]

There were similar statements on phrenology around this time by other heavyweights in science and medicine (e.g., Sir Benjamin Brodie, Sir George Lefevre, William Thomas Brande, and M. P. J. Flourens) as well as articles in significant journals (such as that by the founder of the Edinburgh School of Psychiatry, David Skae, in the *British Quarterly Review*).[100] Taking into account everything that has been said in this chapter, however, it should be clear that only a determined Comtean positivist or an out-and-out Weberian could argue that the endorsement of such statements among former supporters of phrenology had nothing to do with the former supporters changed network of social interests and sense of cultural achievement.[101] Of course, there could be reasons other than social ones to account for changes in the attitude toward phrenology. But since the physiology of the brain had undergone no major change, whatever those other reasons may have been, they cannot be accepted as purely intellectual unless we are willing to endorse that same image of scientific–intellectual purity that phrenologists themselves had perpetrated. Far wiser, surely, to see the irrelevance of phrenology among former advocates as a part of the same social process that had led to the rise of popular bourgeois phrenology, that is, in terms of the accomplishment by the 1840s of what had yet to be secured by the liberal bourgeoisie in the 1820s and what, with the most amazing social tensions and contradictions, had been attained in the 1830s.

Logically, it might have been expected that within and for the reformed bourgeois order phrenology would have become wholly identified as "pseudoscience" and thus have played the same consolidating social function as the attack on hermeticism, alchemy, and magic in the seventeenth century, discussed previously. Since this also would have been a rehearsal in part of the tactics of some of the defenders of the status quo in the 1810s and 1820s, we might have been able to conclude this chapter merely with *plus ça change, plus c'est la même chose*. But such a conclusion would be as mistaken as it would be simple-minded; for, in fact, there is little evidence before mid-century to indicate that phrenology actually did come to be identified wholly as "pseudoscience" and, in *that* way, to function in the interest of the new status quo.[102] Indeed, it only appears logical that this might have happened because we have confined our attention up to this point to the role of phrenology within, and the phrenological reflections of, the early-nineteenth-century struggle against the metaphysics (and metaphysicians) of the unreformed social order. In so doing, we have written at the expense of overlooking the other important side of this ideological struggle – namely, the role of phrenology in the attempted de-naturalization of social and ideological interests different from those of the liberal bourgeoisie. This other, never wholly separate function of bourgeois phrenology depended upon its being received as an authentic science of human nature. Thus, for the reformed urban industrial bourgeois order, phrenology was to maintain its stature as "science," in spite of the fact that by the late 1830s it was clear to most middle-class observers that phrenology as an elitist bourgeois reform movement was otiose and that phrenological societies were, like Lit & Phils, a part of the "debris of an age passed away."[103] As the Unitarian reviewer quoted earlier hastened to add to his explanation in 1836 for no longer requiring phrenology, "We still believe she has merit." That "merit," or appreciation of the use of phrenology for establishing intellectually the legitimacy of bourgeois hegemony, was in fact only beginning to be widely made in the mid-1830s, as we shall see in Chapter 5.[104] Prior to that, however, an acquaintance with George Combe is necessitated since it was Combe who was most responsible for other people's making of that appreciation.

PART III

Popular science

It might be worthwhile, sometimes, to inquire what Nature is, and how men work to change her, and whether, in the enforced distortions so produced, it is not natural to be unnatural. . . . Alas! are there so few things in the world, about us, most unnatural, yet most natural in being so?

Charles Dickens, *Dombey and Son* (1848), p. 750

This whole perspective of a man learning from a separately observed nature is deeply false. The correlative is that in the end it is best if we discuss the problem of social and human relationships in directly social and personal terms.

Raymond Williams, "Social Darwinism," in Jonathan Benthall, ed., *The Limits of Human Nature* (1973), p. 130

4

George Combe and the remolding of man's constitution

We cannot separate personal growth and communal change, nor can we separate...the identity crisis in individual life and contemporary crisis in historical development because the two help to define each other and are truly relative to each other. In fact, the whole interplay between the psychological and the social, the developmental and the historical, for which identity formation is of prototypal significance, could be conceptualized only as a kind of *psychosocial relativity*.

Erik Erikson, *Identity: Youth and Crisis* (1968), p. 23

Science is the most characteristic aspect of our civilization precisely because it provides the mental and physical apparatus for rapid changes in our way of life and even more perhaps in our conceptual views of creation. Indeed, the tempo at which man changes the environment and his views of himself is now so rapid that the rules of conduct for good life must be changed from one generation to the other. In many fields, the wisdom of the father is now of little use to his son.

René Dubos, "Science and Man's Nature," in G. Holton, ed., *Science and Culture: A Study of Cohesive and Disjunctive Forces* (Boston, 1965), p. 252

To phrenology's transformation from an arcane theory of brain and character to that of a socially respectable scientific vehicle of "progressive" ideas on social life and organization, no one was more important or conspicuous than George Combe. The Huxley of early-nineteenth-century phrenology, Combe can no more be omitted from consideration of the social, ideological, and cultural implications of phrenology than Charles Lyell or Hugh Miller could be omitted from nineteenth-century geology. Yet it would be counterproductive to focus on Combe if this contributed to a notion of him as a person of rare and exceptional qualities who, *because of them*, was responsible for phrenology's popularization. Although Harriet Martineau was overstating the case when she described Combe as being neither "a thinker, nor a poet, nor an orator, nor an enthusiast, nor a quack," she was on target in implying that he had no historical claims to great leadership nor claims to being recognized as a social or intellectual visionary.[1] Lacking originality in almost all respects, Combe's place in history is as a moralizing popularizer of received ideas. His phrenology and his ideas on its application were taken from Spurzheim, and his views on education and on criminal and other reforms were reiterations through phrenology of contemporary ideas that were gaining in currency. As a leading philosophical radical once pointed out to him, "There is nothing that you advocate that Jeremy Bentham and James Mill would have hesitated to concur in."[2]

But this is the point of focusing on Combe: He merits our attention precisely because he was *not* a prophet for his times but was a typical product of them. Just as phrenology itself exaggerates the social nature and uses of science, so Combe as a highly representative social type magnifies many of the needs and aspirations of his generation. And as the appeal of Combe's elaboration of phrenology is testimony not to his "influence" but to the experiences that others shared with him at a particular moment in history, so his own interest in phrenology subverts the view that in the realm of ideas individuals are autonomous in all but space and that they receive their ideas in much the same infectious way that the rest of us receive disease. But before turning to his interest in and elaboration of phrenology in order to point to the error of attempting to carve distinctions between intellectual and sociocultural realms, let us heed Combe's immediate context and there take into account, as well, the not unrelated fallacy of attempting to separate personal psychology from society and culture.

BACKGROUND AND IDENTITY

Born in Edinburgh in 1788 into a family of lowland Scots, Combe was one of the thirteen children of the owner of a small brewery and a mother descended from a long line of tenant farmers. Though they lived in overcrowded quarters, they were prosperous enough to employ servants. Only on one occasion, the Scottish famine of 1800, did they have to strictly economize in order to maintain their position in what Combe was to later refer to as "the middle ranks." The children were never held back in their vocational pursuits for which both parents, as good Calvinists, were extremely ambitious. Two brothers became brewers, two were tanners, one was a baker, while George rose to law and his brother Andrew (nine years his junior) rose to medicine.[3]

Combe's father, a tall, burly, and formidable person, appears to have been stern but not unkind. Having himself been severely beaten as a youth, he maintained his resolve never to beat his children, though he apparently held a high opinion of one of George's schoolmasters who was known to "ply the taws" and beat the boys abundantly. "You kept your word," Combe apostrophized in his autobiography, "but you gave us orders; we were remiss in obedience: you threatened severe consequences." The mother offered nothing softer. She was, if anything, more rigidly dutiful than the father and less given to emotional warmth. A cold domestic manager, she never, said Combe, allowed her children to know "the pleasures which a mother's affection sheds over the minds of the young." Precluding "sympathetic tenderness toward her children" and instructing them "never to complain of suffering . . . 'sent by the hand of God,' " she also discouraged emotional warmth between the children. It is not surprising, therefore, that later in life George and Andrew Combe were to admit that an emotional reserve and a certain revulsion to emotional display were the "sad results of the sternness with which we were treated in early life."[4] How far this upbringing was (as the psychologist Silvan Tomkins would predict) accountable for a distrust of solidarity and an inclination to independence and competitiveness it is difficult to say. It is perhaps significant, though, that these characteristics were far more pronounced in George Combe than they were either in Andrew Combe, who was partly raised outside the home by a kind foster mother, or in Abram Combe, the second-born son, who was to involve himself in experiments in community living.[5] George Combe also accords better than his brothers to Tomkins's main finding: that persons thus socialized, while often well suited for human contact, are best suited for that human contact "in which hierarchy, order, and predictability are emphasized."[6] With Scots Calvinism being among the richest, dankest milieux for such socialization, it seems hardly surprising that men better known than Combe for their preaching of the need to comply with the hierarchical and authoritarian structures and relations of industrial capitalism – men such as James Mill, George Birkbeck, Andrew Ure, Thomas Chalmers, Henry Brougham, and Samuel Smiles – should all have been Scots.

Like all in Judeo–Christian culture subjected to the Fifth Commandment, Combe ultimately was to find excuses for his parents' coldness and to repress his feelings of betrayal. In a family of seventeen children (of whom there were thirteen surviving in 1807) it was obviously not difficult to invent excuses for his mother's "general kindness and justices, rather than...endearment." But it was not just the size of the family that was to blame, as Combe made clear when he attempted rationally to account for his brother Andrew's emotional reserve:

The reason was simply this, that, partly owing to the manners of the age, and partly to the incessant occupation of his father and mother in their spheres of imperative duty, little opportunity was left for confiding interchange of sentiment and sympathy between the parents and the children; and moreover, in the family circle, too little account was taken of feelings, when duty was in question.... but, from a dread, on the side of the parents, of spoiling their children by over-indulgence, and the fear, on the children's part, of being misunderstood if they complained, an almost insurmountable barrier to confidential communication then existed between the two parties.[7]

But if aware that his emotional impoverishment was attributable to the socialization of Scots Calvinism, Combe never succeeded in, nor wished to succeed in, casting off the values it inculcated. He was always proud to be numbered among a race renowned for its natural seriousness of character and strong sense of moral responsibility. Described by intimates as "hard," "dry," "cold," and as "tall, puritanical, [and] dissenter-looking," he remained all his life within an ascetic mold, forever preoccupied with the virtues of thrift, industry, and order.[8] He was forty-five and well established in life before he entered into marriage with Cecilia Siddons, the thirty-nine-year old daughter of the famous and respected actress Mrs. Sarah Siddons. Siddons's fortune of 15,000 pounds allowed Combe to retire from law in 1837 and devote himself to the popularization of phrenology. Since Combe was as renowned for his parsimoniousness as for his lack of amativeness, it was naturally joked that he had every reason to overlook Siddons's

unsingular physiognomical and phrenological development.⁹ There
were never any children.

In many ways Combe not only retained the values of his Scots
Calvinist upbringing, but he retained the theology as well. In
daring to express the extent to which as a youth he had detested
the solemn occupations and discipline enforced by the Calvinist
sabbath, detested the agonizing sermons on the sin and misery of
man's estate, and detested the endless memorization of the *Shorter
Catechism*, Combe was not revolting against Calvinist theology,
nor against Calvinist authority per se, so much as he was revolting
against the institutionalizations of Calvinism that made the religion
functionally ineffective for him.¹⁰ The cosmological furniture of
Calvinism seeming to have become nailed to the floor, religious
belief as a mode of action and as a means of continual adjustment
in the personal search for order had become impossible. Or, to
move from the phraseology of Mary Douglas to that of the historian of Puritanism Michael Walzer, Calvinism no longer served
to allay the fears and insecurities induced through Combe's actual
experiencing of exile and alienation.¹¹ Increasingly, as he moved
socially upward, the bleak but "magnificently consistent" doctrine
of Calvin appeared only as a masochistic disciplinary indulgence
for a people with "a tendency to harshness and irascibility" – a
hollow, meaningless religious cultural system offering no means
to self-revelation and cosmic understanding. "Neither in church,
nor school, nor in the family circle," he reflected bitterly, "was
one solitary rational idea communicated to me concerning my own
nature, or the nature of men and things, or my own relationship
to them."¹² Here, classically, was the alienation and moral anxiety
out of which would arise the impulse to reform – the same as
stood behind the efforts of Harriet Martineau, Charles Bray,‡ Henry
Buckle, and Herbert Spencer and behind the popularizations of
"Combean phrenology" by persons such as John Epps,‡ Robert
Cox,‡ Hewett Watson,‡ and W. B. Hodgson.‡ Like them, in their
rebellions against strict and pious upbringings,¹³ Combe experienced an intense aloneness and disorientation, for at the same time
that he was coming to stand outside what might otherwise have
been the institutional comforts of his culture, he was coming to
feel the terrors of being without the support of any logical system
of categories with which to make sense of the world. Features
common to adolescence were thus intensified. As he wrote of his

youth, "There was neither within nor around me any atmosphere of consistency, goodness, and truth; but a constant conflict of emotions and ideas one with the other; *and the world was a chaos.*"[14]

Since it was together with this estrangement from the cultural agencies of Scots Calvinism that Combe became estranged from his family, the latter estrangement is also to be made sense of largely in terms of family-as-cultural-agency rather than exclusively in terms of personal psychology. Although it is true that through his phrenological efforts he did more than most pre-Darwinians to destroy the ultimate father-figure God, and that he only turned to phrenology the year following his father's death, an Oedipal interpretation of his development never quite rings true. Although it was doubtless the case that with thirteen children in the family Combe had to rival his father for his mother's love and affection, and although one might interpret the glandular infection that Combe contracted as a young boy as an instance of a psychosomatic manifestation of such need and rivalry,[15] the fact remains that Combe's mother had no bounty of love to compete for. That, unlike all his older brothers and sisters, Combe sought a career that promised higher social status than that enjoyed by his parents, and that he left his family as soon as he could maintain the barest independence suggests, rather, the primacy of more consciously arrived at social considerations – considerations made in relation to the experiencing of upward mobility. Significantly, in the reminiscences of his early life, Combe never characterized either his mother or his father as in any way wiser than himself; rather, like the physical location of the parental home, the parental intelligence was singled out for its lowliness. Much in the manner of Bounderby and Ralph Nickleby, Combe was thereby able to highlight how successfully he had shaped his own destiny. At the same time he was able to chastise those like his brother Abram who, failing to heed "proper" social values, forced those who did heed them to provide for the destitute families they (the heedless) left behind.[16] (It was Abram's misfortune to have died while trying to establish a socialist community.) It is not difficult, therefore, to see how Combe's disparaging of his parents was a part of a legitimation of certain sociopolitical interests. As Bruch Mazlish has written in reference to James Mill, "the 'self-made man' becomes part of a general attack on ancestry as a justification for potential or social power. One denies one's own ancestors as a preliminary to denying the ancestry of others. 'All men are created equal' when no one has parents."[17]

Another manifestation of Combe's denial of his origins for the purpose of cultivating the self-made image was his adding of the letter *e* to the family name. As with Alexander Tilloch (formerly Tillock), James Mill (formerly Milne), and Combe's nephew Robert Cox (formerly Cocks), Combe's "modernizing" of his genealogy symbolized the severance from and reformist attack upon past authority vested in Church, society, and family. In effect, by altering his name he signified his hope that through change would come a more personally meaningful set of social relations. But just how different those social relations were to be from those being abandoned is open to question. Surely it is significant that men like Combe changed a letter or two in their names but never adopted entirely new names. One wonders if they ever could have gone so far. If on a mother's knee the potential for an alternative society is implicit in the matriarchal ethic of worth, acceptance, and love, how genuinely alternative can the "alternatives" be when they are proposed by those for whom such mothers' knees have been mostly denied?[18] Insights can be gained and further considerations made by turning our attention to Combe's adoption and elaboration of phrenology.

THE ALLURE OF IDEOLOGICAL PHYSIOLOGY

That Combe's attraction to phrenological psychology was intimately bound to a struggle for personal identity and a search for certainty seems as indubitable as the fact that his troubled experience of childhood, adolescence, and early adulthood were part and parcel of the enormous new strains that the Industrial Revolution placed upon both child–parent and social class relations.[19] (Significantly, James Mill, experiencing those same presures and needs with the same Calvinist intensity, also put his greatest efforts into *An Analysis of the Phenomena of the Human Mind*, published in 1829). There is, however, little direct biographical evidence to substantiate the connection between Combe's psychosocial experience and his interest in phrenology. We are not helped, moreover, by the fact that Combe died before the autobiography he was writing reached the twenty-eighth year, that in which he first became acquainted with phrenology.

What the record makes known is that initially Combe followed the lead of the *Edinburgh Review* in mocking phrenology. When Spurzheim came to Edinburgh in 1816 to defend his theory Combe was invited by a friend to meet him and watch him dissect a brain. Since, during the course of his two years at the University of Edinburgh Combe had had occasion to watch John Barclay perform similar dissections and had been exposed to the faculty psychology of Reid and Stewart, he was in a position to appreciate Spurzheim's dissecting skills and anatomical knowledge and, above all, the relative simplicity of a psychology based on physiology. Enthused, but far too level-headed to become evangelical, Combe ordered some skulls from London with which to study the science further. When they arrived he found that he had also captured an audience as anxious as himself to understand the relationship of the skulls to the science of craniology and character. It was inviting to study the science in depth and achieve some little fame thereby. He was soon adept and addicted. In April 1817 he made his first appearance in print with an "Explanation of the Physiognomical System of Drs Gall and Spurzheim" in the *Scots Magazine and Edinburgh Literary Miscellany*. A year later, after visiting Spurzheim in Paris, there appeared in the *Literary and Statistical Magazine for Scotland* the first of his essays on phrenology that were to be collected into a single volume in 1819.[20]

These early publications were important to Combe for, as with the audience drawn to his box of skulls, they earned him some of "the respect of the world" that he coveted. "A desire of fame may be one mark of a mind that deserves it," he had written near the beginning of a diary commenced in 1811, adding, "I have taken the imagination that I have powers of mind sufficient to write some useful book on human nature, and especially on the education and intellectual state of the middle ranks of society."[21] Little did he realize as he wrote these lines that other struggling professionals – Charles Lyell and Robert Chamber, for instance – were penning almost identical aspirations into their diaries; like Combe, they, too, were anxious to achieve fame and to "be looked on as...respectable writer[s] of the middle class."[22] Later in life Combe was to be greatly annoyed on those occasions when that respect was not forthcoming.

It did not take long for Combe to make the connection between phrenology, social reformation, and worldly fame. By the time Spurzheim provided the actual rhetorical and philosophical equipment for doing so – first, through his blend of science, religion, and morality in *Elementary Principles of Education Founded on the Study of the Nature of Man* (1821) and, second, through his ethical catechism, *A Sketch of the Natural Laws of Man* (1825) – Combe had already moved from the purely explanatory and was increasingly speaking of phrenology in connection with politics, society, and religion.[23] Whereas Gall and Spurzheim had lain stress on anatomy, claiming not that it was the source of their discoveries but that it strongly confirmed them, Combe was to rely on anatomy hardly at all. For him phrenology was above all a "stupendous discovery in relation to the moral world," for which the study of the anatomy and physiology of the brain ceased much to matter. As he stated as early as 1823, in his first address to the EPS, the real value of phrenology was as a "mighty engine of expiscation [for] analysis in morals, ethics and political economy."[24]

Spurzheim's *Sketch of the Natural Laws of Man* was to be the incentive for Combe's "On Human Responsibility as Affected by Phrenology," a privately circulated essay of 1826 that was to be the first draft of the *Constitution of Man* published two years later. But, in a sense, Combe's mind had already been prepared for Spurzheim's incentive to link phrenology and social ethics through natural law. The most important preparation was his reading, around 1805, of the works of Paley, Malthus, and Adam Smith. He was then seventeen, was just beginning a five-year apprenticeship in law, and had just finished two undistinguished years in the humanity class at the university. That he was confused and disorientated there is no doubt. Studying in what was the world center of enlightened rationalism predictably did nothing to strengthen his faith in Calvinism; nor was he to gain any settling effect from either the *Edinburgh Review* or Cobbett's *Political Register*, both of which he commenced reading enthusiastically also around 1805.[25] Conscious of an upward mobility, he was in fact largely rudderless, though highly stimulated politically and intellectually. It is not surprising, therefore, that he was deeply impressed by Malthus's revelation of "inevitable" laws of nature; that he found "relief" in Paley's affirming of hierarchy and perfect adaptation in nature; and that (after having taken in Malthus's didactic pessimism about man's imbalanced state in nature) he was bouyed up by Smith's prognostication of civilization's progress through an extending division of labor.[26] As with so many others of his generation, the derivative notion of natural hierarchical divisions of labor in life and society governed over by universal determinant laws increasingly became an idée fixe in the midst of learning to live with change. With Spurzheim's help, Combe was to identify in phrenology the ultimate expression of and means for expressing the "natural law mode of thought." Through the science, it might be said, he was to achieve clear passage to his age – the age that Carlyle was to castigate as "mechanical," wherein everything, "including our modes of thought and feeling," was deemed calculable and able to be ruled over.[27]

There is, therefore, in the historical narrative of Combe's life more than merely coincidence to explain why he should have gratified his rationalism, liberalism, and egotism through phrenology in particular. There is in fact a great deal more, but to unearth it properly we need to turn to the substance of phrenological knowledge itself: not merely to the rhetoric surrounding the science, but to what was fundamental to that rhetoric, the symbolic and metaphoric significance of phrenology's basic form and contents. To fully understand Combe's attraction to phrenology we must ask what it meant for a person of his background and his social context to gaze into Spurzheim's map and guidebook to cerebral reality. We need, that is, to try to reconstitute his gaze by decoding the science's signs and symbols and discovering how they rationed, limited, and filtered access to reality at the same time as they disclosed it.[28]

Like all the substantive features of the science, the first to be noted, that this was a doctrine about the *head*, is so obvious as to normally pass without comment. It is only when we stop to consider that in cultures other than our own other parts of the body are often regarded as more important that a celebration of the head takes on significance.[29] Conceivably, had Western culture taken a very different turning at some point, palmistry, not phrenology, might have been the most popular science in the nineteenth century. But it was not to be. The head, not the hand nor the genitals nor the breast nor the heart, was the part to be celebrated; elevated in the body hierarchy was the seat of the intellect, not the signifiers of human labor, love, emotion, or soul. Was it coincidental that

Gall, increasingly distant from Catholicism, established beyond all doubt that the brain was the organ of the mind? It hardly seems so when we realize that with the mind reposing in the brain, sin was displaced from its religious stronghold in the soul and given an entirely biological secular dimension. Gall's strategy, if we may call it that, was to enshrine the seat of reason so as to discredit the institutions of power that depended on blind faith, superstition, and spontaneous irrational behavior. Impinged thereby was the credibility of eternal damnation as the ultimate weapon for social control in the arsenal of the ruling class. An exaltation of the head therefore can be seen to symbolize the victory of reason and rationality over superstition-based repressions of the past. Inseparably, such exaltation can also symbolize the struggle to understand and to control or exert power over natural as opposed to supernatural forces; can symbolize the struggle against privileged interests based on property and inheritance rather than on intellect; and, not least of all, can symbolize the struggle to establish the dominance of mental over manual labor.[30]

But the phrenological head was obviously not just any head. It was a unique representation of the human cerebral interior that disclosed a particular ideal view of the nature of mental reality. Not unlike gazing through the open front of a Victorian doll's house, gazing at a phrenological head confronts one not only with order and classification par excellence, but also (just as with the actual domestic workings of the middle-class Victorian home) with a clear hierarchy of spaces for specialized functions and duties. No aspect of human behavior and no action is incapable of allocation in the classification scheme; everyone can be seen to have his or her proper place and duty. Like the horizontal stratification, symmetry, and regularity that the Hutchinsonian found in the earth's crust and that allowed him to see disorder, confusion, and irregularity as reflecting back upon God's order in nature,[31] phrenology allowed the chaotic, the ambiguous, and the arbitrary in the environment to reflect back upon nature's rational order in the human mind.

Since human experience was quantified and forced into logical categories in the phrenological head, we can also think of it as functioning in ways analogous to the mechanized factory dealing with its raw material and labor. Indeed, the way reality is presented in the phrenological head bears a resemblance to the way the factory interior is illustrated in Andrew Ure's classic *The Philosophy of Manufactures* (1835): There, too, symmetry (in phrenology all the organs were duplicated), order, a sense of mechanical complexity rationally understood, as well as purposeful function through division of labor emerge as the conspicuous features. As much as in the factory interior, the phrenology head was an advertisement for a less confusing and more automated reality in which character itself reduced to digits on a graft.

But although mechanical function was an important part of phrenological imagery and rhetoric, the dominant metaphor for describing the diverse functions of the brain (and within which was contained the the metaphor of the machine) was that of the body. The brain after all was not an engine but an organ, a malleable living instrument for service and success. Characterizing the brain as the organ or "body of the mind"[32] could facilitate, to far better effect than the metaphor of the machine, the description of holistic development with diverse function. It could also deflect denials of free will implicit to assumptions of man as an elaborate machine. Moreover, it allowed everyone to participate in understanding the "laws of organization" – regular movements, nourishment, exercise, exertion, absorbtion, balance, harmony, and so on. Absent from the phrenological scheme of mental functions were those planetary and corpuscular billiard-ball models and metaphors rooted in mechanics, physics, and chemistry that had suited the rhythms and social needs of an earlier age.[33] Supplanting the wholly predictable, eternal cyclical return of the planetary system or the competitive colliding social atoms of the corpuscular philosophy were the organically based laws of life – of growth and development, of biology, adaptation, structures, and functions – of organisms living and growing not chaotically but according to the harmony of regulated natural laws. Regularity yet change, order yet progress – this was the service of the organismic metaphor celebrated by phrenology. It is thus less ironic than at first it seems that mankind should have been transported into the mechanical age not by a predominantly mechanistic explanatory model but by an organic one. In part because it subsumed mechanical function within a vitalistic framework,[34] the organismic metaphor offered shelter from the frightening social and intellectual reverberations arising from the new technology and commercial growth; but at the same time, precisely because the metaphor lacked the

hard-edged, causal, reductive, materialist dimensions of Newtonian mechanism, it more readily facilitated a toleration of and a
coming to terms with the emergent structures and relations of
industrial capitalism. It was not that phrenology "justified" the
emergent social system nor, even less, that its version of organicism mollified lingering revulsion against a universe of "dead matter" governed over by an inanimate and wrathful God (though
on occasions it could do either or both).[35] Rather, phrenology
naturalized the emergent structures and relations of industrial capitalism by casting them into the descriptive and explanatory language of mental organization and mental function. Thereby those
structures and relations came to seem "as of ourselves," or as
corresponding with the known "facts" about the innate nature of
man, while deviations from them began to appear as pathological.[36] Here, in fact, were the roots of what would come to be
known as functionalist social theory; and it should come as no
surprise that the seminal theorists of functionalism all owed large
debts to phrenology. Herbert Spencer drew from the science his
concept of man's adaptation of faculties to organic, psychological,
and social needs; Henri de Saint-Simon justified his biological
categorizations of society; Auguste Comte did the same, maintaining, as well, that Gall had (among other things, such as "proving" the inferiority of women) perceived the innate sociability of
man.[37] Extending from these theorists, and in an unbroken tradition of biological extrapolations articulating organicists' models
(most notably by Durkheim and Radcliffe-Brown in the 1930s),
the organismic metaphor emerged dominantly and pervasively in
the reigning theory of sociology, social anthropology, and industrial psychology.[38] George Henry Lewes, who was no partisan of
phrenology, was quite right to conclude, as he reflected in the
1850s on Comte and Spencer's debts to phrenology, that Gall's
"bold assignment of definite functions to definite organs" was
revolutionary and that Gall therefore merited to be known as "the
Kepler of Psychology."[39]

But other than in a superficial way, it is not easy today to
understand why Gall's "bold assignment" in human psychology
should have been considered as "revolutionary." While we can
remind ourselves that before Gall there was no psychology in the
modern analytical sense – discounting Hartley's associationism or
sensationist psychology, which was not analytical, there was only

the classical humoral distinction between the lymphatic, sanguine, bilious, and nervous types – we have become so accustomed to the specializing and fragmenting forces of modern life, and have made the presuppositions of the economic system so much our own, that Gall's basic idea does not strike us as in the least "revolutionary." Since the idea itself that there should be such a thing as a *science* of human character is not likely to strike us as ridiculous (until we think about it), how much less so is the idea that such a science should be based upon the fragmentation of personality into specialized cerebral parts? Even an outraged contemporary such as William Hazlitt can only begin to remind us what was startling about phrenology in the early nineteenth century: that it "professes to account for the differences of talent and disposition in a simple and unequivocal manner by making a *division of labour*, or distributing the different sorts of cleverness and capacity respectively among the different organs."[40] It was this and more than this, however, that was appreciated by Lewes and those endeavoring to erect sciences of society in the nineteenth century. They appreciated that Gall had done more than merely step quantatively beyond the classical humoral classification scheme when he identified his mental functions; they divined and welcomed that he had in fact made a qualitative leap in the understanding of human psychology when, Adam Smith–like, he elaborated a division of mental labor. For by thus revealing the physics of mind, Gall brought the mind within the categories of capital that had come to seem "natural" to those erecting or commenting upon sciences of (capitalist) society. What was appreciated, then, even though it was not politically understood as such at the time, was that Gall had made mind a part of the bourgeois concept of nature.

But it was in a way that was particularly appropriate for the early nineteenth century that Gall located mind in "nature." For what he revealed of the relations between mental parts in intellectual production had its counterpart in the relations between people in industrial production. In industry the division of labor that Gall depicted in the brain was depriving workers of access to the totality of production and (if we hold labor as the essence of being) was disassociating them from themselves. Thus the way in which industrial capitalism was coming to alienate laboring people and to denigrate them by reducing their labor to a mere wage commodity can be seen as mediated in the phrenology head where human psychology – the thinking and emotional essence of being human – was reified into so many interacting clumps of brain tissue, none of which had access to the whole except under the *abnormal* condition of monomania. Reified, mind–humanness was drained of its essence or subjectivity, and into the vacancy were parked the "objective" relations of capital. The social relations of industrial capitalism thus having come to define the terms for conceptualizing humanness, the imagery of the human mind came to contribute to the reality of human degradation. At root, therefore, phrenology was to humanness in the psychological abstract what capitalism was to human labor in the real. And historically there is no distance between the viewing of the human mind in these objectivist terms and the treating of humans as mere objects; in terms of the historical development of industrial capitalism, the perceiving and the treating were mutually constitutive. However "natural" it may appear to some anthropologists that in periods of rapid change people seek to relate more to things than to other humans,[41] the early-nineteenth-century enthusiasm for mere phrenological plaster casts and symbolical charts of heads cannot be separated from the *kind* of socioeconomic change then taking place. Of course, once the social relations of industrial capitalism were naturalized in "cerebration" (a term invented by phrenologists), the science of character could be put to use in a more or less overt way as a justification from nature of those relations. The social theorist Charles Fourier, for example, was to preach that "labour is only an image of man's internal faculties."[42] The social and political implications of such preaching will concern us in later chapters; for purposes of better understanding Combe's attraction to phrenology, it is only necessary to observe here that phrenology's physiological organization of brain addressed within man himself exactly that division of labor that was discerned by Carlyle as being "the problem of the whole future, for all who in future pretend to govern men."[43]

It has been noted that the phrenological faculties were not only neatly classified, but were also hierarchically arranged. It needs adding that it was according to their location in the physical hierarchy that the faculties were valued and numerically assigned: from the animal propensity of Amativeness (no. 1) at the lowest point at the back of the head to the perceptive and reflective intellectual faculties (nos. 22–35) territorializing the forehead. The arrangement gave new form to the ancient concept of the *scala naturae* and to its eighteenth-century derivative the "Great Chain of Being" as depicted by Arthur O. Lovejoy. As with the older forms of the concept, the phrenological form both reinforced the idea that "some are, and must be, greater than the rest"[44] and, at the same time, made the naked fact of hierarchical distribution of power less naked and more justifiable through an emphasis on the cohesive social and psychological benefits to be derived from such an arrangement.[45] Through the phrenological arrangement each person and each social class could be understood necessarily to fulfil a natural determinant function within a unified whole.

But in other points of significance the Great Chain of Being and the hierarchical division of mental faculties in the phrenology head differ fundamentally. Whereas in the Chain of Being relations were fixed and static, in the phrenology head the relations between the parts were functional, the perfect operation of the whole depending upon the parts' harmonic inter*action*. Although Spurzheim (and Combe after him) was to extrapolate from Gall's physical model the notion that the intellectual and moral faculties were *functionally* superior to the others, such superiority was not held as arbitrarily assigned through some special and mysterious relationship with God, but as attributed consistently and justly by nature. Moreover, in spite of the phrenological claim that the faculties were inherited, the science was never to be perceived by traditional retainers of status and power as confirming their "natural" inherited rights and privileges. On the contrary, largely as a result of the way in which Spurzheim popularized the science in Britain, phrenology was seen as radically attacking inherited power and wealth through an assertion of the prior claims of an "inheritance of talents," theoretically fluid and endlessly progressive. Further, at the same time that phrenology replaced the "artificial," "mere parchment-based" inheritance of property with the "real" biologically based inheritance of mental ability, it partly displaced the whole idea of inheritance with the idea of self-effort and industry. Again, as a result of the way Spurzheim promoted the science, it emerged that only those who worked hard to fully exercise and/or develop their moral and intellectual faculties could hope to be socially superior. Indeed, among the organs that Spurzheim added to Gall's list were "Conscientiousness," "Time," and "Order"; it was only left for Combe to add "Concentrativeness."[46] The concepts of time and work discipline were thus biologized through the very *qualities of character* that phrenology held nature as revealing; through the scientized Smilesian nomenclature the Calvinistic concern with industriousness was made secularly good while more relaxed agrarian values were challenged. A groundplan for the reformation of humankind was thus laid out in the physiological certainty that just as the true understanding of man's neurobiology allowed people to apply themselves to the full development of their talents and propensities, so a natural motive had been supplied for a reorganization of society on the basis of those talents rather than on the basis of inherited and divinely sanctioned social station. Broken over the phrenological head, therefore, were not only the agrarian aristocracy's traditional intuitions about character, but also, inseparably, their most powerful, time-honored legitimations of hierarchical social power.

The final substantive feature of phrenology requiring special attention is the fact that it was only from the *surface* of the cranium that human psychology was to be read. This, too, could signify a total assault on traditional thought and society, in which what really matters is held to be implicit or obscure to all but the privileged. The notion that character could be read from the surface of the head was frightening to established elites not simply because it exposed peoples' heads to the mercy of others' observations (though the doctrine was often attacked for this reason). Rather, it was, as suggested in the previous chapter, that the "reading off" from the surface of matters hitherto considered profoundly mysterious and requiring deep study signified a mockery of the intellectual activity and productions of the elite through which the elite justified its position. What the "insiders" in the intellectual, social, and religious elites held to be sacred was thus profaned and their social dominance challenged. Steven Shapin is undoubtedly correct in asserting that it was for this reason that Edinburgh antiphrenologists endeavored to expose, among other things, the existence and importance of the frontal sinuses that intervened between the surface of the cranium and the brain.[47] A science that led people to believe through its insistence on observable reality that *anyone* could understand nature and human nature and, at the same time, characterized the knowledge that had been hoarded by the privileged few as "mere barren speculation" that was "built in the clouds" was obviously ideologically potent.[48] To men of Combe's background, the immediacy of understanding promised by phrenology's surface revelation was no less revolutionary than Calvin's ambition to have men know the moral state of their souls and the wishes of God without recourse to confessors or scholars. As Calvinism and Puritanism cut out the interventions between God and man (or as anarchism cut out those between man and man, and mysticism and spiritualism those between soul and self), so phrenology in claiming that the nature of man could be read from the surface of his skull did away with what seemed to be the obfuscations between people and the truths about themselves. Bunyanesque, phrenology laid the thing "truth" down as it was.

From this demystification of self through revelations on the head's surface came also rationalizations for emotional shallowness. For those socialized to fear and repress emotions, it was an attractive science that maintained that what was literally out of sight was out of mind. But in emptying the head of its secrets by engraving them on its surface, the feelings of confusion, anxiety, guilt, and impotence that went into Victorian *Angst* were only disguised in order to be disqualified from consideration. As Combe's recorded biography makes clear, phrenology allowed the darker side of the conventional middle-class Victorian mind, the profound ontological insecurity, the emotional turmoil, the aesthetic and sensual, and all other aspects of reason and humanity that could not be reduced to rationality to be, indeed, rationally reduced. By "surfacing" character, legitimacy was given to the repression of deep feelings, of abstract and speculative thought and metaphysical concerns with the soul, and of the body's anarchical sensual parts. These, the concerns of humanists, neoplatonists, and romantic rebels in particular, were not the concerns to harmonize best with the needs of an industrial capitalist society of disciplined producers and consumers. Thus, although phrenology was never designed to celebrate humanity's desensualization, by teaching that the book of human life was to be judged entirely by its cover, it served covertly to authenticate and naturalize both the dehumanizing forces in industrial society and the social reality they fostered. The irony of phrenology ever being regarded as a form of psychology is manifest: Like social history badly done, phrenology had everything to do with outer reality and nothing at all to do with inner structures of thought.

As with the other distinctive features of phrenology, then, its cranially superficial way of divining character brings together aspects of evident psychosocial and ideological significance. The provision was thus not simply or even necessarily that of the means to justify early industrial economic and social conditions, but rather the sense-making structures for comprehending that reality. Given the basic human need constantly to seek "a meaningful inner formulation of self and world," so that actions, and even impulses, have some kind of "fit" with the "outside" world, phrenology can perhaps best be understood as a multifaceted symbolic resource that enabled people to establish some kind of consonance between their inner and outer worlds under conditions tending otherwise to anomie and dissonance.[49] In acting as both compass and map for self-orientation in the fragmenting social world, the hierarchical physics of brain permitted an exchange of impressions of senselessness, purposelessness, and anarchy for those of order, pattern, and control. In a way that would appeal to a Dickensian character, all was made plain: The mind was no longer Pope's "chaos of Passion all confus'd," it was a set of physiological structures functioning in an orderly way. Relative to this, it was merely a bonus point that phrenology also spelled out and rationalized the mental and physical superiority of bourgeois males, the special roles and duties of women, children, workers, and other races, as well as the punitive requirements for social deviants.

As certainly as George Combe experienced dissonance was he to find a satisfying consonance through this pseudointrospective means of understanding the external world. The title alone of his famous book *Of the Constitution of Man and Its Relation to External Objects* (1828)[50] gives a clue to this inner–outer rapport, while the book's contents can be seen as the superimposition upon Combe's psychosocial insecurity, searing doubt, and sense of chaos of the framework of certainty, order, and meaning manifested through the phrenological head. As Winston Churchill and Isaac Newton are said to have transformed their prevalent personal neuroses into powerful social and intellectual forces, so Combe may be said to have transformed his neurosis into a powerful secular–theological means of gaining mastery over the chaos of modern life: Reversing the terms, he explicated the theme that Wordsworth in 1814 felt was

> ...but little heard among men –
> The external World is fitted to the Mind.[51]

THE CONSTITUTION OF MAN

Merely to discern the manner in which Combe moved from one form of reality to another in translating the map of mind into explicit social and moral terms would be reason enough for our turning to the study of his opus. For the social and cultural historian of ideas, however, there is a further compelling reason: the fact that the *Constitution of Man* was one of the most esteemed and popular books of the second third of the nineteenth century. By 1847 total sales amounted to over 80,500. By 1860, some 100,000 copies had been sold in Britain and some 200,000 more in America (where it passed through more than twenty editions).[52] In terms of popularity (and profitability) the *Constitution of Man* hardly compares with the *Origin of Species*, which sold a mere 50,000 copies by the end of the century; hardly compares with Robert Chambers's *Vestiges of the Natural History of Creation*, which sold over 25,000 copies in eleven editions between 1844 and 1860, or with Hugh Miller's *Testimony of the Rocks* (1847), which is said to have sold 42,000 copies. By its sales as by its real and apparent meaningfulness, better comparisons would be with, on the one hand, Samuel Smiles's *Self Help*, which sold 258,000 copies between its publication in 1859 and 1905 and, on the other hand, with the book with which the *Constitution of Man* was sometimes bound and often simultaneously condemned, Tom Paine's *Rights of Man* (1791), alleged to have sold 200,000 copies by 1793.[53] Certainly there was some truth to the claim that for the second third of the nineteenth century, after the Bible, *Pilgrim's Progress*, and *Robinson Crusoe*, the *Constitution of Man* was next in circulation and, what is as much to the point, that it stood on bookshelves where no others but these were to be found.[54] "If in a manufacturing district you meet with an artisan whose sagacious conversation and tidy appearance convince you that he is one of the more favourable specimens of his class," wrote the *Spectator* in 1841, "enter his house, and it is ten to one but you find COMBE'S *Constitution of Man* lying there."[55] For this reason Harriet Martineau put Combe beside Von Humboldt in the "Scientific" section of her *Biographical Sketches* (1865). To her, as to others involved in retailing bourgeois ideology and political economy to working people, Combe was envied as "the agent, if not the author, of a great revolution in popular views"[56] – in effect, the successful salesman of the world view presaged in the philosophy of David Hume and Adam Smith and naturalized by parsons Malthus and Paley. Combe's great book, so Martineau believed, led the multitude to their first glimpse of "man's [proper] position in the universe." Later in the century other leading polemicists of bourgeois liberalism and positivism raised the same hosannas to the author of the *Constitution of Man*, though, like Martineau, they either avoided or dismissed Combe's phrenology and seldom let on that in their lives, too, the reading of the book had been something of an "era." As John Morley put it in his biography of Combe's friend and correspondent Richard Cobden, "Few emphatically second-rate men have done better work than the author of the *Constitution of Man*," the principles extolled in which "have now in some shape or other become the accepted commonplaces of all rational persons." Although there are grounds for doubting both the effect and the benefits of the effect of the book "on the health, morality, and intellectual cultivation of the people," it cannot be doubted that from the point of view of Martineau & Co. the book "fell in remarkably with the needs and desires of the time."[57]

Though ostensibly an objective description of the natural relations between man and his environment, the *Constitution of Man* was in reality a scientistic prescription for daily living, modes of conduct, and social relations – a literal "constitution" *for* social behavior based on a politically symbolic constitution of mental organization. Among the virtues it preached were temperance, cleanliness, regular habits, work discipline, the nuclear family, individualism, property rights, and free trade; while proscribed was everything from the eating of spicy foods and living by stagnant waters to lack of industry, absenteeism, insubordination, licentiousness, early marriage, and excessive breeding. The laboring classes – depicted as living only to gratify their inferior propensities and as "rather organized machines than moral and intellectual beings" – are seen, on the one hand, as holding to "erroneous notions" about the "pleasures enjoyed in past ages" and, on the other, as forever flying to dreams of future happiness as the compensation for their miseries and as attributing to the system "evils which result from their own gross errors in conduct."[58] Among the book's proposals is the idea that mating should be based on the best-developed brains and that criminals, instead of being hanged or exploited for their labor, should be kept in solitary confinement so that their evil thoughts, desires, and passions would break down and new moral influences could be fed into their evacuated faculties.

Rationalizing and explicating all of this were the moral laws of nature. Like Comte and Spencer after him, Combe was attempting what hitherto had not seemed possible (nor so necessary, or desirable): "a demonstration of morality as a science."[59] What rendered the demonstration possible was of course phrenology – "the clearest, most complete, and best-supported system of Human Nature" – for true knowledge of the organization and functions of the brain permitted actual scientific laws of human nature to be derived. As Combe saw it, phrenology gave scientific proof that "proper conduct" was "*that which is approved by the whole moral and intellectual faculties, fully enlightened, and acting in harmonious combination.*"[60] It therefore followed (since harmony was "synonymous with enjoyment of existence") that the maximization of happiness depended upon the cultivation of the intellect and moral sentiments and upon the repression of animal desires. Thus were constituted Combe's natural laws of morality. But whereas in the natural philosophy that Combe drew upon "law" was normally a metaphorical attribution applied descriptively to uniform physical phenomena (such as the "law" of gravity) and had nothing to do with free will, since such law cannot help but be obeyed, in Combe's writing the "laws of nature" became moral prescriptions that, if transgressed, would lead to consequences "formidable and appalling."[61] For Combe, failure to subordinate oneself to the natural laws of morality by trusting to some other standard of right and wrong is as consequential as attempting to fly from the top of a building or attempting to breathe under water.

Notwithstanding that from the time the *Constitution of Man* first appeared there was considerable criticism of its conflation of prescriptive moral law with descriptive physical law,[62] it was largely from the book that this use of natural law spread throughout the English-speaking world. In *Vestiges*, for example, Combe's friend and fellow phrenologist Robert Chambers was to assert:

It is hardly necessary to say, much less to argue, that mental action, being proved to be under law, passes at once into the category of natural things. Its old metaphysical character vanishes in a moment, and the distinction usually taken between physical and moral is annulled.[63]

It was against just such a conflation that William Whewell had remonstrated as early as 1833. But it was not until the last third of the nineteenth century that it was seriously taken to task, notably by Lewes, William Carpenter, and Huxley – the last seizing upon it in the 1880s as the distinguishing mark of pseudoscience.[64] Crucial to these end-of-the-century critiques was John Stuart Mill's essay "On Nature," which, although written in the 1850s, was not published until 1874. Mill's object was to expose the subjectivity of nature when relied upon as an external criterion for morality, and he singled out Combe's writings as having been very largely responsible for the confusion between *naturam sequi* and *naturam observare*, "from whence it has overflowed into a large region of popular literature, and we are now continually reading injunctions to obey the physical laws of the universe, as being obligatory in some sense and manner as the moral."[65]

But what Mill and others were at liberty to examine logically, Combe could only consider practically. As a member of the legal profession he needed no reminding that the law, by proscribing and sanctioning, was *the* instrument of domination and the means by which social relations were fixed. From his interest in dismantling traditional authority and reordering the world, it was expedient to have nature don the garb of neutral justice and through science decree and police an absolute moral code. Since his opponents relied upon God as their ultimate legitimator of truth and authority, it was essential for Combe to attribute a physical law–like power and authority to his purported moral laws. Thereby he had what all who seek to morally reform society require in the face of their opponents, an ultimate touchstone of truth – a touchstone, moreover, that, in stemming from nature, could be held to be uncorrupted by the culture and customs nurtured arbitrarily by the traditional retainers of power.[66] It is thus hardly to be wondered at that Combe, in defending his work, always managed to evade the criticisms of his handling of the concept of natural law.

Nor is it so surprising, given the antiestablishment task of Combe's natural laws, that the *Constitution of Man* was enthusiastically received by the reform-minded in both the middle and the working class. To fully understand this, however, one must add that it is only in the hindsight of normative urban industrial bourgeois values that the *Constitution of Man* appears as a blunt instrument for the inculcation of those values. In context, the book appeared in quite a different light – appeared to many, indeed, to be, as the Swedish translators retitled the book, "The Doctrine of Happiness on Earth." For while Combe's phrenology showed "it to be a law of nature, that until the intellect is extensively informed, and the moral sentiments assiduously exercised, the animal propensities bear the predominant sway; and that whenever these are supreme, misery is an inevitable concommitant," the science also rendered certain the health, prosperity, and happiness of the individual and the "superiority of civilization."[67] For happiness, all that was required was that people come into harmony with and abide by the natural laws of mind and morality. Had not the philosophers of the Enlightenment optimistically predicted that once nature was properly understood society would arrange itself harmoniously? Combe, it seemed, through phrenology, had supplied the necessary key to that understanding. Henceforth humankind would be free from the false secular and religious restrictions of the past and be free from the "conditions of savage and barbarian life in the present day." Humankind, located (at long last) in a *natural* evolutionary process, could now be propelled into a future of unbounded progress, perfection, and harmony.

Thus it was that humanitarianism, not repression, that liberty and freedom, not subjugation, appeared as the distinctive features of the *Constitution of Man.* And it would be wrong to suppose that Combe was not sincere in espousing these virtues – even in connection with the treatment of criminals. In fact, with respect to criminals in particular, Combe had every reason to believe that his approach was radically benevolent compared to the reigning "animal system" of brutish punishments. Just as with the reformation of humankind in general, Combe's "moral system" for reforming the criminal mind had as its object the restoration of mental harmony and the establishing of the supremacy of the moral and intellectual faculties. Since the activity of these faculties was supposed to be the "fountain of pleasure," Combe's (brainwashing) means for making them operative seemed justifiable. The "moral system" of punishment having no other object than to bring the criminal "*back to obedience for his own welfare,*" Combe believed that the offender ought to have every reason to be grateful for the treatment.[68]

Of course, it might be said that the whole of Combe's interest in criminal reform only reflects the urban bourgeoisie's mounting fears for private property in the early nineteenth century and that Combe's humanitarian reform gestures were but a means of obfuscating fundamental social inequalities. Certainly such fears existed in his mind, as witnessed by the fact that it was the section on punishment in the *Constitution of Man* that expanded most over editions.[69] And just as surely as Combe's writing helped to obfuscate the class realities behind crime and its treatment, his humanitarian interest in criminals served to reinforce the controls to deal with them.[70] But Combe did not perceive his interest in that light. Nor was he aware, in the sense that Foucault has made many aware, that in focusing on criminals and to a lesser extent on lunatics he was engaged in a process of redefining social solidarity.[71] Combe was not to know (though he would have appreciated had he known) that all societies need deviants because their exclusion gives everyone else, and especially those performing the acts of excluding, the feeling of social belonging. In his redefining of the criminal mind and its rehabilitation requirements – as, indeed, in the whole of his interest in phrenology as the means of extolling normality and abnormality – is to be seen not just the bid of the social "outsider" for "insider" status but, as well and inseparably, the antitraditionalist expression of the need to modernize the nature of social cohesion. Perfecting punishments for individuals was both a means to and a symbolic expression of perfecting an individualist society. But this was no more apparent to Combe than it was to Jeremy Bentham; as far as Combe was concerned the reform of the treatment of criminals was simply a necessary part of the wider program to create, in the name of humanity, a more rational society. The same can be said of his interest in the working class.

Although Combe's heavy investment in American railways might be taken as highly symbolic, the author of the *Constitution of Man* spoke neither as a capitalist nor as one whose primary objective was to reconcile workers to an exploitative and dehumanizing economic system.[72] Quite unlike his minor contemporary Andrew Ure, Combe did not apologize for the manufacturing system but criticized it as "tend[ing] constantly to increase the evils of which it is the source."[73] Manufacturers he accused of suffering from enlarged faculties of Acquisitiveness and Self-Esteem and of violating the laws of nature by rendering their laborers incapable of anything other than gratifying their baser faculties. Political economists were likewise condemned for assuming and asserting that the accumulation of wealth was the great end of human ambition. Strikes, as Combe saw them, offered "natural checks" to the proceedings of greedy manufacturers, and he therefore asserted a natural place for trade unions in a well-adjusted society.[74]

Naturally we cannot jump from the expression of these opinions to the opposite conclusion, that Combe therefore held to some kind of proto-Marxian critique of industrial capitalism – no more than we can arrive at the same conclusion about Adam Smith on the basis of his similar incidental negative comments on the industrial division of labor and capital accumulation in the *Wealth of Nations*. In the history of ideas the more correct jump would be to Plato's *Republic*, for central to Combe's (and Smith's) deploring of the greed of manufacturers was an ascetic deprecation of the sensual satiation that Plato saw as the ultimate object of money lust.[75] In any case, Combe's was not a critique of industrial capitalism, but an exposure of those technical imperfections of the system that, if remedied, would make the system healthier.[76] Behind the advocacy in the *Constitution of Man* for shorter working hours and better working conditions lay no interest in the working class for their own sake, but rather the hope that the working class might be brought to share the author's own rationalist mindscape: after all, by spending less time on factory floors, workers would have more time to study phrenology and the "laws of nature"!

In the final analysis, then, it was not the socioeconomic system that the *Constitution of Man* rationalized in an immediate sense, nor simply the values of the emerging-as-dominant urban industrial bourgeoisie. It was Enlightenment rationalism itself that the book sought to propagate; and in Combe's mind there was no recognizable ideological relationship between that rationalism and the structures and relations of advanced capitalism. No more than Condorcet or Destutt de Tracy was Combe ever to call into question the power of the rational thought he celebrated; no more than they was he aware that the Reason he was celebrating was born of the urge to dominate others, obscured in the urge to know and control nature and human nature.[77] Which is not to say that Combe was not as capable as Condorcet of recognizing that nature is often made an accomplice in the crime of political inequality. Nor is it to say that he himself did not seek to justify specific social, political, and economic views.[78] Obviously he did. It is to maintain, rather, that like most of his contemporaries, Combe had no awareness of how anthropomorphic and historically constituted was his conception of what was "natural." That "nature is a societal category," politically constituted and historically specific, Combe had simply no idea;[79] he had no idea that the phrenological revelations of human nature that he took as neutral were socially constituted and ideologically predetermined; and he had no idea that the moral laws he based upon that version of human nature – that mediation of reality – were merely scientistic impositions permitting a reciprocal confirmation between his phrenology and (in general) the political philosophy of David Hume and Adam Smith. Because Combe also had no idea that Hume and Smith's philosophy had been developed in opposition to Hobbes and those who held to the notion that society derived from social contract, we may say, finally, that just as Combe had no conscious understanding of the ideological nature of the world view he was naturalizing, so he had no awareness of what that world view ideologically *denatur-alized* through its omissions. It may safely be said that had he had such awareness while writing the *Constitution of Man*, the end product would have been far different, and so too its reception.

What Combe *was* aware of, and what the readers of the *Constitution of Man* most often consciously responded to because of Combe's challenging of it, was the power of orthodox sectarian religion. Relative to that, the book was either famous or infamous. Yet it was not an entirely godless book. Although Combe tended privately to a Hume-like agnosticism, publicly he professed deism.[80] This convenienced his interest in eroding the "legacy of Gall" – the association between phrenology and a politically dangerous radical atheism. Like almost all of his contemporaries, both to his left and to his right, Combe viewed atheism as something outrageous, dangerous, and offensive to moral instincts. To repudiate it, he implied that it was the retarded development or malfunction of the faculty of Veneration.[81] The profession of deism also permitted Combe, in the anthropomorphic manner of Paley, to deploy God as a final authority enforcing compliance with the order being naturalized. Accordingly, as he informed the "industrious classes" of Edinburgh in the 1830s,

The Creator has arranged the spontaneous division of labour among men by the simplest, yet most effectual, means. He has bestowed the mental faculties in different degrees of relative strength on different individuals, and thereby has given them at once the desire and the aptitude for different occupations.[82]

In the *Constitution of Man*, God biologically certifies social and economic inequalities as He biologically certifies that poverty lies in the minds and morals of the poor and may be remedied by the poor's own efforts. In this respect there is only a difference of style between Combe's book and Thomas Chalmers's Bridgewater Treatise on *The Adaptation of External Nature to the Moral and Intellectual Constitution of Man*, which was published five years *after* the *Constitution of Man*. Whereas Chalmers (exchanging "mind and morals" for "hearts and habits") delivered his sermon in the style of the Old Testament and expected his reader to comply with his injunctions because they came from on high, Combe expected his reader to comply by coming rationally to understand the reasonableness of doing so.[83] (It is, incidentally, only this greater degree of ratiocination that distinguishes the *Constitution of Man* from Spurzheim's *Sketch of the Natural Laws of Man*.)

In context, the difference between Combe and Chalmers was more than merely one of style, however. Although Combe was in step with other early-nineteenth-century natural theologians in that he identified God with the laws of nature, he was naïvely on his own in thinking that through that identification he and they together were marching toward a more rational Christianity in which "God's will and man's duties" would be clearer and less complicated.[84] Almost wholly, he failed to appreciate, first, that the orthodox natural theologians did not just identify God with the laws of nature, but teleologically directed those laws to God; second, that the natural theologians were careful not to deny Providential interventions in nature, nor to doubt the relevance of Scripture; and, third, and most important, that the whole natural theological enterprise of the early nineteenth century (as sponsored by the earl of Bridgewater and others) was an effort to prove, in the face of late-eighteenth-century and early-nineteenth-century radical atheistic social uses of science, that science was not necessarily in conflict with religion and could, therefore, safely be used by the establishment in intellectual arguments for social repression.[85] Combe, thinking that he was attacking only the irrational and dogmatic authority of sectarian religion – his Calvinist past – inadvertently undermined the subtle niceties and deliberate ambiguities of the natural theologians: his God was not only incapable of working miracles, but was so far back into the "Baconian heaven of first causes" as to be virtually interchangeable with nature;[86] the Scriptures were more or less relegated to the status of fairy tales; while his natural laws, rather than being teleologically directed to God, located man within an evolutionary scheme in which God's wisdom and will were irrelevant. It was after all, not to God that the constitution of man was related, but to mere "external objects." Thus Combe did more than challenge religious sectarianism through a deistic rationalism that denied the hereafter and denied sin as the result of the Fall. He also exposed how readily the social legitimating resource of nature could be expropriated and severed from that of God.[87]

Predictably, therefore, the *Constitution of Man* provoked the "bewilderment, horror and indignation" of the religious.[88] This was particularly the reaction of the Scottish Evangelicals led by Chalmers and the Reverend David Welsh, some of whom (Chalmers and Welsh included) had previously taken a deep natural theological interest in phrenology.[89] At a time when deism (the faith of Tom Paine) was still regarded as socially and politically dangerous, Combe was seen in much the same way that Gall had been seen in the context of Vienna in the 1790s: as one who had driven a basically sound and safe body of natural knowledge too far in a direction that was not just mistaken and ungentlemanly, but was downright dangerous. The whole character of the book was French, lamented William Scott, an early member of the EPS, the French of the revolutionary philosophers, of Voltaire and the *encyclopédistes* and those avowed infidels Volney and Mirabaud.[90] As more temperate critics pointed out, the book was simply "too much about the laws of Nature, and too little about the laws of God."[91] But what made Combe's scientistic refinement of heresy worse was the popular attention it received – attention that was only increased by the religionists' efforts to counteract its impact. Very largely, it was out of the religious controversy over the *Constitution of Man* that was born the so-called nineteenth-century conflict between science and religion – the increasing unreality of which conflict as the century wore on and as power moved secularly from parish church to town hall was eventually to result in the apparent paradox of the conflict's hypostatization.[92] In its real

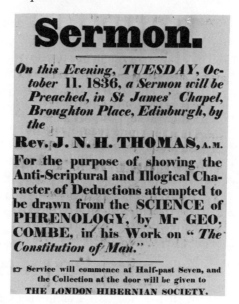

Sermon.

On this Evening, TUESDAY, October 11. 1836, a Sermon will be Preached, in St James' Chapel, Broughton Place, Edinburgh, by the

Rev. J. N. H. THOMAS, A.M.

For the purpose of showing the Anti-Scriptural and Illogical Character of Deductions attempted to be drawn from the SCIENCE of PHRENOLOGY, by Mr GEO. COMBE, in his Work on " *The Constitution of Man.*"

☞ Service will commence at Half-past Seven, and the Collection at the door will be given to THE LONDON HIBERNIAN SOCIETY.

Figure 5. Handbill for the antiphrenological sermon of the Rev. J. N. H. Thomas, Edinburgh, 11 October 1836.

as in its hypostatized form, however, the conflict only served positivistically to further establish science in and of itself as autonomous objective truth, separate from subjective human interests and, pari passu, to deflect attention away from the fact that both sides in the conflict were fighting on and for control over the same socioeconomic terrain. By thus publicly opening out the conflict between science and religion, the *Constitution of Man* represents a watershed in the social legitimation of power in industrial capitalism. It was largely through the similar but lesser reactions to Chambers's *Vestiges* and Darwin's *Origin of Species* that that secularized social and cultural power was to be consolidated and the positivist "religion of science" affirmed.[93]

The *Constitution of Man* was on the rationalist side that ultimately won the war, though it lost the phrenological battle. It is easy, therefore, to see the controversy over the book simply in terms of science versus religion, or in terms of reason, rationality, scientific naturalism, and freedom pitted against superstition, supernaturalism, and dogmatic and authoritarian sectarian repressions. In large measure that is how the book was written and how it was responded to. As Combe recapitulated his position in 1847 in what was intended as a new chapter of the *Constitution of Man*:

In the present time the leaders of the Calvinistic sects are strenuously exerting themselves to bring back the public sentiment to the opinions of the beginning of the seventeenth century; and if they do not succeed, it is science alone which prevents this consummation of their labours.[94]

What we have preferred to argue here is that the mere contextualization of Combe's writings (as also the phrenology they are based upon) is in itself historically insufficient. Obscured is not only the general point that both science and religion may serve similar social, ideological, and psychosocial functions,[95] but also, the particular point that the *Constitution of Man* was less an *alternative* to the Calvinism that Combe rebelled against than a secular *revival* of it, sacralizing the social norms and values most appropriate to the industrially modified and modifying economic order. Upsetting the throne of the ultimate father figure, the book ushered in a new authority in secular natural law to which the new bourgeois individual man could relate directly and "rationally." In effect, God's controlling laws as codified by Calvin were modernized or made to seem more reasonable through Combe's appeals to ultimate authorities in nature and the cosmos. As in Calvinism, so in Combe's philosophy, man stands alienated from man but in harmony with a supreme and ostensibly neutral, universal, and eternal authority. Class interests are likewise disguised by a concentration on individual responsibility for salvation. The blame for the problems of the mass of the population – poverty, ill health, ignorance, intemperance, and so on – are shifted away from the exploitative social structure and to the conscience and industriousness of the individuals exploited, who had disobeyed nature as they had formerly disobeyed God. In Calvinism as in Combe's system, entry into the Elect was in practice closed to all except those born into the more respectable and prosperous classes, or born with the "best"-developed brains (though the blatant double standard of Calvinism, where the Elect were also the saved, was muted by making salvation secular or worldly and therefore theoretically open to all who were willing to work to put their cerebral house in order). Persons such as the brothers Chambers, Hugh Miller, and the heroes of Samuel Smiles were visible proof of how "anyone" could enter the earthly kingdom of the saved, and visible proof of how secular salvation or happiness could only be achieved through hard work. To achieve happiness – or at least to stave off suffering – it was imperative to come into harmony with the social, political, and legal external relations laid down by the new secular priesthood, to find your social niche and make the best of it.

As the *Constitution of Man* emerges as a secular Calvinism, so we might conclude with the observation that Combe, once armed with the biological certainties of phrenology, became a secular Calvin reproducing many of the same structures of thought and values. Weber carefully pointed out that the Calvinist mind had to rationalize the life cycle into an ever more methodical and single-minded movement toward the glorification of God for the assurance of a place in Heaven.[96] Phrenology, the pursuit of the natural science of mind, was another form of that "methodizing" process – not, however, for the glorification of God but for the abstract future kingdom or ideal rational order. Through the phrenological image of and insight into that kingdom, Combe, like Calvin, became a regenerating evangelical of what, from the perspective of traditional structures and relations, was a revolutionary ethic (even though the individualist values celebrated in the ethic reached centuries deep into the roots of capitalism).[97] "A second reformation in religion is imperatively called for, and is preparing," Combe wrote, as always couching his instructions for the transformation of the world in the image of his antitraditionalist ideal.[98] In the process of rationalizing the life cycle, however, Combe, like Calvin, amputated everthing that appeared to him as irrational ritual and obfuscation, since these represented enslavements of the past and obstacles to reform. Both Calvin and Combe were in turn reduced to enchantments with material forms and sensuous *surface*. Once Calvin had deritualized life, he then reritualized it with a set of formal and explicit rules. In the *Constitution of Man* Combe repeated the process and appealed as effectively as Calvin to an ultimate authority to legitimate a moral necessitarianism. Finally, Combe acted the part of Calvin in undermining filial piety and idolatry to intensify an ascetic drive for self-effort in an ever more "rational" world. "The only difference," Cobden wrote to Combe a month after the repeal of the Corn Laws, "is that John Calvin and George Combe act upon different theories, and rely upon different motives, and start from very different premises, but they recognize the self-same ends, secularly-speaking, and I cannot quarrel with either."[99]

But then, not everyone read Combe as Cobden did, nor necessarily perceived phrenology as Combe did. As indicated in reference to certain of the science's early supporters, an interest in phrenology connected to religiosocial experiences different from Combe's could lead to quite different impressions of its use and meaning. Thus one of the questions that lies before us now, as we turn to phrenology's popular audience, is who among them *could* quarrel with Combe and phrenology?

5

The poacher turned gamekeeper: phrenologists abroad

[The] probable effect [of science education] on the average human being would be to narrow the range of his thoughts and make him more than ever contempuous of such knowledge as he did not possess: and his political reactions would probably be somewhat less intelligent than those of an illiterate peasant who retained a few historical memories and a fairly sound aesthetic sense.

George Orwell, "What Is Science?" *Tribune* (London), 26 October 1945, in *Collected Essays* (Harmondsworth, 1971), vol. 4, 29

Science is not only valuable for what it makes us do, but for what it prevents us from doing.

Report by the Committee for Arranging the Preliminary Details of the Courses of Lectures on Geology, Chemistry, and Phrenology (Edinburgh, 1832), p. 3

The extent to which English society by the early Victorian period had been penetrated by "rationalist" influences was a question to which Alfred W. Benn could propose no firm answer in his 1906 *History of English Rationalism in the Nineteenth Century*. He could only suppose that the considerable supply of those influences would not have been such had not some real demand existed.[1]

Nearly a century later it is difficult to say that the ground upon which Benn stood has become more solid. Indeed, certainty about the penetration of rationalism in the nineteenth century has tended to lessen due to increased historical awareness of the persistency in that century of religious evangelicalism, popular millennianism, spiritualism, and a variety of other seemingly nonrationalist concerns.[2] What is odd, however, is that while these latter considerations have contributed to the eclipse of the Whig perspective entertained by Benn on the "inevitable triumph" of Enlightenment rationalism in the nineteenth century, they have not generated new interest in the basic historical issue: the eventual emergence into dominance of the rationalist mode of cognition facilitating social management through individual self-regulation of behavior. Whereas one might have thought that the historical process by which this characteristic mode of cognition and control came to predominate would have become all the more worthy of investigation *because of* its *non*inevitability, in fact, the fundamental historical question has itself entered into eclipse.

Obviously, to a problem of this order – at root, how we have come to think as we think – no solution can be expected from the consideration of merely a single historical phenomenon, not even when, as ironically is the case with the "pseudoscience" of phrenology (in its Combean form), the phenomenon is virtually the epitome of Enlightenment rationalism. As the foremost "People's Science" at the dawn of the Age of Capital, however, phrenology can reinvoke and shed light on Benn's more modest inquiry into the timing of rationalism's popular spread and into its nature and growth. It is thus that our discussion is directed in this chapter, where the main forms and historical contours of phrenology's popular diffusion are taken up as an essential preliminary to the cultural assessment of that diffusion.

THE POPULAR SPREAD

As early as as 1826 "craniological mania" was said to have "spread like a plague ... possess[ing] every gradation of society from the kitchen to the garret." Assessed in 1834 as "a science of more rapid growth than any in the catalogue ... a species of intellectual mushroom or scarlet-bean," thereafter, to an extent declared (in 1845) to be "strikingly observable," the science infused itself into common language and thought. In its heyday in the 1830s and 1840s, recalled Harriet Martineau, "No power on earth could stop it."[3]

The *Constitution of Man* was at the center of much of this enthusiasm, the opinion of the *Spectator* in 1841 being that directly or indirectly Combe's book was responsible for the seepage of phrenology into every chink and cranny of public opinion.[4] But equally important, indeed scarcely separable from the science's intellectual inroads, was its virtually inescapable visibility. As pointed out by a visitor to London in the mid-1830s, it was difficult to walk along the streets and "not be struck with the number of situations in which *phrenological busts and casts* are exposed for sale." To this particular commentator, it was

truly remarkable that, whilst most other articles of sale are confined to some one or two lines of business, the instruments of *Phrenology* are articles of *universal* sale, and, of consequence, of very general purchase. But a still more convincing proof of the same circumstance is found in the fact that you cannot walk the streets, you cannot turn into the Bank or Exchange, but you are accosted with the well-known phrase, "Buy immaches," and observe, not the least conspicuous among the said "immaches," the bust and dissections illustrative of Phrenology. These are strong facts, and tell vastly more than a host of mere verbally expressed opinions.[5]

Similarly telling are reports such as that of an Irish beggar claiming clemency in a Dublin court in 1832 for whacking a miserly gent on his faculty of Benevolence, or that of farriers in 1828 delineating their horses phrenologically. That the *Golden Farmer* in 1831 would applaud Lord Kames for his "mass of Frontal brain" and that a speaker in the Manchester Athenaeum in 1837 would feel the need to title his paper *A Non-Phrenological Essay on the Philosophy of Education* testify further to the science's general invasion of common culture and consciousness and makes unsurprising the frequency with which unselfconscious use of phrenology is to be found in the writings of the nineteenth century's self-educated.[6]

Certainly by the 1840s – by the time the daily press was being accused of being the "vehicle for conveying the poison of Combe's system of philosophy through the length and breadth of the land"[7] – the claim that "the general dissemination of some amount of knowledge of phrenology amongst all classes . . . [was the] striking feature of the present times" had long since ceased to be mere braggadocio on the part of phrenologists. Yet, as further revealed by the correspondent to the *People's Phrenological Journal* who made this observation, it was the operatives more than their factory masters who tended to be familiar with the science.[8] By then, in fact, phrenology had largely found its popular niche among a literate and self-improving stratum that, while extending as far as an enlightened ribbon manufacturer such as Charles Bray,‡ was for the most part composed of sober artisans and workers in danger of revolt. In Dundee these Adam Bede and Felix Holt types had come together to form their own Mechanics' Phrenological Society in 1826, and within a decade similar study groups had sprung up all over the country.[9] By 1836 there was scope for all manner of fond accounts as to how it was

no unusual thing to hear the mechanic discourse of it [phrenology] as he handles the implements of his trade, or to see him, in his hours of recreation, appreciating by its laws, the capacities, and hopes, and prospects, of the laughing children who disport around his knee. In the associations of artizans, it forms a subject of popular, and frequent occupations, and the books, and lectures, concerning it, which have been addressed to that part of the community, have been in an eminent degree widely circulated, and well attended.[10]

IDEOLOGICAL DESIGNS

Although it is doubtful that phrenology's cultivation by artisans was ever so rosy, there is no doubt that the interest was genuine and enthusiastic. But as suggested by the reference to phrenological books and lectures specifically directed at this audience, "voluntary demand" for phrenology by working people was more often than not the result of sustained efforts made by persons outside plebeian and artisan culture. Following Combe and anticipating J. S. Mill, such persons were often strongly opposed to all forms of that culture's independence. Though rarely making it explicit and public, most middle-class phrenologists held with the Edinburgh advocate and phrenologist James Simpson[‡] that the laborer was really "an overgrown child" who rarely knows

how to better his lot in life, by rational reflection on causes and consequences ... [since] he is the creature of impressions and impulses, the unresisting slave of sensual appetites, the ready dupe of the quack, the thrall of the fanatic, and above all, the passive instrument of the political agitator, whose sinister views and falsehoods he is unable to detect.[11]

Ultimately it was for the purpose of imparting the rational (antianarchistic and nonegalitarian) reflection necessary to fit these otherwise "brutal and ignorant" workers "for friendly intercourse with their superiors" (or, as Combe put it, to fit them to be trusted with the power of arbitrating their own destinies)[12] that various middle-class persons clung onto the science well into the 1840s and 1850s, long after their own needs of the science for cultural assertion against the old order had been satisfied. Quite literally in some cases they transported their lecterns, their phrenological paraphernalia, and their administrating selves from the Lit & Phils to the mechanics' institutes.[13]

Yet it would be wrong to try to distinguish too sharply between, on the one hand, use of the knowledge for purposes of rationalizing ambitions in the face of the collasping old social hierarchy and, on the other hand, use of the knowledge for instilling in workers bourgeois normative values. In reality, both the socially upward-directed and the socially downward-directed enterprises were a part of a single exercise in naturalizing emergent values and interests for the achievement of social and cultural hegemony. It is because in practice these enterprises were not separate that discussion of the activity of the phrenological ideologues of change cannot be conducted exclusively in classless terms of "marginality," social "mobility," and generational shifts – at least not without there being a serious political distortion of history. However, given the extent of these men's efforts to reach out to the working class and impart rationalist notions to them, it is entirely possible and not inappropriate to pay particular attention to the history and nature of what in retrospect can be abstracted as the phrenological motion to consolidate the emerging (or newly emergent) social relations of power.

EVALUATION AND CHANGE

Significantly, the elitist interest of British phrenologists in molding the supposedly sensual, irrational, and fragmented minds of "the lower orders" can be dated from the time of Peterloo. In his *Essays on Phrenology* published in that year, Combe wrote:

If we can cultivate the moral sentiments of the mechanic, his lower faculties will be controlled in proportion as the energy of those is increased. If we cultivate his knowing and reflecting faculties, we open up to him sources of gratification of a higher nature, and give him an increased power of usefulness, and a capacity of adopting means to an end, which will not only benefit the individual himself, but make him a much more useful member of society.[14]

Phrenology aside, expressions of this sort, reflecting interest in the socialization of workers (or lunatics, criminals, and children) were regarded as extremely liberal in 1819 in the face of the then more prevalent direct forms of coercion. That it was to be another four years before this approach to behavior manipulation was seriously applied through the middle-class-directed mechanics' institute movement, and that it was to be another seven years before the Society for the Diffusion of Useful Knowledge (SDUK) was established, reminds us that Combe's ideas, while never original, were always in the vanguard. That he read out his essay on the *Constitution of Man* to the EPS some six weeks before the appearance of the first of the tracts issued by the SDUK further reminds us that he was in early on what was to be rapturously referred to by middle-class liberals as the "grand experiment upon human society."[15]

It was not, however, until after the publication of the *Constitution of Man*, and after the political settlement of 1832 in particular, that Combe's phrenology began to be widely appreciated as an educational device. Prior to then the efforts of phrenologists were regarded with suspicion by the leading promoters of "useful knowledge," in spite of the fact that many phrenologists by the mid-1820s had come to share the objectives of Lord Brougham and his colleagues. Whereas the latter's efforts were calculated (however inaccurately) to gain the support of landlords and clergy seeking to reassert paternalistic authority, the labors of Combe & Co., emerging out of an often naïve faith in the power of Enlightenment rationalism to undermine traditional social attitudes and relations, served mostly to alienate the establishment and on that account among others to win for them the support of workers. The problematic status of phrenological knowledge, moreover, served to threaten the godlike image of science that Brougham and his colleagues were attempting to convey in order to exploit science as an ethical arbiter.[16] If phrenology was "science," then Morality and Truth might themselves appear as impermanent and open to *human* negotiation. Thus in the eyes of authority in the period prior to the passage of the Reform Bill, phrenological educators appeared closer to those in need of "education" than to those heading the March of Mind. To the latter, attempting to eradicate workers' disposition to "idleness, anarchy, and dissension" and to instil in them a complacent acceptance of bourgeois political economy (hence to preserve through moderate reforms the social order in which they exercised power), the naïve do-gooding purveyors of phrenology seemed the worse upsetters of the applecart. Thus when Combe offered in 1825 to give a course of lectures on phrenology in what was one of the earliest mechanics' institutes, the Edinburgh School of Arts – a school in the pocket of the university and jurisprudential elite of Edinburgh and run by the Whig functionary Leonard Horner – his application was "politely declined." Similarly, when Sir George MacKenzie[‡] offered to submit an article on phrenology to the SDUK's *Penny Cyclopedia* in 1832 he was told that "the opinion which they [the editors] entertain of phrenology, and its connexion with the moral and intellectual sciences, is not such as would justify them in adopting the offer so kindly made."[17] With Brougham at the SDUK's helm and with his friends Jeffrey and Roget on the provincial roll, this reaction was all too predictable.

By the time the *Penny Cyclopedia* reached the letter G in 1838, however, the tables had completely turned. By then it was predictable that an entry on Gall would appear and that his life would be appropriated into the entrepreneurial self-help mythology: "invincible perseverance and industry" in the face of great adversity, and so on.[18] Many reasons may be adduced to account for this change in phrenology's fortune. None, however, is mutually exclusive, and all are constitutive with the economically rooted changes in the social relations of power that brought the liberal bourgeois order into being in the 1830s. Arbitrary, therefore, must be any attempt historically to separate the various bearings upon phrenology's popularization.

The initiatives taken on behalf of promoting the *Consitution of Man*, for instance, while clearly important in accounting for the wider appreciation of Combean phrenology both as a rationale for engaging in workers' education and as wholesome commodity for workers' consumption, were initiatives that, in themselves, were as much reflections as causes of that appreciation. The Edinburgh printer William Fraser was reflecting that appreciation when, as secretary to a central committee of mechanics' societies in 1830, he issued a circular drawing the attention of mehcanics to Combe's book and the *Phrenological Journal* as "works highly calculated to give them sound practical views of their own nature and duties."[19] In a like manner William Ramsay Henderson,[‡] upon his death in 1832, left five thousand pounds for phrenology's propagation, a part of which sum was directed to the publication of the *Constitution of Man* "in a cheap form, so as to be easily purchased by the more intelligent individuals of the poorer classes and Mechanics' Institutions, &c."[20] It was to the fulfilment of that purpose that some of Henderson's money flowed (appropriately and not by chance) into the book factory of the two friends of Combe whose own rise to riches on the proceeds of mass-produced "useful knowledge" was illustrative of the self-help philosophy extolled in Combe's book – William and Robert Chambers. Of Chamber's stereotyped "People's Edition" of the *Constitution of Man* (costing 1s 6d), sixty four thousand copies were sold between October 1835 and October 1840, thus making up the largest proportion of the sales referred to in the previous chapter. Henderson's money also went toward reducing the cost of the standard edition of the *Constitution of Man*, some eleven thousand copies of which were sold between 1835 and 1837 alone.[21]

How Combe's phrenology might have fared without this backing of the *Constitution of Man* is impossible to tell. Significantly the first edition of the book (1828) did not exhaust its fifteen hundred copies until Henderson's subsidy began to be applied in 1835. But in view of 1835 also being the year in which Chartist organization began, it would be shortsighted to argue that merely lowering the book's price accounted for its high sales and heavy impact. Plainly, like the writing of the book, its promotion and bourgeois appreciation were not events sui generis; additional and necessarily dialectical circumstances are there to help explain why middle-class persons who might have had little interest in Combe's phrenology in 1828 (had they known of it) and who, for different reasons, might have found it inappropriate in 1848 could be found in the wake of the Reform Bill and the Bristol Riots writing glowingly of it in their press and hawking cheap copies of it in working-class districts.[22]

Centrally important was the fact that by then phrenology could be seen to have become a popular staple in the intellectual diet of the self-improving. Educational efforts were thought to be imperiled by its omission, and journals of popular instruction and entertainment came to fear that identification with antiphrenological sentiments would put their patronage at stake.[23] The popular success of the science clearly bred successful popularization, but at the same time there was, as it were, a win by default for phrenology and phrenologists in the widespread realization that the efforts of the SDUK had been singularly unsuccessful. The instance of over two hundred "mechanics, shopkeepers and clerks" soliciting Combe for phrenological instruction in Edinburgh in 1832 (and receiving in return three months of twice-weekly evening lectures) is only one of many instances of enthusiasm for phrenology that starkly contrast with the apathy and hostility that greeted the propaganda efforts of the SDUK.[24] In the face of these relative fortunes, it is not suprising that Combean phrenology began to command the attention and respect not only of increasing numbers of functionaries for the new order but as well persons more closely wedded to the traditional elites. The Whig judge Henry Cockburn, for example, noted in his journal in 1836,

this excitement [over phrenology and "kindred dogmas"] will do infinite good, for although there is much ignorance and conceit in it, there is, at least on everything physical or mechanical, a great proportion of sound valuable matter both in lectures and in the books, and even [the phrenologists and others'] moral views and educational systems, however defective or even absurd in philosophy, tend powerfully to awaken the attention of the people, to direct their thoughts to intellectual subjects, and to convince them of the value of self-improvement.[25]

Eventually even the *Edinburgh Review* (of which Brougham was a cofounder) could not help acknowledging "the useful service to humanity" that Combe was performing in popularizing "truths which, if not absolutely new, are yet new to many, and too little regarded by all." Since, by 1823 Combe had already brought the weight of phrenology against Owenite collectivism, it was perhaps out of this recognition of the science's Broughamite educational usefulness that Francis Jeffrey (whose fear of the multitude was excessive) was prompted in 1826 to concede that, at least, "Phrenology in [Combe's] hands, has assumed, for the first time, an aspect not absolutely ludicrous." That in the 1840s Combe himself was to write for the *Edinburgh Review* marks well the cause and course of orthodoxy's shifted opinion of phrenology, as well as the shifting of orthodoxy.[26]

That some middle-class phrenologists made no secret of the fact that their ultimate interests were scarcely different from those of the SDUK naturally contributed to the appreciation of phrenology's educational worth. Richard Beamish,[‡] for example, in his phrenology lectures in the Cheltenham Literary and Philosophical Society in 1841 related tales of Lancashire cotton manufacturers who, by setting up schools for their workmen, proved to them the utter folly of attacking the industrial structure "from which they were then deriving an ample livelihood."[27] Anecdotes like this, which denied any legitimacy to working-class grievances, were to be heard with greater frequency in phrenology lectures as industrialization speeded up. With greater frequency, too, came overt naturalistic defenses of bourgeois political economy and anti-trade union propaganda. For instance, Jonathan Barber[‡] in his lectures in Bristol in 1841 (shortly after a highly controversial debate between Robert Owen and the antiphrenologist and anti-socialist John Brindley[‡]) stressed how man had been endowed with the organ of Inhabitiveness (or the propensity to remain in one place) and how God had so designed this to facilitate the accumulation of capital and hence industry, civilization, and effective colonization.[28] A few years later in Edinburgh, James Simpson[‡] devoted a separate lecture to political economy in order to make it perfectly clear to his mainly working-class audience that "the laws of God and man are violated the instant a working man, either singly or in combination, presumes to prevent another from working or not working according to his pleasure." "One fact should be engraved on the working man's memory," he added: *"All the extensive strikes recorded have failed in their object, after producing great suffering. They have failed, because they have worked against the laws of nature."*[29] Owenite socialism was frequently the impulse behind these overt declarations, and although there were many Owenite phrenologists (see: Chapter 8), most followers of Combe would have agreed with the writer in the *Analyst* in 1837 who claimed that "such a work as the *Constitution of Man*, or Gall's immortal *Fonctions du Cerveau*, will benefit mankind more than a dozen New Lanarks; for the former will put the people in the way of procuring these latter by their own exertions, independent of any individual."[30] Truly, as the renegade phrenologist Arthur Trevelyan pointed out to his phrenological friends in the early 1840s, there were many among them who were only too anxious to use the science "to prop up a doctrine which has led to the greatest misery and injustice." Trevelyan was referring mainly to the applications of phrenology to Christian doctrines (the relevance of which will be seen below), but as a financial patron of Owen's Harmony Hall, his comment can also be seen as including the wider application of phrenology to the needs of industrial capitalism per se.[31] William Hunter‡ had no doubt: "The principles of Phrenology applied to the science of Political Economy," he told Combe in 1836, "were found strikingly useful, as the gentlemen who attended a Course of Lectures I lately delivered are ready to testify."[32]

These latter remarks do not, however, constitute an explanation for the heightening of the middle-class appreciation of phrenology. Functioning mostly only reciprocally to confirm the social orthodoxy of phrenologists to an already appreciative audience, such remarks were also largely incidental. In no way do they characterize phrenology's general presentation, which was (as in the *Constitution of Man*) not a direct apology for industrial capitalism, but rather a practical means to the self-help/self-serving ideology upon which the system flourished. Fundamentally, it was not in the terms of Andrew Ure's call to "subdue the refractory tempers of work-people accustomed to irregular paroxyms of diligence" that phrenologists perceived their role, but rather, humanistically, in terms of inculcating in people the "rational" self-interest necessary for success in the competitive capitalist society.[33] Celebrating liberal faith in the right of the individual to fulfill his or her own destiny and not be made to submit either to the intellectual or physical force of others, phrenologists could be seen to be promoting the most effective and permanent protection against dissent from bourgeois industrial capitalism: the internalization of the attitudes, responses, and duties most appropriate (most "natural") to the progress of that order. Without usually being conscious of the fact, they pursued the philosophy that the way to effect "real" subordination (as distinct from merely "formal" or shop-floor subordination) was to remake people's "image of reality," thereby to mystify domination in the minds of the dominated.[34] Thus, as Combe put it, to effect "considerable changes in many of the customs and pursuits of society," and to bring "even civilized nations into a condition to obey systematically the natural laws," no pressure was needed.[35] All that was required, as William Ellis made unusually explicit in the "Dedication to Teachers" in his *Outlines of Social Economy*, was that one teach people (in this case schoolchildren) to observe for themselves how misery, suffering, and discomfort, are almost always traceable to a disregard of these [natural] laws. . . . Let nothing induce you to suffer them to be blinded to the "nature" of their duties. The laws of creation are what must "rub against them at every step."[36]

Literally knowing the minds of those one was "called to act upon and mould" was of course a good reason for enquiring into phrenology,[37] and as far as most phrenologists were concerned this was the reason why they were first and foremost among the "schoolmasters abroad." But to most other educators (especially to utilitarians like Ellis who were experienced with the less successful tactics of the SDUK), it was not phrenology itself that inspired, so much as Combe's use of natural law to rationalize and inculcate a cerebrally reified version of *self*-discipline. Natural law both mystified phrenology's bourgeois behavioral basis and justified its dissemination on humanitarian grounds.

Withal, then, it would be wrong to suggest that recourse to phrenology by would-be instructors of the working class was the result of any particular logic or calculated process. However they might appear in hindsight, bourgeois educators did not rationally assess the SDUK's shortcomings and then, in view of the popular enthusiasms for phrenology, arrive at an appreciation of Combean phrenology as a convenient and expedient means of achieving "social control." As always, tactics took shape in a piecemeal fashion without anyone's witting understanding of what they were adding up to.[38] Although to many educators the *Constitution of Man* was the book of revelations (on the practical ideological value of deploying phrenology), it appeared so only in the course of the formalizing of liberal bourgeois power and in the context of increasing popular interest in phrenology. Noticeably, it was not until 1847 that Ellis said of Combe (in specific relation to seeing "man taught and trained to place himself in harmony with the laws of Nature"), "I admire – I revere him."[39] Earlier, most educationalists, including most phrenologists, were largely groping in the half-light of the new industrial order; though ideologically motivated, ideological strategists they were not. The point is illustrated and amplified by the place and role that phrenology came to assume in the mechanics' institutes.

MECHANICS' INSTITUTES

In general the space occupied by phrenology in the curricula of the institutes set up for mechanics (that is, skilled laborers or artisans) expanded in proportion as the middle class expropriated control of the institutes from the mechanics: A frequent topic of discussion in the mechanics' institutes by the late 1820s, phrenology was more or less institutionalized in them by the mid-1830s.[40] In 1827 – two years after Brougham and George Birkbeck had wrested the control of the London Mechanics' Institute from its founders and custodians, the economic radicals Thomas Hodgskin and Joseph Robertson – a mechanic from the Rotherhithe and Bermondsey Mechanics' Institute complained (in Hodgskin and Robertson's widely circulated *Mechanics' Magazine*) that "the lectures announced at the general meeting last month, for the ensuing quarter, were on the subjects of Naval Architecture – Phrenology! Botany!! and Ornithology!!!" and added that this situation applied "to all the Mechanics' institutions in and near London."[41] The same was becoming true in the provinces, although there, in most cases, the middle-class had control of the institutes from the outset.

But phrenology did not enter the curricula in the 1820s simply or even necessarily because middle-class managers had an interest in displacing the customary ideas and rights of artisans with new and/or expropriated and trivialized knowledge. As witnessed by the presence of articles on phrenology in the struggling and opportunistically orthodox *London Mechanics' Register* in 1825 and 1826,[42] the wholesale introduction of the subject in the mechanics' institutes, reflects, at least in part, the nature of the rescue operation of the institutes that was by then already underway.

Although Brougham had foreseen that it would be self-defeating to pull the reins of control too tightly in the mechanics' institutes (since attendance in them was entirely voluntary),[43] most middle-class managers initially did just that in their anxiousness to drum sound knowledge into the heads of mechanics. Too late did they realize that their pupils were neither passive nor idiotic, but, on the contrary, were quite capable of making, for instance, *An Exposure of the Sophistry that the Promoters of Our Knowledge Are Endeavouring to Thrust down the Throats of Us Unintellectual Geniuses of the Loom.*[44] Voting with their backs to such condescending chaff as the SDUK provided (as well as to nondemocratic managements and high costs), many artisans abandoned the institutes forever. Typically, at the institute at Rotherhithe, which the radical shipwright and labor organizer John Gast had helped to establish in 1825, membership slipped in 1826 from three hundred to one hundred, thus necessitating an increase in the cost of subscriptions to a prohibitive 16 shillings per quarter and resulting in a further decline in membership.[45]

What concerned institute managers first and foremost in the second half of the 1820s, therefore, was not *which technique* to use in the aculturation of workers but, more basically, how to attract and/or retain members and keep the institutes alive without seriously compromising ideological directives. It was this fundamental problem of survival that lay behind the flow of revisionist rhetoric on the most appropriate methods of instruction and subjects of study – rhetoric that, by directing attention to the symptoms of class antagonism and their treatment, unintentionally served to keep the antagonisms themselves thoroughly concealed. Thus the concerns of the mechanic from Rotherhithe and Bermondsey were neatly reversed in the much-heard sentiment (often shared by mechanics themselves) that "after working at wheels all day [workers] ought not to be made to study wheels at night."[46] The trouble, as Combe plumbed the matter phrenologically, was that in the working class in general the intellectual faculties had not been cultivated "either in their school instruction or practically in their trades," so that when confronted with "pure science addressed to the intellectual faculties only" they soon lost all interest[47] (although, in truth, middle-class interest in science also fell off in the late 1830s and in the 1840s[48]). It followed from this consideration of the minds of workers in relation to educational provision hitherto that what was required for the success of the institutes as places of workers' education was exactly that which middle-class educators were coming to see fit to provide them: ideally, with instruction that while elevating was yet not arid; while entertaining was yet practical, rational, intellectual; while diverting was yet morally uplifting; and, above all, while not appearing as intended to meet urgent needs for social stability, yet directed the attention of individuals to themselves and the benefits of *self*-reform.[49] Understandably, perhaps, since this ideal was in large part defined by the popular progress of phrenology, Combean phrenology came closest to fulfilling it.

The only obstacle to the wholesale introduction of phrenology into the mechanics' institutes was its doubtful relation with religious orthodoxy. For the most part, however, this problem had been solved in the gravitation of the "thinking classes" toward the knowledge as a relevant sociopolitical symbolic expression of their views. It is a measure of that relevance (and of the place of phrenologists in adult education)[50] that within the institutes a Christian phrenological view of the knowledge's harmony with Scripture and faith was allowed rapidly to erode all opposition. Indeed, in accord with the inexorble logic of bourgeois need, phrenology was turned into a boon for counteracting infidelity. Dr. John Fife[‡], for example, in his two-hour lecture to a capacity audience in the Newcastle Literary and Philosophical Society in 1836, was much applauded for his exposure of phrenology as "a science which taught the system of moral philosophy, most practically useful the purposes of education, and most satisfactory, as affording a *philosophical defence against the doctrines of materialism.*"[51] President of the Newcastle Mechanics' Institute, Fife had four years previously led the armed attack on the Tory opposition to the Reform Bill. Three years later, he was to be knighted for his part in crushing Chartism in Newcastle. How acceptable was his and other phrenologists' view of the knowledge as an antidote to working-class infidelity is well reflected in the appearance of popular "professors" of phrenology such as Henri Bushea[‡] only too willing (for a price) to reveal phrenology's harmony with Scripture and to refute the claims of republican atheists and secular socialists.

Armed with the social rhetoric of religious orthodoxy, educators could safely lay aside the kind of opposition to phrenology that had been raised by men of the stamp of Brewster and Brougham. But again, it was hardly a matter of choice: At the Hitchin Mechanics' Institute, for instance, every educational device had been tried in an effort to recruit and retain members. Faced with closure in 1840, the management decided to rent the Town Hall and hire professionals to lecture on elocution and on phrenology. So successful was this that the institute was able to struggle on for another four years until the practice of mutual instruction was begun (when, after once again relying on a phrenologist to give lectures, the managers found membership increasing substantially). The Sheffield Mechanics' Institute similarly ran aground in the 1830s. Witnessing the evident attraction of phrenology in the town's other more commercial and proletarian-orientated institutions, it introduced the science in order to have a hand at all in the development of the people's "moral and intellectual faculties." Until the 1850s phrenology remained the most successful subject of instruction at the Sheffield Mechanics' Institute; indeed, the science achieved that distinction throughout the Yorkshire Union of Mechanics' Institutes (established in the late 1830s) where, in 1842 alone, a total of thirty-two lectures on the science were delivered in six of the larger institutes.[52]

Needless to say, financial solvency was part and parcel of some institutes' struggle for survival, and part and parcel too of their need to turn to phrenology. "What has ruined four-fifths of [mechanics' institutes]," stated the SDUK's *Journal of Education* in 1831, "is getting involved in debt: making a very brilliant commencement, they get embarassed, and every one's zeal is cooled."[53] Since the problem was worse among those institutes not sponsored by the middle classes, it was there in particular that phrenology was often to be considered in the most naked commercial terms. Although when Hawkes Smith,‡ the vice-president of the Owenite-controlled Birmingham Mechanics' Institute, stated in 1835 that "a Mechanics' Institution vigorously conducted becomes a school of Phrenology," he was far from meaning that the survival of an institute demanded the financial exploitation of phrenology, his statement might easily have been interpreted that way. In fact, only a few years later that interpretation could have been based on Smith's own example since, for the sake of the institute's depleted coffers, he hired the antiphrenologist Brindley‡ to follow a course of lectures given by Combe.[54] Scottish workers had recognized this financial potential of phrenology as early as 1827 when a committee for the Relief of Distressed Operatives capitalized on the controversy between Sir William Hamilton‡ and Combe by selling tickets at two shillings sixpence to hear Hamilton lecture against phrenology. A week later the committee rented the Town Assembly Rooms and issued new handbills announcing Combe's "Popular Demonstration of the Evidence of Phrenology," for which the same entry fee was charged.[55] Fully twenty years later the science's popularity and the allure of its financial exploitation were still in evidence when the managers of the secularist Finsbury Institute, faced with "falling into the hands of a religious body" if funds could not be found, staged a debate between Peter Jones‡ and the antiphrenologist and Christian apologist W. Baker.‡[56]

The same financial incentive also lay behind the public exhibitions that began to be held in mechanics' institutes in the late 1830s, in many of which phrenology featured centrally. Over five thou-

sand visitors attended the Dumfries Mechanics' Institute in 1842
to see the phrenological exhibition set up by the secretary of the
Dumfries Phrenological Society; and over one hundred thousand
were drawn to the special phrenological exhibition set up by the
resident phrenologist of the Manchester Mechanics' Institute, William Bally,‡ during the Christmas holidays in 1844.[57]

For many institutes the real kiss of life came in 1843 with the
advent of phreno-mesmerism. Fittingly, the first institute to gain
was the one in Sheffield, where the major popularizer of this hybrid
science, Spencer Timothy Hall,‡ demonstrated its principles in
November 1842. Thereafter, hailed as "the New Science," "the
new philosophy of life," it spread to every corner of Britain with
amazing speed. Though it exhausted itself nearly as rapidly for
want of finding a recognized place in the culture of self-help (its
second wind coming later in the century), it nevertheless proved
to many to be phrenology's ultimate vindication. Except to men,
such as Thomas Wakley and Friedrich Engels, who had strong
motives for scepticism, touching the individual phrenological organs of a mesmerized person and having him or her perform the
behavior associated with the mental faculty seemed a persuasive
demonstration of phrenology's truth. As Elliotson pointed out
(with only slight exaggeration), where formerly *one* had been converted to the truth of phrenology, now, through mesmerism, *one
hundred* were converted. Managers of mechanics' institutes could
likewise have said that phreno-mesmerism enhanced their propects
enormously, even if it also contributed to modify their perception
of their function.[58]

From the point of view of both the institutes' survival and their
ideological function, then, phrenology made practical sense, as
managers recognized from the late 1820s onward. As emphasized,
however, these managers had little option but to go with phrenology's popular tide, if only in some cases because of the curiosity
of their patrons. As the *Spectator* remarked,

the question, whether a man's character could be read by the conformation of his head, had so much of novelty, and the plaster-of-paris
casts [were such] ... amusing toys, that no mechanics' institution, however hermetically sealed against morals and politics, could refuse their
scholars the relaxation of hearing one or two lectures about these strange
crotchets.[59]

The implicating of phrenology with "relaxation" on the one hand, and "morals and politics" on the other reminds us, though, that the managers' arms needed little twisting. Clearly they understood that without breaking taboos on idleness nor bans on overt discussion of politics and religion, the science operated to satisfy both needs for recreation and demands to broach matters of contemporary social and religious significance. The perfect token gesture, in other words, phrenology met these needs without facilitating any real reunion of science with radical politics and religion, nor sponsoring anything that could be criticized as self-indulgent. Thus managers, unprepared for the most part to follow Brougham's advice and allow for some discussion of politics in their institutes, considered that they had found in phrenology the ideal alternative. When in 1837 the newly formed West Bromwich Institute for the Advancement of Knowledge made as one of its first purchases a copy of Combe's *System of Phrenology*,[60] it was reflecting what had by then become conventional educational wisdom: not to resist popular demand but to appropriate and exploit it.

LECTURERS

Nothing reflects so well the success with which that demand was created as the number of lecturers that phrenology called forth. Over two hundred have been identified as active before 1860 (most of them between 1825 and 1845). It seems unlikely that these numbers were ever at any time in history surpassed by lecturers on any other science subject;[61] indeed, they suggest that the more appropriate comparison would be with religious evangelicalism. Nor is it just their numbers that suggest this comparison: Although the annals of science and medicine are packed with aspirants of one sort or another, nowhere in those annals (compared to those of evangelical religion) do we find so large a contingent of the seedy, the radical, the thunderstruck, the vain, and the opportunistic. Devout Combeans, as previously pointed out, claimed that they would gladly have done without these others. But that was hardly a possibility, since to become a phrenology preacher required neither deep study, nor ordination, nor affidavit. With a little cheek almost anyone could do it. And they did, or at least tried to.[62] Among them were shoemakers, shopkeepers, teachers, dentists, bank clerks, fustian cutters, exiles from Harvard, swindlers, Catholics, Methodists, Swedenborgians, freethinkers, Chartists, Owenites, feminists, men with limps, and persons inscrutable, simple-minded, and with "flaming pretentions."

The majority were volunteers from the ideological vanguard of the professionalizing lower middle class – the same who acted as directors or leading promoters of mechanics' and literary societies. If they differed at all from the zealous Combeans to whom we have already referred, it was only in that many of them believed the more passionately in the need (as Bray[‡] aptly described his function) to "convert" by the "Spoken Word" "those not given to reading."[63] Like Combe, and unlike Bray, most of them had no real experience with or understanding of the industrial production that formed the base of the social order they championed; the most zealous and best known nationally (besides Combe) were a judge (Simpson[‡]), a madhouse administrator (W. A. F. Browne[‡]), an educationalist (W. B. Hodgson[‡]), and a physician (John Epps[‡]) – true functionaries whose relationships with the world of production were, as Gramsci would have it, " 'mediated' by the whole fabric of society and by the complex of superstructure."[64] Along with such local representatives as William Lowe,[‡] a wholesale chemist (later bankrupt) and town councillor of Wolverhampton; William Cargill,[‡] a Newcastle merchant for the East India Company; T. S. Prideaux,[‡] a Southamptonian of independent means; Joseph Lacon,[‡] a solicitor and author, and president of the Liverpool Philomathic Society; and Marmaduke B. Sampson,[‡] secretary to the Treasury Committee of the Bank of England and then financial editor of the *Times* (before being exposed for fraud), they constituted a kind of cultural mafia. Driven on by a paternalistic ruthlessness connected often to the insecurity and uncertainty in their lives (like Combe, many of them were climbing out of backgrounds in which the father had been a tradesman or skilled artisan), they propagated through phrenology the ideology for a "regulated order" of self-interested persons.

Like all persons bent on extending their hegemony, generosity was a commodity never in short supply among these godfathers of the phrenology movement. Nevertheless, by the mid-1830s one was less likely to hear phrenology preached by them than by itinerant "professors." Evangelists to be sure, the peripatetic lecturers differed from the ideologues in that most of them depended upon their preaching as a means of livelihood (the majority seemingly struggling to keep up lower-middle-class appearances). Excepting those who had a particular political point to make with the science, most were less concerned with or aware of the knowledge's political and cultural significances. Although no less ideological for that, their primary consideration, like that of the mechanics' institutes where many of them lectured, was most often survival. For that, a minority of them had few scruples against appearing more as popular performers than as science lecturers. Particularly inclined to the entertainment end of the spectrum were those involved with lecturing on and demonstrating the effects of phreno-mesmerism – a subject that, besides occasioning attendance at private parties and seances, also afforded countless opportunities for branching out into such medical sport as painless tooth extracting or the curing of palsy, blindness, painter's colic, uterine complaints, and lumbago. By the 1850s phreno-mesmerism was routinely billed as "wonderful, amusing and astonishing" and was frequently staged, with other side-show attractions: "Dr." Owen's[‡] lectures on the subject in the Cosmorama on Regent Street in 1850, for example, being accompanied by "a Few Gymnastic Feats of Mr Reynoldson's Celebrated Cripple."[65] Less in a performing way, several other peripatetic lecturers (H. W. Dewhurst,[‡] William Richardson,[‡] and W. H. Crook,[‡] for instance) included phrenology among scientific and elocutionary subjects they were already teaching. Others branched out from phrenology into physiology and mesmerism or matured as lecturers on temperence (such as J. L. Levison[‡]) or on the repeal of the Corn Laws (such as Sidney Smith[‡]).[66] Matthew Allen,[‡] the first itinerant in Britain after Spurzheim,[‡] was a fast-talking, slightly eccentric spendthrift and womanizer who took up the science in 1816 purely for pecuniary reasons. Capitalizing at first on the science's novelty, he later (according to Carlyle) began to introduce his own cosmological fantasies and scientific wonders. By 1825 he had retired from phrenological lecturing and invested in a private madhouse in Epping Forest (a madhouse that, said to be informed by progressive phrenological principles, was regarded as a model of its kind).[67]

Allen was not the only person to try to get rich quick on phrenology, nor the only lecturer to lead scoffers to describe the science as "the folly of the many for the gain of a few."[68] Most, however, stuck truthfully to the details of the science and worked hard for

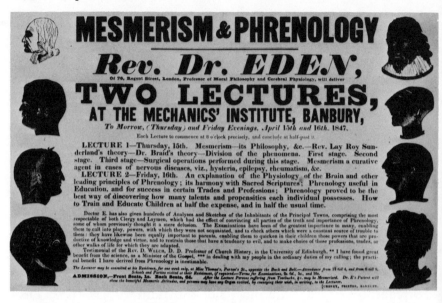

Figure 6. Handbill for the Rev. Dr. Eden's lectures on mesmerism and phrenology at the Mechanics' Institute, Banbury, April 1847.

meager livings in a field that became increasingly competitive in the 1840s as the demand and support for other kinds of science lectures fell away. J. J. Garth Wilkinson, the Swedenborgian homoeopath who began lecturing on the "Physics of Human Nature" in the mechanics' institutes in the late 1840s, considered himself exceedingly fortunate in having Emerson go before and recommend him to managers. Even so, the competitiveness of the business contributed to Wilkinson's view that there was no task more difficult than that of popularizing science to make it apprehensible by the world at large "unless it be that other task of propagating the current notions and doctrines of Christiandom among heathen nations."[69] It is hardly surprising, therefore, that many itinerant phrenologists (perhaps many more than we know of) did not succeed; that many succeeded only for a short while, to be superceded by advocates of herbalism, homoeopathy, temperance, and so on;[70] and that many more did poorly. Even with added incentives and slick showmanship (as, for example, the chance to view the Stadhausen lens and Bielfeld Aphanascope after W. J. Vernon's[‡] lectures at the Royal Adelaide Gallery, or the man and

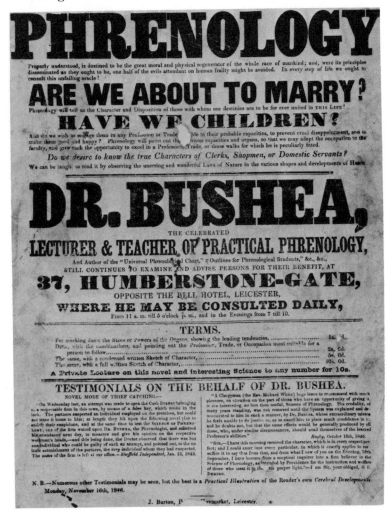

Figure 7. Handbill for Dr. Bushea's practical phrenology, 1846.

wife performance of Aitken and Aitken,[‡] with Mrs. Aitken doing
the lecturing), few of these lecturers could expect the three-figure
takings of Combe.[71] Although W. H. Crook[‡] (who, like Allen,
did well by being on the lecturing circuit early) could charge a
half-guinea per person for a course of three lectures in the Crown
and Anchor in the Strand in February 1827, by the 1840s as little
as a penny was being charged for a phrenology lecture, and itinerants such as C. Donovan,[‡] D. G. Goyder,[‡] and A. Falkner[‡] could

expect no more than a guinea per lecture from the managers of mechanics' institutes.[72] By the latter date the largest part of the income of popular professors of phrenology came not from lecturing but from what the lectures afforded: the opportunity for hawking phrenological charts, manuals, and pamphlets and, above all, for soliciting customers for phrenological delineations (at two shillings six or more a head).[73] For these purposes, and especially the latter, at least six of the itinerants carried on a tradition associated with eighteenth-century quack medicine: of operating shops with window-front "museums" to attract custom.[74] Certainly, for a phrenologist to cut a reputation in the 1830s and later, it was insufficient merely to evince what in the 1820s had been deemed the universal and necessary characteristic of the "sturdy phrenologist" – the insatiable desire to dispute;[75] it was now necessary to be a skilled delineator as well.

As for the contents of their lectures, there is little to choose between Combe's and those of such indefatigable itinerant phrenologists as E. T. Hicks,[‡] Goyder,[‡] Donovan,[‡] E. T. Craig,[‡] J. L. Levison,[‡] F. Bridges,[‡] and J. W. Jackson.[‡] Legitimately, all of them could be accused of uttering "a mere transcript" of Combe and Spurzheim's views, since it was from the latters' printed works that they chiefly borrowed.[76] Not until mid-century when the cheap publications of the American phrenologists Orsen and Lorenzo Niles Fowler began to flood the British market (through depots such as William Horsell's) was there much change in the style of the presentation and elaboration of the science. And it was not until L. N. Fowler[‡] commenced his highly successful British lecture tours in 1860 that the science fully acquired that nonintellectualist, healthean – watered, fruity, and farinaceaus – almost fundamentalist tone that was chiefly to characterize its popular presentation ever afterward.

Most of the lecturers referred to thus far lectured conventionally in middle-class and working-class institutions. Obviously, however, there were other places for lecturing both up-market and down, though, unfortunately, little is known of these, and even less of the kinds of discussions that they might have inspired. While it is not hard to guess what the Glasgow phrenologist and zealous educator A. James D'Orsay[‡] might have said in the lectures he gave in Forfar in 1836 at the invitation of the town magistrates, one is left wondering where the emphasis might have been placed by the sixty-year-old Sir George MacKenzie[‡] when he lectured at the Royal Yacht Club in 1840. Nor do we know exactly what it was that brought tears to the eyes of the Midland listeners of the phrenology lectures of the Owenite social missionary John Green.[‡77] Close to Green's patch, and at the other end of the spectrum from MacKenzie, was Mrs. Hamilton,[‡] who lectured for free in public places in Scotland and England. Combe's friends described her as a "Speg wife" (or fortune-teller), and the diarist Elizabeth Eastlake thought her a "dirty old wretch," "illiterate and common" (though this did not stop her from putting her head into Hamilton's hands in 1843). Owenites applauded Hamilton as an uncompromising popularizer of women's rights: With a bunch of marbles wrapped in a handerchief to illustrate the human brain, she gathered large crowds as she argued that, by confirming the mental equality of males and females, phrenology gave "the power to break the chains of the [male] tyrant and the oppressor and set [woman] completely free."[78]

While it is doubtful that there were many other itinerant phrenologists of Mrs. Hamilton's kind, the institutional dragnet is obviously inadequate for finding out, just as it is inadequate for discovering the impressions left by such lecturers. Redeeming in this respect (and suggesting that the impressions left were far from superficial), is the unique account of the efforts of a phrenological lecturer in a rural location given in the autobiograhy of "the Dundee Factory Boy," James Myles. In this instance the lecturer was the secretary of the Dundee Phrenological Society, William MacGlashan,[‡] who arrived in Myles's Forfarshire village in the mid-1830s. The introduction of the village to phrenology, wrote Myles, was

the crowning event in our history.... It was a perfect epoch in our village, so much so, that the farmers even to this day [c. 1850] are often heard say, "It was a guid year that year the Phrenology came here!" It was strange ... that the proclamation of the science of brains should have caused such a stir in our clachan.

I yet recollect the eventful night, the parish school was the theatre, the lecturer was a lank bare-boned tailor named M'Glashan, and Dundee was the birth-place of the philosopher of bumps.... When he entered the schoolroom laden *cap a pie* with busts and human skulls, he looked as if he had deserted from our ancient graveyard, and the rustics were awe-struck at his presence. His prelection on organs and skulls made us all gape in amazement, and nearly overturned our vulnerable notions of the dignity of man.[79]

The account is all the more valuable for reminding us that in the 1830s there was still a public not yet sunk in scientific rationalism and who might be stimulated by phrenology not because they saw it as daringly rationalistic but, on the contrary, because they perceived an association between it and subversive mystical and irrational forms of knowledge. The account also reminds us that in the final analysis it was not the lecturers themselves that mattered, whether they were in the country or in the town, or whether they were timid or raving, radical or deferential, sincere or opportunistic. What mattered, and what mirrorlike captured and held audiences' attention, was the subject(ive) matter itself, "the HUMAN MIND" – the source (as few lecturers failed to emphasize) of all man's happiness and misery: oneself in the abstract.[80]

STUDY GROUPS

Once interest in phrenology had been aroused it was not unusual for it to be nourished in a mutual instruction class. These were frequently set up in mechanics' institutes, often with the managers' encourgement. In Newcastle it was after the lectures by Fife and Combe that the directors of the institute (Fife being chairman and Arthur Trevelyan being on the managing committee) announced in their annual report that "along with other proofs of the advancing spirit of enquiry amongst members, it must be mentioned that a portion of them have formed a class for the study of Phrenology."[81] In Derby, Donovan was "induced to remain [after his lecture] ... for some time longer, in order to meet the wishes of a number of the members of the Institute, by instructing them in the art of practical observations in the phrenological science by manipulation, etc."[82] In Southampton in 1833 J. R. Stebbing[‡] suggested at the conclusion of his course of lectures at the Mechanics' Institute that a phrenological society be established within the town's Literary and Scientific Society – with the result that the members of the Mechanics' Institute "in a spirit of emulation immediately formed a phrenological class of their own" to which only members of the institute could belong. Characteristically, it was the mechanics' phrenological society that continued to thrive while the one in the Lit & Phil "fell off for want of punctuality in its members."[83] As in the formation of the class at the Cleckheaton Mechanics' Institute in 1846, or the phreno-mesmeric one established in Northampton after Hall's lectures there in 1843, it was frequently remarked that all the members were working-class.[84]

Such study groups are known to have been formed after lecture courses on phrenology in nearly all the mechanics' institutes. Setting them up was clearly another of the means by which itinerant phrenologists could supplement their meager incomes. Goyder was doubtless thinking of future returns from the science when, in the 1840s, he advertised gratuitous lectures to any group interested in forming such a class.[85] The classes themselves were usually composed of from ten to sixty members, each paying a few shillings' entry fee and/or a few pence per weekly or fortnightly meeting.[86] Members – most often adolescent males – attended as many of the regular sessions as they could afford or until they had an adequate knowledge of the science and its practical applications and some skill in manipulation. In the London Mechanics' Institute the phrenology class was established after J. L. Levison's lectures there in 1830, and over the next decade it was estimated that the class had been responsible for teaching over three hundred persons the rudiments of the science, "most of whom," wrote their class secretary and leader, the Islington law-stationer E. J. Hytch,‡ "steadily adhere to its doctrines, and the names of some are not unknown in the phrenological circles as expounders of the science."[87] Apparently the largest class in the institute after the music class, it had an average attendance of thirty-four members and was responsible for advising the directors on the hiring of phrenological lecturers.[88] In a room in the institute crowded with casts and books on phrenology the class met on Saturday evenings to discuss such topics as Shakespeare's *Macbeth*, the principles and mental organization of Robert Owen, applications of phrenology to self-government, impediments to the progress of phrenology, insanity and civilization, and so forth – rehearsals for the most part of what had occurred in the elitist phrenological societies and what was being discussed in the *Phrenological Journal*.[89] Usually, what students could not solve with Combe's *System of Phrenology* they resolved with his *Constitution of Man*. As in Bible classes, the purposes of phrenological study groups was not to question the dogma – Combe's liberal philosophy (including the dogma of not submitting to dogma) – but to discover the joy of harmonizing with it. The endless debates on "Is Phrenology True?" sustained an illusion of enquiry, of not giving "blind credence to the dogmas of other men," while reaffirming the particular social outlook of the leading propagandists.[90]

THE PASSION TO CULTIVATE: A PRELIBATION

It is generally agreed that mechanics' institutes and other middle-class educational provisions for the working class failed to achieve their social and ideological objectives because they failed to reach the artisan audience for whom they were originally intended. Recent assessments of the institutes, while making it clear that natural knowledge was a far more important part of the curriculum than political economy, grant only that they extended the audience from whom legitimation and support for urban industrial bourgeois values and interests could be sought, and that the natural knowledge disseminated in the institutes provided a kind of framework of rationalist discourse "upon which the culture of a stabilized re-integrated society might eventually be built."[91] As we have observed, prior to and during the promotion of phrenology in the institutes, managers lost the patronage of many traditionally and politically minded mechanics and gained a large audience from the lower middle class. By the 1830s it was often more appropriate to refer to members of the institutes as emerging from "the people" than from any more discrete social or occupational stratum. In a few instances it became appropriate to alter the name "mechanics' institute" to "literary and scientific institution." Arguably, therefore, managerial enthusiasm for phrenology was (especially in the face of some workers' recognition of the class ambitions of managers) a means of compromising with the unpleasant reality of failure: Through the people's response to phrenology, bourgeois educationalists could convince themselves that their efforts had not been in vain, that their labors had been above "selfish motives of class."

Yet the point *is* arguable, in part because it is wrongly premised. It forgets that the early nineteenth century saw a tremendous expansion in the numbers of skilled and semiskilled workers both in mechanized and unmechanized trades and that, because of this and because of the expansion also in the kinds of their employment, a great many artisans had no strong political sense of customary rights or of the need to protect them (which is not to say, however, that such workers were necessarily political eunuchs). What evidence we have of the membership of mechanics' institutes suggests that toward the mid-century they were very largely filled with these "nontraditional" artisans ("the superior order of the working classes, receiving wages from 1£ to 30s a week"), along with (and including among them) a great many young persons.[92] For much the same consideration of tactics as noted earlier, it cannot be said that the managers of mechanics' institutes conscientiously sought out such persons thinking that they would make good fifth columnists among the laboring masses. It can be said, however, that, because of the greater familiarity of these artisans and youths with the urban industrial order and its dominant values and social relations, the knowledge provided in the institutes could lead them more readily than it could lead their fathers to accept the new order of things as natural. Considering, too, that there were apparently over seven hundred "Literary and Mechanics' Institutions" in Britain by 1851 with a total of over one hundred twenty thousand members, their "failure" seems less unequivocal.[93] It is also worth recalling that among the graduates of these institutes were such spokesmen for workers as E. T. Craig,[‡] A. R. Wallace, and G. J. Holyoake[‡] – students of phrenology all. Hence the belief of ideologues such as Combe, Buckle, and Spencer that by making an impact in the institutes they were effectively reaching the minds and lives of the people seems less an instance of self-delusion than may be at first supposed.[94]

In any case, it does not follow, from the assumption that phrenological efforts on behalf of mechanics' institutes did more for the psychological quiet of their bourgeois managers than for the political quiet of traditional artisan leaders of the laboring class, that there was therefore no support for these efforts from below. As the mechanics' institutes themselves were at no time simply pushed at an unreceptive and deferential public, so neither was phrenology.[95] The phrenology class, like the Sunday school, was entered voluntarily by "the great unwashed," even if there was plenty of encouragement. The laurels that working-class audiences bestowed on phrenology lecturers (to the extent of a silver tea service for Browne from the mechanics of Montrose) were freely given and sincerely meant, even when it was the high sheriff of County Durham, Henry Witham,‡ who had taken the pains to "instruct the poor, and to put within their reach the means of moral and intellectual improvement."[96] Perhaps the most extreme example that can be given here is the Owenite hosannas raised to Simpson – Simpson, who made no secret of the fact that in nothing should the middle classes "reap more every day satisfaction from judicious education, than in the improvement of our domestic servants," and who held the lower classes to be dirty, uncivilized, unfit for free admission into parks, cursed with drink, and indulgers in "Sunday orgies."[97]

The voluntary involvement with phrenology by working people is witnessed repeatedly in their autonomously constituted places for learning – the breakaway mechanics' institutes, the "people's colleges," Owenite Halls of Science, cooperative evening schools, and, most numerously, the mutual instruction or mutual improvement societies – those spontaneous working-class orgnaizations that have been seen as "either explicitly or implicitly, adverse judgements on the mechanics' institutes and other education societies established under middle-class patronage."[98] When in 1839 in his *Hints to Mechanics on Self-Education and Mutual Instruction*, Timothy Claxton, the artisan founder (in 1820) of the first society for mechanics in London, recommended the teaching of phrenology to workers as a means to their independent development, he was arguing for what by then had become commonplace.[99] For, as Thomas Cooper reflected on teaching phrenology to Leicester Chartists, it was taken for granted in mutual instruction societies that a knowledge of phrenology was basic to every man's education.[100] In the Owenites' Hall of Science in Sheffield where (ironically) discussion of science was conscientiously avoided in order to stimulate discussion on politics and social morality, the only permitted exception was phrenology.[101] Alexander Bain discovered a very different sort of "strict orthodoxy" in the mutual instruction society formed in Aberdeen in 1835, but there too a number of men "were inclined to speculations that the others viewed with suspicion ... chiefly upon Phrenology."[102] Quite unlike the contempt in which the science was held by the mechanic from Rotherhithe and Bermondsey in the late 1820s, members of mutual instruction societies in the 1830s and 1840s looked upon it as a philosophy that was as ill suited for the brutish lumpen and the idle aristocrat as it was for working-class "flunkeys and lickers of trenches" (*v.* the phrenologizing Chartist Sandy Mackaye in Kingsley's *Alton Locke*).

Variously interpreted across religious and political boundaries (but never altered in its fundamentals) phrenology was one of the few subjects pursued by nearly every mutual instruction society – and by the 1830s there was hardly a village in Britain that had not at least one of these societies.[103] Some in fact were set up solely for the study of phrenology or became preoccupied with it after someone had come along to spread the gospel. This was the case in Myles's Forfarshire village after MacGlashan's lecture: Myles's employer, a true-to-stereotype radical shoemaker, as a result of the lecture and a "correct" delineation by MacGlashan, became the local "phrenological monomaniac."[104]

All over Britain persons like Myles's employer, as well as others less politically minded and less well off, were similarly moved upon encountering the science in mechanics' institutes, mutual instruction societies, Sunday schools, radical clubs, and pubs. A minority of the working class to be sure, they made up the thousands who parted with a shilling-six for the *Constitution of Man*. It was their cash, too, that allowed Hewett Watson[‡] to claim in 1838 that the "sale of elementary books on phrenology was greater than the sale of books on any other science not constituting a part of professional education."[105] The several popular journals on phrenology also had their public in these self-educators, as did a journal such as *Chambers'*, which leveled off at a weekly circulation of ninety thousand in the 1840s after the doctrines of the *Constitution of Man* had been "covertly" introduced (so Robert Chambers later explained).[106]

As with the difference between a mechanics' institute and a mutual instruction society, it does not matter, as far as phrenology's popularization is concerned, that many of those who called the SDUK publications "juiceless chaff" of "Whig benevolence" also called the publications of the Chambers brothers illustrations of the middle-class liberal "Run-a-head and Stop-Short Philosophy."[107] Working-class journals with no intention of apologizing for middle-class values espoused the science as well: Joseph Livesey's *Moral Reformer*, for example, or the weaver Joseph Barker's *The People* – the latter (subtitled "A Journal Devoted to Phrenology") being read weekly by apparently thirty thousand persons humble in occupation and fearless in the spirit of rebellion against opression and hollow rhetoric. Since in *The People* one may read workers' letters declaring that their getting hold of the *Constitution of Man* was the greatest event in their lives, "Barkerites" as much as "Chamberites," it might be argued, made worthwhile those "remarkable pains" (as *Fraser's Magazine* called them) that went into disseminating phrenology and having cheap copies of Combe's book circulated among the laboring population.[108]

We will see that this enthusiasm for phrenology could be quite differently motivated than that hoped for by the bourgeois ideologues of the knowledge. Nevertheless, it cannot be denied that ordinary people's enthusiasm for the subject was everywhere apparent. The only laments seem to have come from those cut off from phrenological sources. A correspondent to the *Edinburgh Chronicle* in 1834, for instance, spoke of the operatives in the south of Scotland as beginning to appreciate phrenology's merits, and added that

nothing but cheap information on the subject is required. A public lecturer upon that interesting science would meet with certain and deserved success. Many of the readers of your journal in this quarter, have faint perception of its doctrines, and the expression of your opinion would be an unspeakable benefit and pleasure.[109]

The editorial reply, when it came four years later, was typically expressive of the liberal opinion on phrenology that had meanwhile gained ground:

We (the editors of this paper) have had personally the means of observing and estimating the effects of lectures on Phrenology, addressed to the working classes, as a means of opening up their minds to a perception of the necessity of education, and of the advantages of studying physical and all other sciences that may conduce to their moral and intellectual improvement, and we have seen nothing that can at all be compared to its quickening and enlightening influence.... where the working classes had been instructed in Phrenology, the effect of it in enlarging their view of the human faculties, and in conveying deep impressions of the advantages of knowledge, were most conspicuous, and that its direct fruits were an eager attendance on scientific lectures upon other subjects, and a general interest, of the most valuable description, in human improvement.[110]

In other words, amid the inequalities thrown up by the new manufacturing system and the blatant hypocritical rhetoric issued by its overt apologists there appeared no finer means than phrenology for capturing the attention of that part of the workforce thought capable of formulating economic critiques and of revolutionizing the rest of the working class. Phrenology's success, Cobden had said in one of his weekly letters to Combe, was bound up with having people's "preconceived notions superseded";[111] arguably the science's triumph was in having so many, who were normally wary of the schoolmaster abroad, stride willingly and enthusiastically into this pursuit of reconceived human nature.

AN INTERLUDE IN UNDERSTANDING POPULAR PHRENOLOGY

Here at any rate is laid bare what must be one of our main concerns in the chapters that follow: If phrenology functioned with increasing conservatism in the interest of consent to bourgeois liberal rule, how and why was it cultivated with alacrity by working people of even the most radical complexion? In advance of that discussion it is worthwhile to spend a moment elaborating the kind of historiographical enterprise being entered into and the point of view for which we are arguing.

Essentially, our premise is this: that to understand the mid-Victorian bourgeois hegemony what is required is a deeper-than-normal ideological demystification of the ideas and institutions of the early Victorian period. The trick of demystification itself is now of course routinely applied, and nothing is perhaps so frequently heard as the sounds of crumbling Victorian saints and their immaculate institutional conceptions. Humanitarian robes so admired in the past hang about the ankles of those once quoted for their murmurings of love and charity. But the denouement is characteristically unsurprising: a whip in one hand, a purse of gold in the other. With reference to the SDUK, for example, as recently as 1964 it was still being seriously argued that the society's interests were purely altruistic and that it was "mere conjecture" that the society was interested in preaching morality to disguise class antagonisms and provide a permanent anodyne for socially disruptive thought and action from below.[112]

But by halting at the latter point more is endangered than recovered: Ideology being equated with political and economic interests, it occurs that where these interests are not apparent (as in the lesson on brain anatomy) ideological interests are thought to be nonexistent. Sociopolitical analysis, in other words, extends as far as, say, the SDUK's sponsorship of useful knowledge, but not as far as SDUK tracts on chemistry, botany, or hydrostatics (which are still to be seen as value-neutral and as having been capable *only* of scientistic and/or deviational use). Abetting such restricted analysis are those "revisionist" historians in whose wisdom Marxist analysis is based on the crude notion that economics is the standardbearer of ideology, and who then seek to attack "Marxists" because of their (the revisionists') inability to locate any of the crudity![113] But there are many historians on the left whose view seems equally myopic. Implicitly accepting the "vulgar Marxist" equation, these historians tend to seize upon any evidence of workers' exposing the rhetoric of the schoolmasters as indication of working-class ideological autonomy.[114] (This follows Engels in believing that the places of proletarian education, as opposed to mechanics' institutes, were "free from all the influence of the bourgeoisie.")[115] Of course, if the historical aim is simply to portray the nobility of the working class in the early nineteenth century, nothing is easier or more pleasing than to cite instances of working people unmasking the rhetoric of Ures, Broughams, and Shuttleworths. But if the aim is to explain the origins of mid-Victorian stability or, indeed, the continued survival of industrial capitalism, this configuration of ideology is inadequate, since among the things upon which that stability depended was the acceptance of the dominant ideology or at least an accommodation to the routines it demanded.

Now to say that workers suddenly accepted the ideology that degraded them and that they had earlier partly rejected is obviously untenable.[116] But this is no reason to seek elucidation in the manner of John Foster, for example, by plunging further into vulgar Marxism and opting for its last refuge, as it were, by claiming that the working class must therefore have been defeated after a class struggle conducted solely on the economic front. Foster would lead one to believe that social stability at mid-century was entirely dependent upon the almost Machiavellian manipulations of capitalists: "The revolution" did not take place because the capitalists were always in control, always knowing when to compromise with and concede to the working class, and when to critically divide them. Though stimulating is Foster's use of Lenin's thesis on the key divisive role of the "aristocracy of labor," as an explanatory basis for the disappearance around mid-century of working-class aspirations for social structural change it falls as short of the mark as would the effort to seek a monocausal link between economic distress and the rise of radicalism earlier in the century.[117]

Naturally economics or, more specifically, the history of capital's control over various forms of labor in production is fundamental to understanding the origins of mid-Victorian stability. But revolution or its absence is a matter of more than bread alone. What the emphasis on economics underrates is the degree to which capitalist ideology, mediated and mystified, as in the diagram of the phrenological head, may in its own right become a signficant force in the determination of consciousness *within* the "superstructure." Not that "superstructure" is the term we would choose to use; as many have pointed out, the distinction made between it and an economic "base," along with the idea that the economic "base" is reflected in the "superstructure" that in turn reacts back upon the "base" (as is assumed by Foster), artificially dichotomizes historical reality and categorizes inertly through mechanical causality processes that are better understood, dialectically as constitutive. If we accept something closer to the Weberian perspective, that in the beginning was the value and that values are enclosed in ideology, it is the "superstructure" that will be seen to determine the "base"; and it is in the "superstructure" that are to be found the values and assumptions behind the ideology of bourgeois capitalism.[118] In short, the assumption that the economic can be separated from the total "lived experience" of which it is asymptotically a part is a misleading historical abstraction.

For our purposes it is better to think of ideology more in terms of religion: as a shared reality, or as a system of ideas about reality and the means by which they are communicated.[119] Since Combean phrenologists, on the basis of their methodically catetorized understanding of human nature, spelled out a theology for self-discipline and self-restraint and for the individuated duties most conducive to the routines demanded by the new economic system, it is wholly appropriate to regard phrenology in these terms, as, indeed, did contemporaries.[120] More specifically, we might regard the science in its popularized form as a secular Methodism providing an intellectual passageway into a value medium that could inhibit the forming of anticapitalist logic and solidarity. *How far* we can regard the science in this light, and to what extent this may allow us to parallel phrenology to E. P. Thompson's depiction of Methodism as a form of psychic exploitation, remains to be seen.[121] It only needs remarking here that the relevance to phrenology of what Thompson has to say on Methodism in relation to the working class derives not simply from his appreciation of the "consolations" that were to be had from a form of worship that weakened people from within and made them into their own slave drivers. The relevance derives as much from his recognition that the need for the consolations – the spiritual orgies and the promises of the hereafter – was specific to a socioeconomic context – one in which other temporal and political aspirations were meeting with defeat.[122] To approach Methodism and, more generally, the quiescence of the mid-Victorian English working class in this way is to fall neither into economism nor into intellectualist abstraction (as if Methodism's theological tenets had a power in and of themselves). Rather, it is to approach religious systems as socially constituted mediations of ruling ideology and to perceive their popular support in terms of specific contexts of class antagonisms and negotiations.

In a like manner, we can approach the popular cultivation of phrenology in our effort to understand better how the emergent ruling class could achieve social stability by achieving the consent of those they would rule. In much of what follows, therefore, we will put aside ideas of unmediated relations between economics and ideology, and we will discard as well, for the most part, the notion that there is necessarily malicious cunning or conspiracy involved in some people's engagements with other people' consciousness.[123] In "religion" mystified and mediated through the structures of a life science, we wish to show, the system's bread becomes and *is* its eucharist.

6

Secular Methodism

Marx's famous saying that "religion is the opium of the people" is habitually wretched out of its context and given a meaning subtly but appreciably different from the one he gave it. Marx did not say, at any rate in that place, that religion is merely a dope handed out from above; he said that it is something the people create for themselves to supply a need that he recognized to be a real one. "Religion is the sigh of the soul in a soulless world. Religion is the opium of the people." What is he saying except that man does *not* live by bread alone?

> George Orwell, "Notes on the Way," *Time and Tide*, 6 (April 1940), in *Collected Essays* (Harmondsworth, 1970), II, 33

Ideology is believing what you experience to be the truth and the only truth.

If social relations were self-evident there would be no need for social science. One can accept the appearance of things and relations as if they were self-evident or one can search for a reality behind the appearance. The difference between doing the one or the other is the difference between justification and investigation, the more or less ideological. Ideological discourse makes of appearances the category of reality.

> Stephen Feuchtwang, "Investigating Religion," in Maurice Bloch, ed., *Marxist Analysis and Social Anthropology* (1975), pp. 70–1.

To suggest that a fuller understanding of popular science depends upon our penetrating beneath the empirical surface of history is not to suggest that we abandon that surface for some deeper realm alone. Rather, in agreement with Fernand Braudel that "any . . . history that is not written on two levels – that of the well's rim and that of the depths – runs the risk of being appallingly incomplete," it is to suggest that we pursue well and rim together.[1]

Quite simply, this need exists because there is often a significant difference between what is popularly thought to be gained from scientific information and what is actually (or additionally) received. Well-packaged ecological information, for instance, though appearing only to encourage the saving of the environment from pollutions of one sort or another, implicitly beckons simultaneously the protection of the "natural" system being polluted. Likewise, endorsement of well-meant research by geneticists aiming to raise the habitually low "intellectual performance" of black Americans is endorsement of both the racial boundaries and the ethics of the competitive achieving society that has in fact created, defined, and maintained "the problem."[2]

So it is when we turn to examine critically any scientific movement or scientistic popularization at levels beneath manifest professions of "humanity" and "progress." Hence, in the case of popular science, merely to reveal the benefits perceived or experienced by the recipients of the knowledge is to only half-pursue the historical task. Called for as well is an understanding of how and in which specific ways such bodies of knowledge, in conjunction with their perceived benefits, function(ed) in the interest of less evident social and ideological interests.

This will always be a complex task, especially in the life sciences, where biological disinterest is forever muddled with people's interest in their own social lives. In the case of people's phrenology the problem is compounded by the structural fluidity of the society at the time when the knowledge was having its heaviest popular impact, during the critical period for bourgeois stability from the mid-1830s to the mid-1840s. The shifts in the social structure at that time are reflected in the tensions, contradictions, ambiguities and ambivalences to be found at every level and in every aspect of life and thought. Understandably, this confusion manifests itself when we seek to address the question of why people embraced a protean science that claimed among other things to be *the* science of mind. No single answer can be expected; nor should we be surprised at contradiction and inconsistency in people's explanations. All things do not dovetail, nor should they be expected to in a contradictory society in the making. People's motives and their explanations differed insofar as their backgrounds, experiences, and expectations varied and continued to vary over these turbulent years.

Yet to a degree, the "people" of people's phrenology were no more or less disparate a body than those who cultivated rock music in the middle of the twentieth century, or astrology, or Althusserianism. We have seen that phrenologists were able to make their deepest impression in a particular niche of society: among a predominantly young and self-improving section of the working class, many of whom thought of themselves and were seen by others as a "connecting link between the lower and middle classes of society." In 1840 they were depicted as among "that new and numerous class which has arisen within the last quarter of a century, and which is composed of the more intelligent members belonging to the operative order."[3] While the majority of these persons might have preferred to have had *Pilgrim's Progress* next to their copy of the *Constitution of Man* rather than *The Rights of Man*, no such distinction can really be insisted upon. After all, in the early industrial period (as previously) *Pilgrim's Progress* as much as *The Rights of Man* was a book for common people hoping with the aid of a higher power to burst through the barriers of poverty, ignorance, and contempt.[4] Moreover, while on the one hand there were those such as "the true infidel" who wrote to the *Reasoner* in 1847 declaring himself "an ardest disciple of George Combe, but no disciple of either Voltaire or Owen,"[5] on the other hand there were many advocates of phrenology from among the politically active and often more class-conscious Carlilians, Owenites, and Chartists. Although it is more convenient to deal with the latter minority separately (Chapters 7 and 8), in reality all these persons shared much the same culture – a culture whose roots were still deeply embedded in the traditions represented and protected by Paine and Cobbett, but that, by the mid-1830s, was no longer as centered as it had been on the independently minded, horny-handed artisan. The rise of the new political economy, on the one hand, and trade unionism, on the other, had sharpened the boundaries between manual and mental labor while lending a new and heightened importance to property and capital. Along with the growth of a more factory-dependent artisanry, which had diminished control over production, was the erosion of the former integrity of the culture of the "horny-handed" with their pride in workmanship and mystery of craft. Thus in many ways the former certainty of the artisan's place in society was thrown into question.

Although it is dangerous to overgeneralize (since "artisans" remained a far from homogeneous group, and the impact of industrialization was far from even),[6] it is not entirely unwarranted to
conceive of artisans in the second quarter of the nineteenth century
as among (or as becoming) the first psychological casualties of the
arbitrary industrial world. Unlike the unskilled, whose struggle
was simply against naked exploitation, the artisan was engaged in
a struggle against the loss of human autonomy attendant upon the
process of deskilling – a struggle less physically tragic, but all the
more anguishing for its social imprecision or lack of a discrete
enemy.[7] Though most often remaining proud of their identity as
workers, and in some cases developing a political outlook com-
mensurable with the "horizontal" consciousness of the emergent
"mature" industrial working class, artisans or mechanics in general
(and/or operatives and journeymen) found themselves caught essentially between the developing consciousness of the two major
conflicting classes of industrial capitalist society.

Phrenology, while not "designed" or deliberately intended to
exploit the ambivalences in the artisan's situation, nevertheless
played effectively upon them and in this way contributed to the
sectional exploitation of the working class. Issued by radical ideologues of change, the science was, as we have seen, specifically
directed at artisans – at those setting the tone for all working-class
behavior, and who were, claims Iorwerth Prothero, "the most
numerous and most important of all the organized groups of workers in the first half of the nineteenth century."[8] Phrenology celebrated their separateness in a naturalized hierarchy of labor, and
through its biological sanctions encouraged the socioeconomically
constituted shift from traditional artisan "respectability" based on
status attainable through craft or skill to respectability based on
status attainable through the display of personal or moral worth.
By making the latter appear as a natural concern determined by
the very structure of the human brain, phrenology provided artisans with what in retrospect can be seen as a rationale for accepting more individualist-orientated forms of self-improvement,
the overall effect of which was to render the gap in values between
artisans and other manual workers wider than the gap separating
artisans from the middle class.[9]

But it was not in order to be thus instructed that artisans went
to phrenology. Rather, at the same time that phrenologists were

beginning to reach out to them, artisans were reaching for the proferred knowledge as a means of understanding, improving, and rationalizing the situations in which they found themselves. Increasingly the science was to make sense in their own terms. Hence centralized in the period between the Reform Bill and the repeal of the Corn Laws, in the midst of the confusions and displacements caused by the enormous changes, there was beginning to be a confluence of interest in the knowledge: the ideologues' efforts to popularize it among literate artisans coinciding with the latter's greater needs of it.

It is against this general backdrop that we can fill in the process of acceptance itself.

FACETS OF APPEAL

However compelling phrenology became to those anxious to solve the mysteries of human psychology, most people were initially attracted to it (as in Myles's Forfarshire village) out of curiosity and with a view to being entertained. In this sense, as novel and accessible entertainment, phrenology was hardly different from G. A. Stevens's celebrated "Lecture on Heads" that enjoyed enormous popularity throughout the latter half of the eighteenth century. Lavater's physiognomy, though bearing little resemblance to Stevens's comic satire, may also have contributed at a popular level to heighten interest in the subject of heads.[10] Phrenology, however, in treating the internal structure of the head and relating that and its functions to external form, was intrinsically a subject of far greater fascination. Indeed, the phrenological motif is still very much alive in the advertising world because this notion of external conformity to internal order remains arresting (and at the same time amusing and faintly satisfying).[11] Nineteenth-century audiences were clearly titillated by the subject, if for no other reason than that it claimed to offer new and intimate insights on the famous and infamous.[12] Always there were the skulls (often in rows illustrative of animal and human cerebral progression) and occasionally, too, medically macabre specimens in formaldehyde.[13] Sex was also there, thinly disguised in discussions of the faculty of "Amativeness" (on the supposed cerebral seat of which whole volumes were written);[14] and while a new dimension was given to lechery, by the merest casual glance at a passing pate, phrenological delineations provided unheard-of opportunities for otherwise impermissible physical contact.

Attentions gained, the ease and simplicity with which phrenology could be learned contributed to its appeal. "As logically consistent as any problem in Euclid," phrenology took just enough application to a few basic principles and just enough investment in books, casts, and classes to make one feel the knowledge was earned.[15] Thus, sneered the critics, "Barbers, carpenters, joiners, artisans of all sorts, 'swell the throng with their tumultuous throats,' and run gaping after [the] lecturers"; phrenology "flatters the superficial with telling them that they too may become philosophers, and 'at so small a cost!' " "To 'know thyself,' " remarked Sam Sly, "is a a hard task, and the search is not accompanied by much amusement or satisfaction. But to 'know they neighbour' is not so difficult, and not at all unattended by pleasure and relief."[16] Such condescension was deserved so long as one forgot the backgrounds of physical and intellectual privation, the dogging and dulling effects of manual labor, and the generally restricted space for ego function in the lives of workers. For every serious-minded autodidact such as James Myles, Alexander Bain, or Joseph Gutteridge who, in the face of extensive privations, would devour the works of Gibbon, Voltaire, Bentham, Mill, Lyell, Condillac, and so on, there were dozens of "gaping mechanics and beardless apprentices" who, like Myles's shoemaker boss, lacked the stamina for such study, yet were as anxious as Combe to be taken with philosophical seriousness.[17] Such persons "of strong and ardent minds, delighted with any new ideas that are presented to their recently awakened powers,"[18] believed that in an age of scientific miracles they had indeed struck upon the true principles of human nature. Why should they doubt it? Robert Chambers, among others, reassured them that phrenology was "eminently ... the system of mental philosophy for the unlearned man." From his own experience he understood that in being "much less abstract than any other [system] ... ordinary people feel, for the first time in their attempts at psychological investigation, that they have ground whereon to rest the soles of their feet."[19] Likened to the Newtonian theory – "the *simplest* which science has ever unfolded" – phrenology's lack of complexity and its accessibility seemed to confirm its veracity.[20] Since implicitly this truth = simplicity equation was a critique of the exclusiveness of other intellectual systems and of private elitiest accumulation in general, alongside all pretentions to *break into* the "intellectual estate" must be set the republican desire to *break down* the walls protecting such estates and to open out the land of privileged learning. Phrenology was one area where it seemed possible for common people to storm the walls and regain the participatory right that had not been unknown to some of their forefathers.[21]

Inseparable from the above and from all other aspects of phrenology's appeal was its basic message – that there was nothing in the vast confusing complex of human emotions and jumbled facts of existence that could not be explained and made sense of through the precise mapping of the mental faculties. The sense of exhilaration that autodidacts derived from this is captured in T. S. Prideaux's reflections on his discovery of Gall and Spurzheim's system, around 1806:

such revelation of the constitution of humanity seemed like the discovery of a new world; such a key to the character and motives of the beings by whom I was surrounded, – a new Aladdin's lamp, which revealed treasures of knowledge more precious than gold. I immediately became possessed with the most insatiable curiosity to know my own development and that of everybody by whom I was surrounded.[22]

In the "new world" that phrenology opened up through its cerebral microcosm what had formerly seemed disparate now seemed pulled together. As suggested in reference to Combe's attraction to the knowledge, its patterning of the anomalous through classification, and its making the intangible world of emotions tangible, contributed to give a sense of precision to experience, order to reality, logic to contradiction. To Emerson there seemed no doubt that it was "the pleasure arising from Classification that makes Calvinism, Popery, [and] Phrenology run and prosper."[23] With mental reality thus reduced, unified, indexed, and ordered, life could be slipped from its social moorings and become utterly comprehendable psychologistically. Not until the writings of Herbert Spencer later in the century (themselves dependent in part upon phrenology) were people to feel – or feel the need to feel – so drunken with comprehension.[24]

Another major aspect of phrenology's appeal lay in its apparent practicality. Much in the manner of astrology (which had also

been within the grasp of the tyro, and had also been all-explaining),
phrenology in treating a subject upon which everything else could
be said to depend excluded nothing from the realm of its applicability.[25] Shifting the heavens to the head, as it were, and reading
bumps as stars, works of practical phrenology – often indeed in
the form of almanacs – addressed themselves primarily to what
has been called the first question of philosophy: "not 'What is the
Universe all about?' but 'What should we do with our lives?' "[26]
In the expanding industrial towns all people were strangers requiring as much sound practical advice as they could get: What
exactly was the one suited for? How could one make the most of
one's talents? Who should one trust and befriend, and how were
these to be separated from the legions of vagabonds, wastrels, and
thieves, obsessives, eccentrics, and maniacs? Who to marry, and
how to raise one's children? By a single consultation with a practical phrenologist, at the touch of an easily tutored hand, all of
these agonizing problems could be solved. Of the 365 recorded
Glaswegians who submitted their heads to Goyder's hands in 1843,
the majority were youthful mechanics; the rest, mostly servants
sent by their prospective employers for character references.[27] Not
until our own time – "by the touch of a computer keyboard" –
would these perennial sources for the neurosis of indecision seem
so open to solution or be handled with such scientific confidence.[28]

To the arduous business of self-improvement phrenology seemed
particularly applicable. It was not just that by placing "a mirror
into each person's hand" to reveal strengths and weaknessess
phrenology enabled one to exploit one's strong points; because
phrenologically "the brain partakes of the general qualities of the
organized system, and is strengthened by the same means as the
other organs," *overcoming* one's weaknesses also came within the
bounds of the possible and practicable. Self-knowledge – "the most
difficult to acquire and the most beneficial to its possessor" – was
thus to be fully and effectively wedded to self-improvement.[29]

Nor was it just for oneself: As the handbills for the lectures of
the itinerant phrenologist Dr. Eden‡ pointed out (see Figure 6,
Chapter 5) here was also the means not only "to Train and Educate
Children at half the expense, and in half the usual time," but also,
to enable parents "to quicken in their children those powers that
are productive of knowledge and virtue, and to restrain those that
have a tendency to evil, and to make choice of those professions,

trades, or other walks of life for which they are adapted." It was chiefly out of this parental worry that the Dundee Mechanics' Phrenological Society had been formed. "From our stations," their secretary told Combe in 1826, "[we] must be content to *receive* [phrenology's] lights, happy if we succeed in rendering them practically useful for restraining the propensities, nourishing the higher sentiments, and training the faculties of our youth into activity, thereby rendering them useful and virtuous citizens."[30] Artisans like Christopher Thomson, who felt that they had been wrongly articled as lads, knew well the consequences of such a mistake. "Doubtless hundreds of men have been led into the same error," he thought, "by the custom of parents apprenticing boys to any thing that promises to pay well, without ever bestowing a thought upon their fitness for the profession selected." Naturally, therefore, "If phrenology, or any other branch of science, can reveal to us the way to avoid such failures for the future, we ought to listen thoughtfully to her counsels." There was, as Thomson was aware, no alternative ethology, while there was plenty of reassurance from honest benevolent men such as Charles Bray that "we may easily deceive ourselves, but not so easily the practical phrenologist."[31]

One of phrenology's most important practical gifts, it was thought, was the information it provided on maintaining health. This could take the form of a lesson on the effects of alcohol on the mental faculties, for instance (specifically on how alcohol deadened the faculty of Self-Esteem), thus revealing biologically the rationale for temperance. Or it might consist of the presentation of seemingly irrefutable evidence taken from necroscopic examinations of the brains of sexual lunatics, in order to show how sexual licence perverted health by sapping energy from the other mental organs.[32] Yet it was not merely or necessarily this kind of specific behavioral proscription that recommended phrenology to the attraction of artisans on the grounds of health. Far more important was the informational framework or general elaboration of the supposed natural laws of health that were here made to seem as if they were as immutable as the laws of mechanics, and as if in a like manner they had just been discovered. This was specifically the task of Andrew Combe's *Principles of Physiology Applied to the Preservation of Health* (1834, and into a thirteenth edition by 1847), a work that extended to the body as a whole the same law-abiding functions that phrenology depicted in the brain, and that inculcated the same need to obey those laws in order to achieve organic harmony and happiness. In this sense the works of the so-called "Locke of Human Physiology" were as much phrenological texts as his brother's *Constitution of Man*.[33] Although more deceptive because they largely confined themselves to physiological description of functions, they were wholly prescriptive socially in that (without excusing the environmental conditions to which much ill health could be attributed) they thrust the burden of responsibility for overcoming ill health (hence health itself) onto the individual. Good health was made to seem mostly dependent upon overcoming personal ignorance about the operation of natural laws and learning to obey them. The message was spelled out so clearly and simply by Combean phrenologists that it was almost inevitable that they (and the brothers Combe in particular) would come to be seen as the independent authors of it. As the atomic theorist Samuel Brown wrote in the *Westminster Review* in 1852:

Who has not observed how effectively the phrenologists have been inculcating the first principles of physiology, and the art of life which depends on that science, into the public mind? Have not those two public spirited brothers, George and Andrew Combe, made the reading portion of this whole nation familiar with the idea of the absolute dependence of health on obedience to the organic laws?[34]

Indeed they had and, directly or indirectly, thereby widened a channel for the easy flow of phrenophysiological literature. Among those who contributed to turn that stream into a torrent was the American Sylvester Graham, whose celebrated *Lectures on the Science of Human Life* (1839) singled out the *Constitution of Man* as having more than any other book excited popular interest in physiology. In Britain one of those early to hop on the popularizing physiological bandwagon was the struggling general practitioner Samuel Smiles, whose first book, *Physical Education* (1838), was correctly described as a "serviceable adjunct or appendix to the works of Dr Combe."[35]

It is not difficult to understand why autodidacts, such as the weaver Bain, "greedily consumed" Andrew Combe's works and studied the natural laws of health religiously. We have only to recall on the one hand the reality of the worsening features of urban life – the bad housing, the alarming levels of infant mortality, the epidemics of cholera, typhus, and other infectious diseases, the venereal disease, chronic tuberculosis, alcoholism, industrial diseases and disfigurements, and much else – and, on the other hand, the kind of financial ruin that ill health could wreak among working people to appreciate why close attention would be paid to any set of seriously proposed rules of health. Far more than merely the fear (expressed by Bain) of the prevailing physic prompted such interest,[36] scientific amulets against illness were literally matters of life and death. Hence even Cobbett, wary as he was of scientizers, expressed a desire to publish in cheap form the work on mental cultivation by the American phrenologist Amariah Brigham, since this appeared to him to provide the rational instruction that mothers required in order to prevent infant mortality.[37]

Hitherto, it often seemed, no one else had made the effort to extend this knowledge outside medical circles. As the *Dublin Medical Journal* pointed out in 1835 in its praise of the *Principles of Physiology*,

Notwithstanding the efforts made of late years by the Society for the Diffusion of Useful Knowledge, and notwithstanding the recent strides of intellect in its boasted march, still mankind are singularly ignorant of that, which of all things concerns them most, viz. the structures and functions of their bodies.[38]

With regard to sexual functions, in particular, where "the moralist is silent, and the philanthropist is dumb" (as Barker put it), "Phrenology mounts the breach."[39] Disseminating their "really useful knowledge" without the usual religious unction and exhortation, phrenologists succeeded in breaking through the prudery barrier. It was clear that cleanliness of mind and body was held in high repute by them not because filth was a mortal sin, but because physiology rationally explained that filth, or sexual indulgence, or intemperance, or – importantly for the cultural origins of the sanitary movement later in the century – foul environment operated in specific ways to induce disease and debilitation. It was almost left for the audience to draw their own morals, although there could be little doubt about which they could be. As one phrenologist pointed out, the science "has awakened us to the connection betwixt a clean skin and a clear conscience – foul linen and foul thought – the indispensability of a

sound body to the production and preservation of a sound mind."
"Mr [G.] Combe did not merely teach that 'cleanliness is next to
godliness,' " remarked another phrenologist later in the century,
"but that 'cleanliness *is* godliness.' "[40]

Finally, while all of this literature on mental and physical hygiene
nudged people to physiological introspection, it was not obvious
(where it was the case at all) that this nudging represented a shift
of attentions away from the body social or toward a denial of need
to be reflective. Although there was hope that physiology would
teach people "to live without groundless apprehensions" and "ignorant fancies" and reconcile people to themselves, seldom did
the literature instruct people to obey the natural laws *instead of*
endeavoring to change society.[41] That was its inference for bourgeois society and its tendency, but to a large extent this was only
because the choice was never explicitly put in the terms of either/
or. The appearance was simply as asocial information with an
immediacy to personal well-being – the precondition for self-
improvement. Thus to working people, conscious that help was
to come from no other quarter than themselves, phrenologists
appeared as offering (with "passionate earnestness") not a resource
for political gelding and acculturation, but a means to purposeful
intervention in their own destinies. The alternative was to remain
passively victimized by circumstances that, individually considered, were otherwise quite beyond one's control.

Control over life and responsibility for one's situation leads on
to a further aspect of phrenology's appeal (the one with the most
obvious religious implications): paradoxically, the blamelessness
that accompanied the belief in cerebral determinism. In this respect, too, phrenology was akin to astrology: If delinquencies were
constitutional – whether predetermined by innate faculties or by
stars – one was clearly not responsible for misdeed nor liable for
punishments. "To the predestinarian," mocked the novelist Henry
Cockton, phrenology "is a source of great comfort: to all who
desire to take themselves entirely out of their own hands – to get
rid of that sort of responsibility which is sometimes extremely
inconvenient – it is really a positive blessing."[42] Desite phrenologists' differing points of view on the socially sensitive subject of
free will and necessity, most working people seem to have been
assured by the science that their weaknesses were not their own

fault, that they were the fault of a system that needed reforming, and the fault of parents who, ignorant of the natural laws of heredity, had visited their sins upon their children.[43] The "tendency" of phrenology was thus, as Combe put it in his earliest writing, "to make us acquainted with ourselves and indulgent to our fellow-creatures, for it teaches us that no individual is a standard of human nature." To the insane and even to criminals, therefore, sympathy could be extended since cerebral malformation was no fault of one's own.[44]

Fatalism did not compromise phrenology as a doctrine of human improvability, however. As with the stars in astronomy, phrenological faculties predisposed rather than predetermined human nature; thereby phrenology, as astronomy, provided insight into the precise nature of the compensation needed to overcome one's cerebral nativity. In spite of inheritance, in spite of the shape of the head, it was thus possible to struggle to alter basic nature.[45] As with the prospect of overcoming bodily infirmities, the prospect of overcoming or improving one's mental endowment also seemed tremendously liberating: life came under one's control when the predictability of science replaced the torment of chance. For what one *was*, one was not accountable (as in Calvinism or Marxism); but for what one could *become*, one was (as in Marxism but not in Calvinism) accountable not to God but to oneself.[46] Since people were therefore no longer to be visited by the sin of Adam, there was to be no retribution for sin.[47] (Indeed, here was the means not only for coping with an agnostic existence in a cultural framework of Christian orthodoxy, but as well for indulging in hope). For one's failing in *this* life (i.e., violations of natural law) one could blame oneself and suffer in this life. But suffering for sin could also be minimized, since secular natural laws, unlike the arbitrary laws of God, could be rationally understood and logically adhered to. Justice could thus cease to be a mirage. No wonder, then, that by putting them "in charge of their own mental and moral health" phrenology "was to ignorant men like entering upon a new state of existence."[48]

Later in the century, when the optimism of working-class self-culture had declined, phrenology became more a solace for those faced with an awareness of their inability to succeed in society. More secularly Calvinistic, it became more a religion of despair, a quietism comforting and reconciling people to their uncomfortable realities in much the same way as some projections of social Dawinism. By 1858 the Sheffield secularist and Barkerite Henry Turner was arguing that phrenology explodes the myth that "man, by his industry, can accomplish everything."[49] But while in the third quarter of the nineteenth century phrenology offered more sense of consolation than of liberation, the real strength of its appeal continued to lie in the fact that it did both simultaneously.[50] It was nicely placed between a fatalistic *tabula rasa* environmentalism and a doctrine of disembodied mind or free will. Biological endowment plus industry avoided those extremes but offered the necessary degree of self-forging solace or "try harder" voluntarism: a meritocrat's charter, an ethologist's rationalization.

The final aspect of appeal to consider is phrenology's overture to democracy. Here, too, the science cut both ways, an essential tension existing between what some people understood the knowledge to say and what, contrastingly, was implied. For the more radically minded, like Henry Turner, it was preferable to emphasize that phrenology made "the declaration that all men were equal," while the less militant, like the Dundee mechanics, preferred to stress that phrenology proved "the truth of the poet's observation, that 'The hand of Nature on peculiar minds / Imprints a different bias.' "[51] In fact it said both: People were equal since they all had the same number of faculties, and they were unequal because each person's faculties had different relative potentials at birth and could be differently developed under different exercising influences through life. But even the explanation of the inequalities seemed democratic and humanitarian since it cut across the usual class divisions and did not proscribe the upward mobility of the poor. As Barker summed up the matter in *The People*:

This science does not deny that a very great disparity exists among men in regard to their mental constitutions. . . . But each man possesses, nevertheless, the faculties and sentiments peculiar to humanity. . . . What the Phrenologist asserts is, that no sane man has a faculty which another has not. – He admits a difference in *degree*, although none in *kind*.[52]

Thus the single framework for assessing a person's worth was to be intellect, not station, nor wealth, nor (theoretically) sex, race, or nationhood. A nearly identical message had been taken by Thomas Jefferson and others from the lectures on the brain by

Cabanis.[53] In other ways it might as well have come from Church or chapel: Were not all men equal in the eyes of the Lord, and had not the Lord bestowed greater physical and mental gifts on some more than others? With phrenology the Elect were appointed by Nature, and the jargon on the differences in innate faculties squared with the commonplace observation that "not every one is fit for every thing."[54] As always, phrenology secularized, refined, scientized, simplified, and made tangible a basic notion, then popularly emerged as the author of it: "the *only* science by which the differences which exist in men . . . can ever be accounted for."[55] As with that other famous rhetorical creation "separate but equal," phrenology's ruling of "equal but different" facilitated such maneuvering between selfish and selfless interests that its appeal could hardly be other than universal. Certainly it is not difficult to see why it would have especially satisfied politically and socially compromised artisans. They could come away smiling from a phrenology lecture where the skulls of the "lower classes" had been spoken of as inferior in *"thickness"* and *"texture"* to those of the "higher and more intellectual classes." Locating themselves among the latter, they would (like the Dundee mechanics) claim on the one hand that these differences accorded with what they had observed in society, while on the other hand agree with the lecturer that the doctrine meant "universal democracy" because it acknowledged "the equal rights of all men to the legitimate use and gratification of all the faculties bestowed by nature on them."[56] This sounded good, even if it only meant that everyone (noticeably males) had an equal right over themselves to improve themselves. But always the *sounds* of phrenology were as important as its sense; perhaps more so, for scrutinized too closely, the science of "common sense" through which so many sought to comprehend and free themselves becomes an overwhelming edifice of contradictions.

THE STRENGTH OF RHETORIC

Emerson, though he believed phrenology to be "foolish," had no illusions abut the bases of its popularity. He appreciated that its appeal lay in the strength of its rhetoric, as "criticism of the Church & Schools of the day . . . [showing] what men want in religion & philosophy which has not been hitherto furnished."[57] Working people, who had less opportunity than the "thinking classes" for doubting that phrenology was the greatest step ever made in mental philosophy, also generally had less reason to doubt. After all, it was primarily those who where most anxious to keep the lower orders in their place who reacted most hostilely to the science. "Subversive of the fundamental principles of all religions," phrenology was seen by the right "as introducing civil anarchy into the political economy of legislation, as substituting disorder for harmony, despair for hope, and eternal darkness for everlasting light." The science's direct tendency, argued another reactionary, was "to render the great mass of the community discontented with their condition, and with the existing relations of society." At "the price of 1s 6d," said another, the phrenologists had put into the hands of "the poor and illiterate ... an edge tool or lancet, with which they are doing great mischief."[58]

Working people could readily appreciate what motivated such condemnations. Had not Combe argued that the master manufacturers brought in the Combination Acts against trade unions only to drive up profits? And had he not urged workingmen to combine firmly and perseveringly in order to raise themselves to a condition corresponding to the nature that the Creator has bestowed on them? Against the Commons' rejection of the Ten Hours Bill phrenologists had united behind the views of George and Andrew Combe that the mercantile and manufacturing population were not only gratifying their Acquisitiveness and Self-Esteem and breaking moral law by forcing their laborers to work more than ten hours, but also were violating the Laws of Nature by reducing the laboring population to human machines capable only of gratifying their base faculties.[59] J. Q. Rumball,‡ by no means the most liberal of phrenologists, was yet as adamant as others that in the new Poor Law "the laws of God had been violated to indulge *acquisition*." The act was, he pronounced, "a disgrace to the land we lived in."[60] Nor was this the most hortatory language of phrenologists: In 1838 the phrenologist Charles Thorold Wood Jr.‡ told Doncaster workingmen that "the time was approaching when the voice of the robbed, despised, insulted Working-man would become more potent than that of Monarch, Ministers, of Parliamentary minion, and that the will of the Palaced Despot would bow in weakness before the will of the half-fed, half-clothed tenant of a hut."[61] While only a minority of middle-class phrenologists actually desired the Chartist backing sought by

Wood and John Epps, many were prepared to stand by the complete suffrage views as put forward uncompromisingly by Hewett Watson.[62] In fact, republicanism, of a Jacksonian sort, was widely endorsed by phrenologists and made cerebrally legitimate by them as a result. Hodgson reminded Combe that the "brain is a republic" in which each faculty was as good as its neighbor and with an equal right to exercise.[63] Though Combe was never to renounce his conviction in the supremacy of the intellectual and moral faculties, he modified his "oligarchical error" to the extent of confessing in a footnote in *Religion and Science* (1847): "I am no advocate of the doctrine of non-resistance. Organs of Combativeness and Destructiveness exist in man, and they have legitimate spheres of activity, one of which appears to be to repel, by physical force, aggression which we cannot overcome by moral means."[64] Perhaps it was sustenance taken from this that caused the former editor of the *People's Phrenological Journal* to be described in 1848 as one "likely to disturb public peace and kindle revolutionary sentiment" and to be imprisoned as a Chartist.[65] It is easy to understand why Charles Wood might have been marked down in some spy's notebook and, conversely, why many working people would have approved of him: While his brother Willoughby lectured on the fallacies of political economy and told the poor to be *dis*content with their lot, Charles challenged that the new Queen

who has one-third of the present power ... does not possess a single faculty more than any of those I am now addressing. The monarch has three lobes – the animal, the moral and the intellectual – so have you; the monarch has the forty mental faculties of the human mind, so have you: the monarch has not turned these to any good account, but many of you have ... and yet the monarch is to be equal to you and all the nation beside! Oh! shame, shame, that this wretched degradation should have been submitted to by Englishmen in the Nineteenth century.[66]

At the same time these and other phrenologists contributed to the artisan's hostility to the stale and dishonest Old Theology. Putting the boot to "the smooth tongued priest, who turns your thoughts to the clouds, that he may get his hands in your pockets, who starves your body and what is worse, starves your mind," phrenologists fed a Jacobin appetite, while giving dissenters to understand that the real targets of their rhetoric were not themselves, but the monopolist State Churchmen. Thus different secular and anticlerical traditions could both be appealed to and exploited.[67]

Hence, in spite of most of phrenology's leading apologists in the 1830s and 1840s becoming decreasingly the radical comrades of "the people" and increasingly their bourgeois guardians, it was nevertheless easy for them to be regarded popularly throughout this period as among a vanguard of radical materialist speculators openly confronting the major political, social, and religious oppressions of the age. Asserting that a Yorkshire weaver or a Northamptonshire peasant had as much right to the secrets of science as anyone else,[68] they did so not only in the face of reactionaries like the bishop of Chichester who were claiming that education, and especially easily learned science, was leading to discontented servants and national ruin but, as well, in the face of SDUK and British Association types who (it could readily be supposed) belittled the science as "presumptuous speculations ... delight[ing] the half-educated and half-witted" because they knew that when "the guinea stamp of rank" was replaced by "the natural nobility" advocated by phrenology the shabby power structure would fall along with all other privileged institutions.[69] It was clear after the betrayal of 1832 that other educators were out to reshape the worker's private life in order (as Kay-Shuttleworth put it) "to promote the security of property and the maintenance of public order."[70] Not so the phrenologists whose simple, empirical, practical science implicitly bespoke equal opportunity and social justice, and who explicitly spoke of lifting the oppressions of the past – of banishing "at once and for ever the remnants of barbarism, the relics of a debasing animalism."[71] With less of the "moral halitosis" of the unctuous do-gooders with their safe morsels of knowledge, phrenologists spoke to working people as adults whom they earnestly entreated to perceive and penetrate the deceptions about them in order freely to improve themselves and escape unpleasantness.[72] Time and again they could be heard to say (as in Combe's speech in Glasgow in 1851), "There is no hope for the working men until they shall become *dissatisfied* with ignorance and dirt, with crowded ill-aired houses, with hard toil and the absence of refined recreation." Forget about prayer, they said (to the chagrin of religionists), and demand, against all the "artificial" obstacles put forward by others, your right to improve your moral sentiments, to control your propensities that will allow you to "rise in the social scale." Surely this was the spread of Reason, not the inculcation of deference; as *Tait's Magazine* said of one of the more popular phrenologists who "attempts no compromise, and seeks no disguise," he shows the science's "inevitable ultimate consequences ... of completely revolutionizing the entire system of society."[73]

To be sure, not all the rhetoric issued by phrenologists sounded radical to all working-class recipients all of the time, as we will have occasion to see in the following chapter. It has already been noted that on occasions some phrenologists deliberately sought to align themselves and their knowledge with overtly repressive capitalist ruling-class interests. But it has also been observed that for the most part the majority of phrenologists had no clear sense of social control strategy. Had they noticed that when the campaign of the Evangelicals against the socialists got seriously under way in the 1830s some working-class radicals began to complain that the working class were being distracted from their true class interests,[74] many phrenologists would have been delighted; but there is little to suggest that they *did* notice, or ever themselves rose above what they so plentifully helped to obfuscate for others. Precisely because they were not misanthropic propagandists attempting to defend the industrial system through a sleight-of-hand that would direct the animosities arising from the problems of industrialization onto the current maintainers of the Norman Yoke, their scientistic attack on traditional power was credible and popular.[75] Much of their rhetoric, it needs recalling, was not specifically directed or intended for the working class. When Engledue, for instance, late in the 1840s, spoke of "discarding completely those narrow and limited views which have so long harrassed and perplexed," he was venting his own assault on the lingering narrow sectarianism that proscribed the fulfillment of the culture he sought.[76] So was Forster in the *Philosophical Magazine* in 1815, or Mackenzie in his lecture to the Edinburgh Royal Society in 1830, or Prideaux in his defense of Gall in 1869. Since the fox-hunting, port-swilling enemies remained real, and the Church powerful, there was no reason why phrenologists should not have continued to be preoccupied with antiaristocracy and antisupernaturalism. Many of them remained thus concerned until their dying day.[77] But even among those of them who directed their rhetoric specifically at workers, there was little conscious deceit and hypocrisy involved. Most were firmly convinced that they were democratizing the revolutionary truths of Nature and were teaching workers to "think and judge for themselves."[78] Of their radical deviancy they could remain convinced by virtue of the often considerable personal and financial expense it involved. Ellen Epps recorded that her husband

was much blamed by some for yielding to the requests ... to give [groups of workers] information; and doubtless the fact of his lecturing to the Socialists did him harm in a circle that might have been the means of doing him good in a pecuniary point of view. His own view, however, was that such an opportunity of spreading what he felt assured was for the benefit of man to know, of enlightening the public mind with respect to God's laws, ought not to be passed by.[79]

One of the main reasons, then, why the voices of phrenologists became resonant among "the people" was because the majority of them, while preaching phrenology, remained largely unaware of the ideological nature of their knowledge, just as Combe had remained while writing the *Constitution of Man*. (Who, least of all Andrew Combe, could mistake what he wrote for anything other than well-meant knowledge to improve by?) Like other zealous but politically naïve bourgeois reformers blindly fulfilling what Marx described as "their mission [of] battering to pieces Old England, the England of the Past," phrenologists contributed to and helped to sustain into the 1840s that conveniently blurred radicalism that was "a kind of cross between Political Economy and theoretic Universal Suffrage – between Ricardo and Major Cartwright – between the *Wealth of Nations* and the *Rights of Man*."[80] Of course the phoenix was rising: Mill's *Political Economy* with its open advocation of class collaboration was on the way, while, more generally, those who were gaining the most in the great social transformation had mounting desires to have those below share their perception of reality – to be (psychically) just like themselves. Inadvertently almost, the facts of what was becoming the class control of the liberal bourgeoisie of industrial society were effaced at the same time that there was the fixing "subliminal flash": "Nature's scheme of social gradation [as] an institution beneficial to all."[81] But most of this was only clear in hindsight, where it was clear at all. At the time, the great majority of artisans could only see phrenology as fitting in and amplifying their own libertarian "battering" tradition. The science, they could echo Engledue, "advocates freedom, and abhors tyranny, ... recognizes the free and unrestained manifestation of thought; it matures all views, and patronizes all schemes calculated to increase man's happiness." As readily they could quote from the *Constitution of Man* that phrenology was leading (albeit "ultimately") to "a great revolution ... in our notions, principles of action, practices, and social institutions."[82] Doubters – above all those in the working class who were beginning to perceive that in the industrializing context there was an air of unreality to the cry "*à bas les aristos*" and a certain sterility to the demand for the "antidote to priestcraft"[83] – had only to witness the spectacle of phrenological literature being cast into the same hellfire that was burning the *Age of Reason* to doubt their doubts and have reconfirmed the belief that Combe's was the true voice of the dissenting populace: antiaristocratic, anticlerical, antimonarchical.[84] The science of phrenology and the *Constitution of Man* in particular crystallized in essence everything the underprivileged had been denied in the past and everything (including absolution from sin) that they may have desired. In the yearning soul, as in the intellect, it struck home.

DECEIVING SIMPLICITY

We have now stated what is trivially true of any religious movement: that phrenology's existence and growth were dependent upon its social and individual functions. Here was what at times was an entertaining escape from reality, but not an escape that allowed one simply to transcend the unendurable. The easily learned rubric of phrenology or the confession to the practical phrenologist allowed a confrontation with the practical problems of everyday life by heightening understanding of self in relation to Nature and in relation to other people; it led to a future path with a coherent rationalized system of ethics. It released people from the bondage of past presentations of reality in Calvinistic religions where wealth and success were the only measures of grace and so heightened individual dignity and worth; it allowed reprobates to know themselves, to confess their guilt and failings and be born again and have the chance to save themselves; it provided people with a natural basis for forbearance, toleration, and charity to fellow creatures.[85] Finally, with the basis for improvement supplied, earthly utopia and self-salvation came within human reach. Here then was a panacea, a blessing, a comfort, a source of all meaning, a sure path to indentity, morality, wholeness, progress, worth.

But conceivably any social movement or any scientism could offer as much. Where phrenology was advantaged was in its central provision of a system of symbols and metaphors, the power and revelational potential of which above all permits our referring to the science as a secular religion.[86] The tangible symbol of the head and its internal symbolic structure we have previously discussed as having reference to the social system, of being external form for an idealized image of social relations, and as providing a template for organizing human action and its experience. These symbols could be consented to readily since, quintessentially, they were personal, intimate, common, flexible, and "real" (because of their external palpably empirical nature). But in so accepting, one consented to interpret experience in certain ways; one consented, if not to wholly endorse certain "objectified" structures and commit oneself fully or in part to a certain "natural" orientation to action, then at least to allow certain other orientations to be obscured. Phrenology was thus a part of what Frank Parkin calls "a public meaning system."[87] The more it was experienced as truth, the further it committed one to its interpretation of reality as the *only* truth. The following conversion to phrenology was typical:

The experience that I gathered, and the facts which came under my daily observation, so entirely corresponded with much that I had met upon [the *Constitution of Man*'s] pages, that I could not withhold the assent of my judgment, or come to any other conclusion than that the science of Phrenology has truth for its basis.[88]

This was the experience of a middle-class woman, a representative of, next to artisans, the single largest category of persons who attended phrenology lectures.[89] Like artisans (or children), the majority of these women also faced a superannuated perfunctory, compromised role in urban industrial society. They wanted to know that there was an underlying order to social relations, to be assured that those relations were natural and unrestraining, and that they were as individuals in their own right integral to and not just appendages to the natural scheme of things.[90] Phrenology fulfilled this religious "quest for lucidity," the need to map the empirical world to combat its disorder, to give through symbols an orientation in nature, society, and daily routine. The anthropologist Clifford Geertz has written,

For those able to embrace them, and for so long as they are able to embrace them, religious symbols provide a cosmic guarantee not only for their ability to comprehend the world, but also, comprehending it, to give a precision to their feeling, a definition to their emotions, which enables them, morosely or joyfully, grimly or cavalierly, to endure it.[91]

But the cosmic guarantees in phrenological symbolism were more than just institutionalized things to be embraced or rejected at will: They were symbols that mediated a particular idealization of differentiated order that became impossible to think against once the symbols had been accepted. They did not function, nor were they ever "designed" to function, as perfect isomorphs for a particular social system; the fact that diagrams of phrenological heads were frequently called "symbolical charts" is an amusing irony; the real cultural work of the symbols – their transcription of idealized social shape and function – was taken up noncritically, unreflectively, as factual knowledge of nature.[92]

It is not therefore to enter into conspiracy theory to claim that the recipients of Combean phrenology could be psychically "manipulated" by the phrenological construction of cerebral reality. In many ways to take up phrenology was comparable to taking up the cross of Jesus or the image of Shiva in societies where those are central symbols. A priori, however, to read this cerebral map as a guide to reality was to accept the authority of the symbol and hence to close off from oneself the possibility of constructing or reconstructing mental–social reality in different, alternative ways. Hazlitt, scathing the science in 1829, touched upon an important truth in this connection when he likened the phrenological head to the woodcuts of model villages that Owen had had printed at the top of the *Times*: "From that instant thought," Hazlitt perceived, "every reader had ocular demonstrations of the truth of his system: the woodcuts were facts, visible and tangible. . . . The bumps on the head are in like manner facts."[93] There was of course textual reinforcement, but the visual impression of the symbol should be seen as having worked subliminally to authenticate the symbol itself. In the unconscious (what has been called "the residue of ideology")[94] the authority of the natural symbol could be taken up – the authority, that is, of a reified psychological metalanguage of idealized capitalist social relations and structures. Along with this went the more basic valorization of the concern with individual psychology, together with phrenology's twofold celebration of intellect (by its focus on the head and by its cerebral hierarchical division of labor wherein the intellectual and reflective faculties predominated over the sensual and animal). In this way working-class recipients of phrenological knowledge could come to accept not directly the naked consciousness of the dominant class, but rather the ideological configurations and priorities dependent upon and implicit to the dominant material relations – an acceptance that at one and the same time powerfully reinforced and norma-tized bourgeois capitalist social relations and imposed heavy per-ceptual checks on working people's ability to determine their own social interests.[95]

Considered thus – as mystified mediation of ideology, rather than as crude ideological rationalization – it is not at all surprising that phrenology was not reacted to as "a tool of bourgeois oppres-sion." Like reality itself, the science existed metaphysically with-out manifesting the alternatives to itself. Its metaphors of function, growth, harmony, order, and so on not only did not appear as the products of social consciousness but, insofar as they remained merely assumptions behind physiological "facts," did not appear as metaphors at all. As a result they were impossible to frame for debate. Likewise, it is only historically that we can see that phren-ology's celebration of intellect was occurring in a context in which previous fusions of mental and manual labor in craft were being sundered. At the time, in the context, neither phrenologists nor any one else could work through the series of abstractions nec-essary to measure the power of ideology mediated by this cultural resource – the idea of cultural mediation itself being an abstraction.

Thus quite apart from its rhetoric, phrenology, by delimiting reality, inclined its recipients to heed certain aspects of the social reality being constructed at the time and to neglect others. It be-came the most "natural" thing in the world for the student of phrenology to strive to fulfill his or her unique individual capacities when the interdependence of specialized parts – the capitalist di-vision of labor – was made out to *be* the nature of things. Similarly, it was easy to forget the old social themes that had been current among common people, of justice, freedom, and violent upheaval, when the validity of human life was seen to derive not from one's relations with one's fellows or class, but from one's individual relation to society as an organismic (class-consensual) whole. Thus immunized against the relevant socioeconomic dichotomies of industrial capitalism, the true light of biology could guide one to recognize as more important such distinctions as those between adaptive and maladaptive behavior, normal and deviant functions, normal and pathological states. Attention shifted to these concepts (their human constructions unperceived) and deflected away from notions of "natural rights" and "social contracts," people could come to evaluate life in terms of their individual adjustment to the natural order of things apperceived in the structure of the brain. To become a part of this self-contained order and defer to the cerebral division of labor "*as the standard of right and wrong*"[96] was not to be a part of a society of working-class solidarity and struggle against exploitation; it was to take on a role adapted to the inherently competitive values of petit bourgeois self-betterment whereby one left the working class behind.

It was with such mystifications of ruling-class ideology that Gramsci was concerned when, in reaction to functionalist social theory, he developed the concept of *egemonia*. Through consciousness-determining encounters in everyday life, he perceived, especially through the everyday encounters with knowledge, class exploitations and conflicts of interests were obfuscated for ordinary people. As Raymond Williams has amplified: "Hegemony" is neither about naked deference to dominant opinions nor about simple manipulations into "false consciousness"; it refers to more than this, to the totality of reality, to the whole body of our practices and expectations – to

our assignments of energy, our *ordinary understanding* of the *nature of man* and his world. It is a set of meanings and values which as they are experienced as practices appear as reciprocally confirming. It thus constitutes *a sense of reality* for most people in the society; a sense of absolute.[97]

Faith in phrenology, it might be said, faith in a religion whose rubric centered on the head and whose sermons focused on a qualified Reason, became a pathway to a qualified reality. If the rhetoric of phrenology exploited certain fractures in the artisan's consciousness, the mediation through the rubric could draw him by his own volition into "false consciousness" rendered no longer "false" by the "real" interest in the new social system. Simply by pursuing a science "characterized by harmony and simplicity," as one advocate put it, students had opened to them "wide fields of usefulness and interest" that, as they proceeded to study, were found "perpetually, novel and increasing[ly] ... display[ing] views the most enlarging, the most delightful, and these *in a ratio perpetually augmenting in proportion to the inquirer's progress.*"[98] Not simply then to social control through psychic *manipulation* did the cultural mediations of the nineteenth century's most popular body of scientific knowledge contribute, but more so to a process of psychosocial maturation rooted in social aspiration. Coming eventually to represent a system of thought totally alien to the working class as a class in modern industrial society, phrenology translated the economically determined reality so perfectly that the aliens could express its truths as self-evident. Thus the reformer's toast to "the people" as the "only source of legitimate power" might cease to be rhetoric and seem to be real in spite of the reality of most people's total exclusion from power.[99]

METHODIST SCIENCE

So the "philosopher of manufactures" was right: Lessons in bourgeois political economy on their own would not instill deference. But he was wrong in supposing that the "sublime doctrine of happiness hereafter" would be necessary to provide "not only the motive to obedience, but the pattern of it."[100] Aside from the fact that in a popular religion such as Methodism it was not just the hereafter that accounted for all the obedience rendered, it is clear that popular phrenology, in supplying a doctrine of future happiness in *this* life, could be quite as effective in establishing those patterns that facilitated the socially appropriate self-control.

To a large degree Methodism and phrenology overlapped. Doctrinally they both accommodated contradictions and, because of it, were able to enhance their appeals: Despite their Calvinistic inheritances, each fulfilled the optimistic implications of evangelical Arminianism, the possibility of perfection on earth. Phrenology, as Wesley said of Christianity, was a "social religion," and the same "good works," improvement, and accumulation of wealth that provided external proof of salvation in the religion applied equally to the science.[101] With phrenology one's moral respectability was to be the external evidence of the internal state of the brain, that is, the soul reified in mental faculties. "Progressive sanctification," the Calvinist doctrine whereby the predestined progressively traced their election, could (as in Methodism) be found by every person through the improvements to their mental faculties, which would be reflected in the state of their happiness or secular salvation through moral rectitude. The doctrine of particular providence, too, which Wesley regretted as "absolutely out of fashion" in 1781, was regained secularly through this system of knowledge.[102] By merely lifting the hair from the brow, some claimed, phrenology gave external proofs of this providence. Others with less worthy foreheads and living perhaps in less worldly comfort might frown upon this fundamentalist habit, though claim that "progressive santification" could be seen in the actual changes that took place in the cranium as one improved.[103] The latter notion, however, besides being too unequivocal, was open to physiological dispute, so increasingly it was simply the good deeds, the hard work, and the effort put into being respectable that were stressed as the true indications of inner morality. Thus, just as Wesley had shifted the emphasis from "walking with God" to having "Christ's image stamped upon the heart,"[104] so through phrenology the ethic of improvement became more deeply rooted – biologically rooted – in the personality. Increasingly, phrenology like Methodism became the religion of finding social security in oneself. Hence the protesting "Thou shalt" in the face of the unreformed establishment's "Thou shalt not" became through this scientific means the same self-disciplined "Thou shalt not" as in Methodism. It is perhaps not so surprising, therefore, that the science and the religion both drew the bulk of their congregations from the same class of artisans and females.[105]

But it was less through appeals to specific doctrines that Methodism and phrenology succeeded than through appeals to experience in a social context where the commonest experience was with change and accommodation to urban industrialization. Like Methodism (as Bernard Semmel contends), phrenology triumphed through its ability to moderate between *Gemeinschaft* and *Gesellschaft*.[106] But it outflanked its sectarian partner by extending the modernizing aspects much further. Moving in the footsteps of Calvin and in the shadow of Wesley, smashing idolatry and dogma

in the interest of plain puritanical and direct understanding, phrenologists encouraged vast numbers of people to become (or feel
comfortable in being) what the Unitarian James Martineau decried
as "mere anti-supernaturalists."[107] To such persons the *Constitution
of Man* was, as G. J. Holyoake claimed of it, "a new Gospel of
Practical Ethics" – in many ways the secular Bunyanesque equivalent of what Wilberforce's *Practical View of Christianity* had previously been to the evangelizing upper and middle classes.[108] But,
alas, the new faith "in the religiousness of man [rather] than in
the reality of God" was to leave people not only frighteningly
committed to "getting on" in the ways defined by the pundits,
but also, frighteningly, responsible to themselves alone for such
improvement, with no hope (as in Methodism) of Godly future
justice. And here was the rub: Although phrenology allowed those
who were too rationalist for eschatology to bestow meaning on
existence and reforge identities, or to contend against urban industrial anonymity and anomie by preserving a sense of ego,[109]
and although in the context this was as consoling as it was liberating, the more arbitrary and anomalous the world became
through industrialization, the more phrenology came to be relied
upon for an explanation of existence within it; while the more
phrenology was relied upon and studied, the more natural became
the alienation.[110] Put otherwise: In spite of the fact that the majority
of persons attracted to the knowledge probably experienced little
actual upward mobility (and therefore had no real reason to rationalize the bourgeois myth of the open society), phrenology by
boosting the ethic of improvement induced the need for its own
rationalization of the consequent alienation. In effect, the science
cerebrally aggravated the problem by leading people to quest after
their "real natures" and fit themselves to them, and then produced
the magical answer that was a mediated reproduction of the prob-
lem-inducing structure. Precursor to Freudianism as a radical form
of self-enlightenment through individuation and reason, phrenology rationalized or made the alienation of modern life intelligible, but offered only the rationalization as the solution.

Harriet Martineau may not have understood this as the provision
of Methodism in secular form, but unlike her brother James she
fully appreciated that people derived religious satisfactions from
the science and that these satisfactions were of a sort conducive to
the stability and progress of the emergent order. In her singular

description of what "ignorant persons" found in the *Constitution of Man* that made them see it "as if a new revelation had come to them" and made them commit themselves to it "as to a Providence," she observed:

they learned that their bodies were a part of the universe, made of substances and governed by laws which it is man's duty to obey. It was a new view to them that by knowledge and self-management, men have their health, and the development of their minds in their own hands. They had before thought of themselves as being outside of the world, as it were, – apart from the rest of creation, – each individual being a single existence, incomprehensible in nature and qualities, and in no way concerned with natural law.[111]

Here, literally in cosmological terms, was the natural universe of the phrenologists, entry into which was to save ignorant men from what was presented as having *always* been their former state of alienation and unhappiness. The tactics were those of the Church: the offering of a key to the only door to salvation from a contrived precariousness. In pursuit of happiness what else could converts to this cosmology do but take up the attitudes and ethics that would further sacralize the norms of "self-management" and thus link themselves as individuals to those who had an interest in normatizing the behavior that maintained their alienation and rendered them unable to gain access to the totality of reality? For some workers this might represent not just an exchange of God for Nature, but the virtual annihilation of a materialist–communal world view for one of utter aloneness in a naturalized capitalist environment. Compensation? – a rationalization of the alienation; a morality more rigid and sacrosanct than anything produced by Old Religion; happiness through rising above disorder, through self-control.

Yet it was seldom that phrenology was negatively experienced as such. If only by virtue of its sheer outlandishness, it took ordinary people out of their ordinary routines, just as through psychoanalysis or rock music or astrology people enjoy themselves in their search for satisfaction through self-discovery. Indeed, the same reasons that have been put forward to explain why other early Victorian "education mongers" hardly reached the working class are those that best explain why phrenologists fared so much better: The greater part of the working class were not interested in learning and wanted to be amused; their ideas were based less on reason than on experience and practical matters; they had an important sense of justice and dignity; and they had a preference for unpretentious knowledge from their own kind or those who seemed closest to them.[112] In reawakening deep-rooted physiog-nomical notions and reaffirming homolitic prescriptions in popular culture, by titillating sexually, by creating bold impressions of order and meaning, by offering seemingly vital but easily grasped practical information for survival and for advancement in life, and by rousing through provocative populist rhetoric, phrenology did not appear to the majority of working people to be religiously affirming and cohering industrial–bourgeois society. If it appeared as exalting or protecting anything, it was only "the right" to possess a true theory of one's own nature, "the liberty" to discover and develop one's potential as a human, and "the freedom" to try to get ahead in an admittedly unjust, unequal world.

PART IV

Radical appropriation and critique

Our lack of knowledge makes it impossible to assess how far the interest in science and the interpretations which were made of its nature and purpose inside the rationalist group have differed from the way in which all those who were broadly favourable to and interested in science have conceived of it.

Susan Budd, *Varieties of Unbelief* (1977), p. 126

Hegemony, even when imposed successfully, does not impose an all-embracing view of life; rather it imposes blinkers, which inhibit vision in certain directions while leaving it clear in others. . . . The question as to whether a subordinate class can or cannot develop a coherent intellectual critique of the dominant ideology – and a strategy reaching beyond the limits of its hegemony – seems to me to be a *historical* question (that is, one to which historical evidence offers many different answers, some of them highly nuanced), and not one which can be solved by pronouncements within "theoretical practice." The number of "organic intellectuals" (in Gramsci's sense) among the artisans and workers of Britain between 1790 and 1850 should never be understated.

E. P. Thompson, "Eighteenth-Century English Society: Class Struggle without Class?" *Social History*, 3 (1978), 164

7

Richard Carlile and infidel science

It is amusing to observe the earnestness with which ... [Jacobin radicals] recommend the study of natural history. One does not readily see the connection of this with their ostensible object, the happiness of man.

> John Robison, *Proofs of a Conspiracy against All the Religions and Governments of Europe* (5th ed., Dublin, 1798), p. 527

It is obvious, that the end for which knowledge was sought and recorded by the learned, and the end for which it is required by the multitude, are not the same, but different ends. I am now speaking especially of knowledge of science, and not so much, of applied knowledge, or of the useful arts.

> J. J. Garth Wilkinson, *Science for All* (1847), p. 3

If the advantage of disseminating scientific over other forms of knowledge is the ease with which it can legitimate specific social and political interests under the guise of value-neutrality, the obvious danger is that others will undermine those interests by directing the same body of knowledge to radically different ends. Those who attempt this have only to echo in their defense the rhetoric of the other side, claiming that science, in being neutral knowledge, belongs to no party except the party of Truth (which they of course claim to represent). Thus, "legitimately" Darwin's ideas were to be pressed into services as divergent as those of the American robber barons, the founders of the German Social Democratic party, and the British Fabians and were to be relied upon by figures as disparate as Mussolini, Ramsay MacDonald, and Peter Kropotkin. Similarly, in the early eighteenth century at the same time that the new scientific culture of the Newtonians was coming to sanction a providential faith in King and Church, radicals less enamored of that faith were utilizing the same knowledge to sanction a naturalistic faith in purely human institutions, republics, and private masonic lodges. Again, at the end of the eighteenth century, in France, various radicals were seeking to divorce mesmerism from Mesmer in order to extrapolate from the doctrine a radical political theory.[1]

Phrenology was likewise used by various nineteenth-century radicals to sanction social, political, and religious objectives different from those of the main body of Combean phrenologists. As observed in Chapter 3, it was partly because of these more extreme, socially contentious deployments that orthodox phrenologists, fearing accusations of guilt by association, sought to police the science's use and to have it more strictly conform to the social norms of early Victorian respectability. In turn, radicals (meaning here primarily artisans who were accepted as representing the interests of the working class) often responded by attempting to distinguish their interest in the knowledge from that of its bourgeois proponents and to contest as reactionary "misapplications" the latter's overtly religious as well as secular methodist deployments. In this and the following chapter we will be concerned with exploring the nature of some of these encounters of radicals with phrenology.

At the outset it needs to be said that, contrary to what is sometimes supposed, at no time during the early nineteenth century was there ever a uniform "radical line" on science. Like working-class radical culture itself in the early nineteenth century, radical attitudes toward science and scientists were diverse, testifying to the mixture of traditional and new outlooks and to the continually changing nature of those outlooks. Some radicals, for instance, mindful perhaps of William Thompson's observations in 1824 on the way in which "knowledge, instead of remaining the handmaid of labour [had] almost everywhere arrayed against labour, not only concealing its treasures from the labourers, but systematically deluding and leading them astray, in order to render their muscular powers entirely mechanical and obedient," were keen to cultivate science among workers largely in order to bring to an end the disunity between head and hand and the consequent degradation of laboring people.[2] Although later in the century it was painfully obvious that "the greater power given us by the thinker and man of science has merely increased the inequality between the possessors and the hordes of the dispossessed,"[3] in the earlier decades many radicals were hopeful that if workers were given access to scientific information in a manner *undivorced* from sociopolitical and socioeconomic struggle and humanist morality, they might be able to assert their dignity and worth and self-reliance and might be better equipped to contest obscurantism and social injustice.[4] Other radicals, however, considered it wiser to stay as clear of science as possible. To some it was clear by the 1830s that science signified the marriage-out-of-wedlock of Jacobinism with bourgeois liberalism. The deradicalizing objectives of some bourgeois scientizers made this clear: "We are anxiously looking for a new system of social organization, in harmony with the lights of the age, and Lord Brougham thinks to stop our mouths with *kangaroos*,"[5] some operatives in Manchester are reported to have declared in the early 1830s. But in other cases the distrust and aversion radiated from the subject itself. As pointed out on the first page of one of the most widely read radical journals of the early 1830s, Richard Lee's *Man*: "Science herself has not been altogether free from the cankering contaminations of custom and pride ... [being] more or less embued with existing prejudices."[6] Yet other radicals (of whom Richard Carlile, the focus of this chapter, is often considered the epitome), while repulsing the efforts of the bourgeois scientizers, accepted science "herself" as a neutral "force ... fatal to that of tyranny and priestcraft,"[7] and were only too anxious to thus exploit it. Still other radicals though, (or the same ones at other times), came to look upon orthodox materialist science as a symbol of spiritual purposelessness and meaninglessness in a hostile industrial–technological capitalist environment. "SCIENCE CREATES WEALTH, BUT IT IS MORALITY THAT PERFECTS MAN," declared the Lancashire radical and Swedenborgian Roland Detrosier in 1831 in a much publicized address to the members of the breakaway New Mechanics' Institute in Manchester.[8] Often closely connected to this Nonconformist-inspired position was a loathing of the bourgeoisie's evermore arrogant, elitist, and humanly abstracted utilitarian conception of science.[9] The early-nineteenth-century radicals who revolted against this conception of science can be seen as following in the tradition of the late-eighteenth-century French Jacobins who executed Lavoisier in 1791.[10] But it was really more in the tradition of the seventeenth-century Digger and pantheistic materialist Gerrard Winstanley that their negative response to bourgeois science and scientists was bound up with deep-seated desires to democratize and to humanize science by reinvesting it with a perceived-as-missing "principle of vitality."[11] Such desires, more especially the antimechanistic vitalist one, were to lead some early-nineteenth-century radicals, as formerly it had lead some eighteenth-century ones, into Neoplatonic, mystical, and esoteric traditions. These radicals, like the others we will encounter here, had no coherent historical understanding of the origins of the division between "science" and the "occult" or between the rational and sensuous and aesthetic that had been socially and culturally imposed by Newtonian mechanists in the seventeenth and early eighteenth centuries. Nevertheless, by their criticisms of these alienating fragmentations of reality, and by their efforts to assimilate the phenomenal world of Nature into the man-made world of society (and so transform Nature herself), they penetrated to the very heart of modern scientific rationalism.[12]

Clearly, then, it cannot be claimed that all early-nineteenth-century radicals had a blind faith in bourgeois positivist science. As in previous times, radicals seldom lived up to the Tory image of them as the wayward children of their science-deceived elders.[13] Not only might their interest in science extend well beyond mere scientism, but also, where and when science was revered scientistically as a powerful tool in social and political debate, the reverence need not necessarily have entailed endorsement of the dominant class's supposedly objective view of the structure of natural reality.[14] (It might only have been used to restrict the influence of other ideologies.)[15] Certainly, much of the radicals' interest in science can be seen as undermining the current assumption that it is only "now all of a sudden, [that] people have awakened to the fact that science and technology are . . . the latest expression of power and that those who control them have become the new bosses."[16]

Yet, awake as early-nineteenth-century radicals were, it would obviously be naïve and anachronistic to attempt to argue that they had anything like a twentieth-century critical awareness of science as the bourgeois ideological embodiment and mediator of capitalist social relations. Assuming that such an understanding might have been acceptable to some of them, it was impossible for them to develop it, since for the most part they lacked the prior necessity for such a critique of capitalist science – historical perspective on capitalism itself. In general, radicals in this period preferred to wrestle with the problem of how to improve social conditions rather than to puzzle over society's origins. As Engels pointed out, even within early socialism, criticism extended only as far as "the existing capitalist mode of production and its consequences. But it could not explain this mode of production, and therefore, could not get the mastery of it." To capitalist science, as to capitalism, the early socialists could, at best, "simply reject it as evil."[17]

It should come as no surprise, therefore, that a mystified mediation of capitalist social relations, such as phrenology, was left virtually critically untouched by early-nineteenth-century radicals and that few inroads were made on the retheorization of received science. Some radicals sought to correct Combe's "oligarchical error" of the dominance of moral and intellectual faculties in phrenology, but none sought to strike a blow to the physiological conception itself. Radicals who rejected the science did so primarily out of a distaste for certain of its applications and propagandists. Like those using (or ignoring) Darwin's ideas, therefore, and unlike either the radical pantheists involved with Newton's idea or the French radicals involved with mesmerism, the radicals who involved themselves with Gall's theory of brain and science of character could not help but reproduce its "official" version of cerebral reality – its mediation of bourgeois structures and relations. Merely to reject certain applications of the science and to substitute others was not only not to reject that version of the mental nature of things but, inadvertently, to reproduce and reinforce it (though this is not the same as saying that users necessarily were manipulated in an instrumental way by that version of reality). Although it remains to be seen just how far radicals actually accepted and internalized phrenology as the true and only science of human nature, as a threat to the establishment of bourgeois hegemony their ursurpations of phrenology were, ultimately, more apparent than real.

But to study the history of phrenology in radical culture only from the perspective of the "ultimate" establishment of the Victorian bourgeois hegemony is to sacrifice much that may be of historical value. In particular, it can cause us to lose sight of what historically is most important about phrenology for the study of science in radical culture: the fact that in two related respects Gall's ideas were quite unlike those of either Newton or Darwin. First, they were neither about the physical universe nor about apes (nor "kangaroos") but, far more important, were about the internal hidden nature of the human mind – the loftiest and most mysterious branch of knowledge. As such, secondly, Gall's ideas remained not just socially controversial but, from an empiricist methodological point of view, scientifically unorthodox. In attempting to provide a comprehensive and unified view of reality and its inner structure, phrenology was always – to employ Comte's terms – more "theological" than "scientific." In spite of there being no other theory of brain and science of character to compete with phrenology in the nineteenth century, phrenology as a "science" (as distinct from the Combean scientism) always remained "alternative," implicitly and explicitly challenging many of the norms and pretentions of conventional science and social science. (In this respect it was more like mesmerism, with which, indeed, it became formally linked and avidly pursued by some radicals.) In a decision such as that of the Owenites in Sheffield in the late 1830s to call a moratorium on all discussion of science in their Hall of Science *except* phrenology, this regard of it as an "alternative" with the potential to contest orthodox science and society seems manifest.[18] Although we shall see that this regard for phrenology was shared in fact by only a minority of radicals (few of whom can really be quoted in evidence of having clearly thought out their position on it as such), for that minority phrenology might be comprehended historically as not unlike Lysenko's agronomy for twentieth-century Soviet ideologues, in that it was a scientific theory and practice that could appropriately be applied to a social structure and set of social relations consciously conceived of as alternative to those emerging in industrial capitalist society.[19]

But if phrenology's scientific unorthodoxy is of primary importance for understanding its place in pre-Darwinian radical culture, the obvious implication is that for understanding the radicals' regard for science in general, in this period, phrenology must be more problematic historically than the study of, say, chemistry or astronomy. Arguably, however, it is *because of* the historical problem posed by phrenology's scientific unorthodoxy that the subject emerges as most useful in illuminating both the overt and the covert social and ideological functions of science in radical culture. As an "alternative" or unorthodox body of knowledge on the structure of mind and the nature of thought, phrenology can be seen as entering radical culture not just as a form of antiauthoritarian rhetoric, but also, socially and epistmologically, as a part of a critique of orthodox bourgeois science and social relations – a critique that included a humanist, antipositivist side. (As we will see, it was into this critique that some radicals saw a need to incorporate phrenology itself.) But at the same time, in the regard for phrenology as the mental counterpart of Newtonian physics, it can be seen as inculcating respect and deference for a positivist conception of science in which science was put above the reach of social and ideological criticism. Thus at different levels phrenology might be seen as simultaneously arming and disarming, liberating and repressing. Consequently, it facilitates an especially good introduction to both the spectrum and the texture of radical engagements with science.

In view of the variegated nature of radical culture at the time, however, the only way in which we can illustrate the multilayered nature of phrenology's involvement is by focusing in detail on specific working-class radical involvements and by attempting to treat them, as we have previously treated the bourgeois involvements, in relation to changing macro and micro material and social circumstances. Only thereby does it seem possible to execute the historical and historiographical justice demanded by the neglected complexities of science's place, role, and meaning in radical culture. The rest of this chapter therefore is devoted to the engagements with phrenology of Richard Carlile, a figure central to the radical movement of the 1820s and one of the first radicals in Britain to take more than a passing interest in the science. In order to approach phrenology's involvement with the radical movement of the 1830s and 1840s, the following chapter will focus on Robert Owen and the Owenites.

RICHARD CARLILE[‡] (1790–1843)

On the face of it, no interpretive problem at all surrounds the interest taken in phrenology by Richard Carlile. For this pugnacious "showman of freethought," who considered the works of Tom Paine of "more value ... than Bacon, Newton, and Locke together" and who believed that the "literary and philosophic world ... alone can perfect society," phrenology was of value as a materialist doctrine that could lend support to an anticlerical intellectual republicanism.[20] For this purpose it was important not that phrenology appear as an "alternative science" but, on the contrary, that it seem a wholly conventional scientifically irreproachable touchstone of truth. Thus, after being introduced to the science by William Lawrence in 1823, Carlile's initial reaction to it was reserved. He was uncertain if it "was a science at all" and was convinced that, if it was a science, then with its "distinct organs . . . for religion," it was being "erroneously stated."[21] Not until 1826, after having read Abernethy's essay on Gall and Spurzheim and Forster's *Somatopsychonoologia*, and having paid a visit incognito to Deville's phrenology shop in the Strand, did he, at age thirty-six, begin to feel that, by endangering the Cartesian duality of mind and brain and by casting man solidly in the scheme of animal instead of special creation, phrenology provided "new and invincible proof of the good foundation of the science called Atheism or Materialism."[22] By 1828 it seemed to him that the answers phrenology gave to fundamental questions on the human mind and on free will and necessity, the solid grounding it gave to a secular philosophy of morals, and the inducement it gave to true forebearance by teaching that men's souls were "not in the moral, but in the *physical* structure," contributed to make it the "most important subject on which a public writer can be employed."[23] Practicing what he preached, Carlile took to the road with phrenology, delivering his first lectures on the subject in Manchester in July 1828.[24]

Orthodox phrenologists could hardly have dissented from Carlile's conclusion about the importance of phrenology. But it would only be by accepting that conclusion at face value and completely divorcing it from the context in which it was uttered that the historian could presume to establish a close affinity between Carlile's interest in the science and that of George Combe (whose *Constitution of Man*, it will be recalled, was published in this same year). Behind Carlile's interest lay a spirit that, if not entirely foreign to that testified to in Combe's book, must be seen as having a different social center of gravity that impelled it in a different direction. Noticeably, the whole of the growth of Carlile's interest in phrenology coincides with the increased success of orthodox phrenologists in making themselves and their science socially accepted and respectable among the emergent "thinking classes." By reasserting phrenology as entirely materialistic, Carlile was flying directly in the face of those changes, protesting, in general, against the watering down by the bourgeoisie of Enlightenment radicalism and the Jacobin critique of Old England and, in particular, against the socioreligious domestication of phrenology for bourgeois cultural hegemony. Thus his interest in phrenology, far from being merely a throwback to the radicalism expressed by, for instance, John Thelwall in his 1793 lecture on "The Origin of Mental Action Explained on the System of Materialism," can be seen, rather, as an alert and sensitive response to the considerably altered social order.[25] Remarking in 1826 on how he had realized the materialist implications of phrenology "at first view of it," but had "thought it wise to be silent for a time, or until it had gained something like an establishment in this country," he confessed the need to now break that silence, for "I have seen it assailed by some sillily [*sic*] religious people; and I have smiled with pity at seeing certain phrenologists attempt to defend their science upon religious grounds ... [whereas, in fact, the science] strikes the very source of religion."[26] He thus began to lash out at the Christianizing phrenologists: first, at the Reverend David Welsh for his phrenological evidences in support of Scriptures and, subsequently, at Spurzheim for going out of his way (in the *Philosophical Catechism of the Natural Laws of Man*) to puff Christianity in order "to meet the prejudices" of those who found, or were now finding, Lawrence's conveyance of Gall's materialist philosophy wholly or partly reprehensible.[27]

It was largely with the intention of further exposing and counteracting the effects of the "incompetent and improper" phrenologists who were "truckling to Christian priestcraft" that Carlile took to the podium. Yet this was not his only motive. By waving the flag of phrenological materialsm in the late 1820, after phrenology had gained "an establishment" in Britain, Carlile was at the same time attempting desperately to retain his influence on the radical movement – an influence that he had achieved in the first half of the 1820s by means of similar atheistical republican polemics. By his celebrating then of the ideas of Tom Paine, and by his republishing of works such as Peter Annet's *Free Inquirer*, Mirabaud's *System of Nature*, Hoggart Toulmin's *Eternity of the Universe*, and Elihu Palmer's *Principles of Nature* (the latter's publication along with the *Age of Reason* leading to his trial for blasphemy in 1819 and his six years' imprisonment in Dorchester Gaol), Carlile did more than merely extend the republican materialist tradition previously represented by certain members of the London Corresponding Society.[28] He in fact did a great deal to revive the radical cause at a time when much of its fire had gone out in the wake of the Queen Caroline affair and the execution in 1820 of Thistlewood for his part in the Cato Street conspiracy. In driving to their ultimate conclusion Enlightenment views on religion which were widely shared but (even among radicals) only privately held for the most part,[29] Carlile had provided orthodoxy, new and old alike, with an irritant, orthodoxy's reaction to which served, in turn, to provide radicals with a new sense of urgency. For a younger generation of radicals in particular – those who, like Carlile himself, had not been much involved with the hard constitutional, antitaxation struggles of the "freeborn," yet were in various ways still attached to what has been called "the old analyses, the old rhetoric of individual and social injustices" developed between the 1780s and the 1810s[30] – Carlile's "life or death" defense of infidelism rekindled an important sense of radical mission and esprit de corps. Although by revivifying this antiauthoritarian rallying point during that "cold season for the London proletariat" in the 1820s,[31] Carlile neither advanced the cause of labor nor advanced the cause of civil liberty, he managed (like his secularist heirs later in the century) to give some coherence to the artisan radical cause and to allow the sound and fury of artisan radicalism to be heard above the din of the construction of the bourgeois establishment.

But by the late 1820s Carlile's scientistic ultramaterialism had lost force and his power base was seriously eroded. Increasingly, after the economic recession of 1826, the tone and tempo of radicalism underwent change. The new radicalism, though rooted in the preindustrial radicalism of small masters and artisans, and still powerfully influenced by agrarian ideals, related more to the swelling mass of deskilled urban industrial wage earners. In general (albeit often more in theory than in practice), this new radicalism had more to do with wages, living conditions, open organization, and large numbers than with political principles, secret conspiratorial associations, theological unorthodoxy, and attacks on aristocracy. As early as 1825 Thomas Hodgskin in *Labour Defended* had asserted that it was "now time that the reproaches so long cast on the feudal aristocracy should be heaped on capital and capitalists."[32]

To this new radicalism and its development, theological unorthodoxy was far from being anachronistic, however; and to pursue phrenology materialistically within the new context for radicalism was by no means reactionary in and of itself. To the radical publishers James Watson, Henry Hetherington, and John Cleave, for instance, it did not seem at all inappropriate in 1832 to publish selections from Lawrence's lectures under the title of *An Essay on the Functions of the Brain* and to advertise this along with republications of Paine, Volney, Byron's *Cain*, and the *Working Man's Friend*.[33] After all, the atheist mission, or more broadly the anti-Christian mission, was itself never merely a strategum: However much religion may have been in decline in the nineteenth century as the real source of social cohesion and division, scientistic attacks on religion always remained symbolically and actually attacks on authority, whether that authority was conceived, as Carlile conceived of it, in terms of "Kingcraft and Priestcraft" or, less traditionally, in terms of an exploitative bourgeois capitalist power structure. Carlile's ill-fated acquaintance George Petrie, for instance, the outspoken advocate of the abolition of private property, perceived science as a force to undermine religion: "Oh heavenly Science!" he wrote in his celebrated poem *Equality*,

> ... were it not for thee,
> Ne'er could our fondest hopes reach Liberty;
> By thee, truth's beams begin to penetrate
> The mind's horizon, and to dissipate
> Those clouds of error hitherto so dense
> That man could not perceive, e'en COMMON SENSE.[34]

But by religion Petrie meant "NOT (as some falsely assert) *an abstract thing between Man and his Creator*," but rather that which "enable[s] the idle, cunning, and voluptuous few to luxuriate on the produce of the toil of the plundered many."[35] To insist, as did Carlile and his Zetetic followers, on denying a First Cause was not merely to replace "God and Providence" with the here and now of "Nature and Necessity" and to identify oneself with opposition to authority. More important, it was to distinguish oneself attitudinally from the merely liberal bourgeois rhetorical use of anticlericalism.[36] Though this distinction was not elaborated theoretically nor articulated in the political and economic terms of social class, it was often implicitly understood as such. In 1845 the former bricklayer William Chilton in his review of Chambers's *Vestiges*, for instance, implied that the "essential and radical difference between the opinions of the materialist and the opinions of those who embrace the [deistic] views of the author of *Vestiges*" was that the latter's sanitized view belonged to "the orthodox party" who apologized for things as they had become.[37] Similarly, Carlile had reacted to Spurzheim's *Philosophical Catechism* (the inspiration for the *Constitution of Man*) as a work in which the laws of nature were insidiously conflated with the laws of the Creator in order to make it appear (as in the classic social apologies by Paley and the authors of the Bridgewater Treatises) that orthodox social morality and Christian religion were interdependent.[38] Carlile fully agreed with Spurzheim on the morally uplifting value of phrenology – its tendency to "increase the sum of human happiness through the medium of moral improvement" – but his reasons differed from Spurzheim's in that they were based on the negation of a First Cause or personal diety. Thus differing, Carlile's criticisms contributed to the *possibility* of creating a very different moral–social order. Far from necessitating acceptance of the bourgeois social order, therefore, or foreclosing on the ability to criticize it, an ultramaterialist deployment of science against religion could pave the way for fundamental critique. Indeed, it might encourage criticism of the ideological function of bourgeois science itself. The biologist A. R. Wallace, for instance, who in his youth in Owenite Halls of Science acquired a lifelong materialist anticlerical interest in phrenology, was able to write in 1913 in reaction to the naturalization of inequalities in industrial society that, *along with religion* "science [had] agreed in upholding the competitive and capitalistic system of society as being the only rational and possible one."[39] Thus the materialism that Carlile sought to advance through phrenology could be said to have contributed to an effect just the opposite of helping workers to rid themselves of what Felix Holt the radical called those "vain expectations and ... thoughts that don't agree with the nature of things."[40]

Yet, in the circumstances of the late 1820s and early 1830s, Carlile's particular use of phrenology arrested, and was seen to arrest, this potential of the science for radical culture. Primarily, this was because directly *in the face of* the new radicalism Carlile sought to use the science to legitimate and conserve *only* the traditional values of the study, independent, freeborn artisan elite. "The great [i.e., primary] moral benefit to be derived from the science," he was to state repeatedly in opposition to the less exclusive applications of the science by Owenite socialists, was its capacity to teach man to "improve himself, where improvement is required."[41] Whereas in the past, in the largely preindustrial context of Paine's radicalism, the effort to preserve these individualist values had constituted a radical threat to paternalistic (Godlike) authority, by the late 1820s this was no longer the case.[42] Carlile's individualist rhetoric too closely resembled that of the new taskmasters, especially since within his rhetoric he suppressed the political thought and economic arguments against private property contained in the second part of the *Rights of Man*.[43] Thus Carlile's use of phrenology to defend the traditional antiauthoritarian creed of artisanal "self-reliance" against cooperators and unionists (those "dreamers and co-idlers" who "never think of putting a shoulder to the wheel" and who would "monotonously tie down the talent or utility of mankind, so as to make the ingenuity of the genius subservient to the dullness of the dolt")[44] was to cause him at the crucial level of economics to be aligned with the orthodox phrenologists celebrating the deradicalizing cult of petit bourgeois liberal individualism. Although Carlile was not in fact arguing for the economic individualism that William Thompson in his *Inquiry* had considered and refuted in 1824, his phrenologically buttressed defense of artisan independence amounted to the same thing since it pushed egalitarianism aside scientistically on the grounds of "differences stamped on each individual by original organization."[45] Asked by Owen to consider cooperation, Carlile raised the objection that "the phrenological inequalities of human disposition rendered any principle of general co-operation for equality, to me, apparently impracticable" (a view shared, incidentally, not only by many working people on his right but as well, though for different reasons, by many on his left).[46] The eventual collapse of the communes established by Abram Combe, Fanny Wright, Owen, and others satisfied Carlile that those who proposed schemes for society that attempted to do "more than assail the superstitions and tyrannies that degrade it" were "persons of excited imaginations, similar to those who have been in search of the millennium of human happiness, or the philosopher's stone."[47] "My opinion has uniformly been," he wrote in 1829, "that man is no further a co-operating animal, than as he is necessitated to co-operate. Co-operation, in Mr Owen's system, implies free agency, man has none applicable to such a purpose, at least, in his present generation."[48]

Against Owen's argument for the power of nurture over nature, Carlile saw phrenology as cementing his own view of man as entirely animal with passions depending not on education but on "the physical construction or quality of the animal."[49] This was not to deny the power of education, especially scientific education, behind which Carlile had always stood.[50] Nor was it to deny the effect on the mind of better environments. Rather, it was to insist that because of the innate differences in cerebral makeup, the only way to morally reeducate people would be to deal with them individually – to "tame the fierce and ferocious [passions], to encourage the inoffensive and weak," as the need may be.[51] The science of phrenology aptly confirmed his belief that it was not wholesale or sudden change that was required to enlarge human happiness, but "the organization or development of the individual that [needed] ... to be acted upon, to work out the ends of moral philosophy."[52]

Accordingly, in 1828 and specifically in opposition to Owen's schemes, Carlile proposed a "New Plan of Reform." Wholly dependent on phrenology for its insights and applications, the New Plan scarcely differed in its basics from the interventionist proposals of orthodox phrenologists. Like them, Carlile called for the utmost care to be taken not only in the matching of parents (according to "phrenological, physical, moral and mental equality, [and] ... equality of age") and in the "time, temper, and temporal means" of their mating, but as well in the maintaining of the good physical and mental health of the pregnant mother.[53] Especially from the moment of the child's birth, Carlile insisted, it was essential for parents to have a knowledge of phrenology – "a science that promises to produce more substantial reforms in education, than all the changes that have been made, or than all the knowledge that has preceded it." Without this knowledge, he argued, parents would not understand how and when the faculties developed or – and here Carlile echoed Cobbett's interest in the science – how and why they should avoid many of the common mistakes of childrearing. If parents were armed with phrenology, however the "child that makes the man" would be perfected and the seeds of permanent reform be sown.

Ostensibly more practical than anything proposed by Owen, Carlile's New Plan of Reform was in reality hardly less utopian. Though he never admitted with Combean phrenologists that "it will require centuries to operate the change," it was impossible for him to deny that to come into effect the New Plan would take "successive generations."[54] Via phrenology, Rousseau's *Emile* was clearly the child of a far-off future – a decidedly less radical prospect compared to Owen's immediately practical ventures into communitarianism. Yet, both in a real sense and by default, the New Plan was not necessarily more "bourgeois" or bourgeois-tending than Owenism. Though entirely individualist in orientation, Carlile's ambition was not the same as that of liberal bourgeois educators, for he was not seeking to reproduce the hierarchical and authoritarian requirements of capitalist social relations by persuading artisans that they were unique or constituted a priviledged minority (though he tended to assume this).[55] Naïvely, perhaps, Carlile's aim was simply the creation of individuals who were completely atheist (implicitly, therefore, not deferring to orthodoxy); and, explicitly, he sought to encourage mental organizations in which all the faculties would be balanced (though he did not specify that this was in opposition to the claims of Spurzheim, Combe, and company, who were arguing for the superiority of the intellectual and moral faculties). On the other hand, though, by the mere adoption of phrenology's reified conception of mental faculties and by the pursuit of a reformism based on the individual molding of those faculties, Carlile was at one with the orthodox phrenologists in abstracting humanness by detaching mind from and putting it above the real social–economic relations of humanity. That the "*organs of the human brain* [are] *created by the human hand* (as Marx was to put it) Carlile wholly failed to see.[56] But then, to enter the argument by default, neither did Owen understand this. Especially during his many years as the industrial paternalist and educator of New Lanark, Owen, too, contributed to the reification and alienation of consciousness. As Cobbett aptly put it after visiting New Lanark in 1832, Owen's educational techniques "made minds a fiction."[57] Thus Owen, as much as Carlile, could be charged with contributing to a bourgeois-supporting idealist perception of humanity as a result, ironically, of having accepted a materialist educational psychology.

There can be no doubt that in his pursuit of phrenology as a means to having "human life studied as a science" Carlile shared and hoped to fulfill the ambition of many post-Enlightenment utopianists.[58] Nor can there by any doubt that Carlile was deliberately exploiting the science's popularity to gain himself a hearing. However legitimate was the need to counteract the truckling rhetoric of orthodox phrenologists, it cannot be overlooked that he only took a serious interest in phrenology after his popularity had waned – after his martyrdom in prison had come to an end in 1826, and after the readership of his *Republican* had dwindled from over ten thousand to one-tenth of that.[59] Almost certainly the desire to retain prestige in radical culture stood behind his attempt at lecturing on phrenology. Thereby he hoped to gain access to working-class educational institutions otherwise closed to him. (Significantly, he left his name off the handbills announcing his lectures and concentrated on lecturing in the provinces.[60])

This opportunist side of Carlile's interest in phrenology also featured in his Allegorical Christianity – the curious millenarian-linked esoteric blend of comparative religion, Eastern mythology, and mystical symbolism in astronomical form that was advocated by the Reverend Robert Taylor, M.R.C.S., the so-called Devil's Chaplain. Carlile's gravitation to Taylor's ideas occurred at roughly the same time as his interest in phrenology heightened at the end of the 1820s. Together with the science, Allegorical Christianity constituted a kind of irreligious religiosity that was similar to the pantheistic materialsm of eighteenth-century freethinkers in being both antisupernaturalist and humanist and bound to a republican vision.[61] Carlile's partner in marriage and freethought controversy, Eliza Sharples,‡ shared these views and encouraged Carlile in them; from her "Ninth Discourse on the Bible" delivered in the Bouverie Street Lecture Room in June 1832 it is possible to sample one of the ways in which phrenology was exploited within Allegorical Christianity:

In the present century, a science has been discovered and reduced to systematic observation, called the science of phrenology. This science of phrenology sets forth proof of the accuracy of this part of the Sacred

Scriptures in the Book of Revelation, which treats of the *mark of the beast* and *the name of God* being in the foreheads of two classes of men. The science of phrenology assumes, upon the strength and test of never-varying comparison, that the absence of brain from the forehead is the criterion of ignorance, not only in man, but in every other animal. Prominency and perpendicularity of the forehead are the signs of God, the indications of knowledge and the capacity to acquire.[62]

In theory, such a fundamentalist blend of science and religion and ancient lore (the "doctrine of signs" in physiognomy) ought to have been a receipe for a popular creed of the Christian Science sort. It is clear that with himself in the pulpit this was what Carlile was seeking through Allegorical Christianity, as he made explicit in a letter to Owen of June 1830. Justifying his religious transformation, he wrote: "If we ... can ... lead that multitude from bad to better principles by such a hold on their noses, why should we withhold it?"[63] Ends were thus seen to justify means, whether the means were phrenological or biblical or phrenospiritual.

And yet it would seem that the religious means were overtaken by the ends themselves, at least for a while in the early 1830s. Perhaps, like Comte's somersault from rationalism to spiritualism in the late 1840s after the death of his lover Clothilde de Vaux,[64] Carlile's turn of mind hinged upon the death, in October 1833, of his and Sharples's only son. Whatever the cause, the consequence is that it is next to impossible to divorce the mere deployment of these religious notions from Carlile's personal faith in them or, as in the lecture by Sharples quoted above, to separate out the phrenology used in their justification. A part of Carlile's sixth lecture to the inhabitants of Brighton in 1836, for instance, was to be entitled "The True Principle of Prayer, Repentance, and Salvation, with an Explanation of the Aid Afforded by the Science of Phrenology," a theme that was further expounded by Sharples in her lectures on "The Philosophy and Theology of Phrenology." In advertising the latter in his *Political Register*, Carlile was to claim that "the religious world has feared that Phrenology is hostile to religion. It is hostile to nothing but superstition. It is in perfect harmony with the origin of the Christian Religion and with all moral and physical science."[65]

Obviously this was to erase the atheist–theist (First Cause) distinction that had earlier been insisted upon and to elevate man from his former consignment to merely animal creation. But this was hardly a concession to the antimaterialist "orthodox party" or a realigning with either the religious-truckling camp of Spurzheim or the natural theological, deistic-cum-secularist camp of Combe. In view of the materialist commodification and reification of humanity in the emergent bourgeois culture (to which deism with its impersonal, alienated God was the best-suited theology), and in view of the fact that utilitarian state administrators and apologists for bourgeois political economy were coming to use arguments based on deistic natural law in order themselves to separate religion from morality and establish themselves as the new priestly overseers, Carlile's altered use of phrenology to give support to the more humanistic theism with its personal deity was conceivably more countercultural than his earlier merely atheistical (anti-immaterialist) deployment. It is likely that Carlile was aware of this, for he is known to have had contact at this time with Muggletonians and other millenarians. He was familiar with the writings of the seventeenth-century radical pantheist John Toland, and he is also know to have acquired an extensive knowledge of Freemasonry – knowledge that may well have included awareness of the radical pantheistic side of that organization's past.[66] It may be, therefore, that his uniting phrenology with mysticism and the occult was actually a calculated radical response to the altered material and cultural circumstances of the 1830s (however much the phrenology and the Allegorical Christianity were at the same time genuine convictions). In effect, by asserting antisuperstitional theistic and mystical views he was not only continuing to protest against the social and political authority of the traditional order as symbolized in orthodox religion, but as well was protesting against the new establishment's deistic rationalization of an antiseptic order of things.

It is impossible to tell the exact nature and extent of Carlile's interest in and contribution to the "radical pantheistic" tradition as it evolved in the nineteenth century (largely as a kind of untheoretical socialist humanism). Nor can it be told whether his interest in the spiritual and the Masonic ever led him to embrace more vitalistic conceptions of nature. (It would be interesting to know, for instance, if he was ever led to reject Paine's acceptance of Newton's view of matter as inert). However, in weaving phrenology into a heretical theistic tradition calling for "universal brotherhood," Carlile (like John Flaxman before him) can be seen as prefiguring many of the Owenites and late-nineteenth-century ple-beian spiritualists after they had come into contact with phreno-mesmerism.[67]

But direct links to Carlile are not apparent. Indeed, in general, Carlile's use of phrenology – with or without the Allegorical Christianity – seems to have made little dent on radical culture. Certainly it did not enable him to reexert the influence over the working class that he had hoped. His attempts at lecturing on phrenology were for the most part thwarted by local authorities. In Halifax in 1829, for instance, the *Commercial Chronicle* warned those who had suitable premises for lecturing "not to be induced to let them off upon any representation that a '*gentlemen, a phren-ological lecturer, is in want of them for a short time*'; and generally, we entreat the public to KEEP ALOOF FROM THEIR MEET-INGS."[68] Although in 1831, Carlile was still referring to himself as "a teacher in phrenology," it is likely that this kind of press exposure cut short his lecturing career.[69] As for his articles on phrenology in his periodicals, most of these appeared in the *Lion*, a journal with a low circulation that was intended mostly as an organ for his imprisoned friend the Reverend Robert Taylor. Let-ters to the editor of the *Lion* indicate, moreover, that even among its readers, not all agreed with the phrenology. There were those, admitted Carlile in April 1828, who "turn round upon us, and say, *your phrenology is a superstition*."[70] A working man calling himself "A Recluse" stated that he had read Gall, Spurzheim, Mackenzie, and others, had attended Deville's lectures, and had read the *Lion* and thought them all wrong. "The thing is carried too far, there's too much dogmatism in it, and if it be true, even in the outline, yet wrong in the detail." Pointedly the "Recluse" cautioned: "*Never invent a cause to explain an effect, when it can be explained without it*."[71] Carlile was perhaps reminded of this warn-ing when he wrote, some time later, that "a scientific system, such as phrenology with some correct general principles, may be strained to an absurdity" (though he seems to have little heeded his own counsel).[72] Another reader of the *Lion* did not dispute the principles of phrenology but was anxious to show that circumstances, not phrenological development, were really responsible for changes in national and individual character. Citing in his support an an-tiphrenological publication by the former constitutional radical James Montgomery,‡ this reader anticipated Godwin's pronouncement on phrenology as dangerously arrogant and dehumanizing by raising an objection rarely made explicit by other radicals: that phrenology did not just "[hold] out the principle that there is superiorily and inferiorily organized beings by nature," but that it located little of that superiority among manual workers.[73] This was close to the recognition that phrenology naturalized the moral and intellectual dominance of the bourgeoisie over the "animality" of workers and that, through its hierarchy of faculties, phrenology naturalized the industrial division and exploitation of labor. Less significant, but much stranger craniological evidence against phrenology was also presented in the *Lion* by the eccentric Pierre Henri Baume.‡[74] Such opposition, doubts, and criticisms were only intensified, moreover, when Carlile enriched his Allegorical Christianity by making it the personification of the mental phenomena of the human race with phrenology at the "root of the science of God."[75] Therewith, as when Comte apotheosized Clothilde de Vaux as the spiritual symbol of the Virgin Mother, Carlile alienated most of his remaining followers and at the same time played into the hands of reactionaries only too anxious to seize upon any opportunity to confirm the alliance between radicalism and madness.[76]

To the extent, then, that Carlile sought phrenology as a convenient means of regaining his grip on working-class opinion, his conceit seems seriously to have misled him. His reputation as a radical republican contributing to the "universal disruption" of the times (as the *Phrenological Journal* charged him in 1829)[77] was too well established to enable him to reach a less radical audience, while to younger men as well as to former Zetetics (many of whom moved into Owenism) the Allegorical Christianity appeared simply as a gross compromise of principles. Dumbfounded, the *Man* wrote of Carlile in 1833,

To hear a man who has suffered nine years of imprisonment, and twice nine of persecution, for the bold and honest expression of his disbelief of religious dogmas, now declare himself a convert to the morality of the most immoral, obscene, and withal uninstructive, of all immoral books that were ever written [i.e., the Bible] ... is ... inexplicable.[78]

But it was with what was considered by many on the left in the early 1830s to be the other side of this same base coin – the opposition to Owen – that did Carlile's reputation the greatest harm.

And it was this that consigned his use of phrenology to a place among the "misapplications" of the science. As late as 1839 in debate with the Owenite Lloyd Jones, Carlile was regarded as "speaking for phrenology."[79] Past recollections of the "bold and spirited manner" in which Carlile had opposed constituted authority (in part by his use of phrenology to legitimate atheism), and memories of the service he had rendered to the cause of free discussion and liberty of the press, only highlighted as all the more deplorable what was seen in 1838 as "his present falling off . . . although he himself calls it progressing."[80]

According to the picture that emerges after it has been filtered through late-nineteenth-century writings on the battle between science and religion, early-nineteenth-century radicals appreciated science mainly as an instrument with which to attack "priestcraft." Supposedly oblivious to the fact that religion was decreasingly the cohering force of society, radicals were consequently hoist by their own scientistic anticlerical petard into a blind faith in positivist science and Enlightenment rationalism. As Paul Feyerabend would have it, "The very same enterprise that once gave man the ideas and the strengths to free himself from the fears and the prejudices of a tyrannical religion . . . [was ultimately to turn] him into a slave of its [science's] interests."[81]

In many respects Carlile's interest in phrenology could be said to support this thesis, irregardless of whether we understand "science's interests" to mean simply an excluding scientific rationalist tradition (as Feyerabend intends) or the capitalist structures and relations sociohistorically constitutive of modern science. Like his mentor Paine, Carlile was not an original or perceptive thinker, and he can hardly be regarded as an "organic intellectual" in Gramsci's sense. His perception of science was in no way akin to that of, say, Ernest Jones, the Chartist friend of Marx, who saw it as a force whose potential to liberate "could only be set in motion through the conquest of power by the working class."[82] Carlile unquestioningly accepted scientific rationality as liberationist, and he opportunistically exploited it as such. Thereby he endorsed, as other historians have said, "a basically liberal individualist 'bourgeois' stance, which looked chiefly to self-improvement within a supposedly eternal, fixed and given framework of 'natural' social, political and economic laws."[83] That he should have trekked to the Anti–Corn Law League in November 1842 and applied to be a lecturer is thus unsurprising. What else should we have expected from this man who, in 1828, opined that "Locke was right, that the phrenologist is right, and that I am right, the difference is only in the degree in which we extend our perceptions"?[84]

Yet it is also clear that it is only by wrenching Carlile's pronouncements on phrenology out of the social, political, and personally opportunistic contexts in which they were uttered, and then statically assessing them solely in the light of the subsequent consolidation of the bourgeois industrial order, that they can be considered simply as supportive of bourgeois hegemony. Likewise, it is only through such histrionics that his pronouncements on phrenology can be seen simply as reinforcing the well known remark of the Chartist Bronterre O'Brien in 1831, that the radical movement had "no ideology beyond middle-class nostrums shouted in harsher accent."[85] While it should not be forgotten that in the immediate context, orthodoxy and unorthodoxy alike regarded Carlile's various appropriations and exploitations of the phrenological resource as hostile to the emergent order and its controls, neither should it be overlooked that there is always a point at which a "perception extended" ceases to be the same perception – or one merely roughed up – and becomes, instead, a perception of an altogether different order. Although socially and politically Carlile's perception of phrenology might be said to have been blocked by his commitment to Painite individualist values, intellectually (especially when regarded from the perspective of his Allegorical Christianity) that perception ultimately extended beyond orthodox Enlightenment rationality. More correctly, perhaps, his phrenology – though never ceasing to be an emblem of reification and alienation – accompanied a spiritual groping beyond that rationality, which took place within a socioeconomic context of increasing human despiritualization. In the light of that groping it becomes impossible to project Carlile's career as if it followed a logical and straightforward trajectory from the scientistic radical materialist to the Anti–Corn Law Leaguer, or to see phrenology within that pattern as "naturally and inevitably" impelling him into the ideological orbit of Combe. It should be clear, in fact, that that approach to his involvement with phrenology can only be taken by eclipsing the historical reality in which a conception of science as divorced from humanity was protested against and by eclipsing the finer dialectics of radical thought and politics during the early nineteenth century.

Carlile's experiences with phrenology when considered in their own context, therefore, rather than filtered teleologically through the hindsight of the last one hundred years or so of developing Western culture, can be seen as in part transcending any immediate appearance of his mystified co-option by the dominant ideology. While at the same time those experiences must be seen as in part reflecting and contributing to the extension of bourgeois modes of thought, "negation" may be said to have existed side by side with "co-option." To Marx this would have confirmed Carlile (as it confirmed Proudhon) as thoroughly "petit bourgeois" – as one who,

by the necessity of his position, acts as part socialist and part economist; ... at once a bourgeois and a man of the people. In his innermost conscience he flatters himself on being impartial, on having found the right equilibrium, which claims to be different from what is common. Such a petit bourgeois defies *contradiction*, because contradiction is the basis of his existence. He himself is nothing but social contradiction, put in action. He must justify by theory what he is in practice.[86]

But to label Carlile "petit bourgeois" in this sense is not to suggest that he therefore is undeserving of serious historical attention or that his phrenological justifications of his actions were aberrant and unworthy of his place in radical culture. On the contrary. Although it remains to be seen just how far Carlile's experiences with phrenology were representative of those of other early-nineteenth-century working-class radicals, his own involvement with phrenology might be seen usefully to serve both history and the present: on the one hand, helping us to avoid anachronism, error, and unnecessary apologetics or condescension when dealing with people's interest in science in the past and, on the other hand, preventing us from falling wholly into human and cultural despair over the impossiblity of reconceiving and remaking the "objective" study of humankind.

8

On standing socialism on its head

> If Faust could have two souls within his breast, why should not a normal person unite conflicting intellectual trends within himself when he finds himself changing from one class to another in the middle of a world crisis? ... Mental confusion is not always chaos.
>
> Georg Lukács, *History and Class Consciousness: Studies in Marxist Dialectics*, trans. R. Livingstone (1971), pp. x–xi

> But their idealism had run to waste in sad futilities. Nothing could be more true, both literally and symbolically, than that they [the phrenological Owenites] had stood the theory of Socialism on its head.
>
> E. P. Thompson, *William Morris: Romantic to Revolutionary* (1955), p. 317

It is a pressing reminder of the extent to which nineteenth-century radicals conceived of science as "the available providence of man" that, at the same time Carlile was utilizing phrenology in an effort to conserve Painite individualist values in the face of Owenite egalitarian ones, Owenites were in such zealous pursuit of the science that some were offering to pay for lectures on it with notes issued by Owen's National Equitable Labour Exchange.[1] This is also a salient comment on the tensions the science could withstand for, on the face of it, the cornerstone of Owenism – the doctrine that character was formed by one's social circumstances – was diametrically opposed to Gall's theory of innate mental endowment. How it was intellectually possible for Owenites to embrace phrenology thus requires comment.

In advance of that, however, it is worth recalling that, although "Owenism" was the first major working-class response to industrialization, at the same time it was an expression of many more traditional and less specifically economic aspects of radical concern. Along with the denunciation of a society based on the principles of competitive individualism, the rejection of bourgeois political economy and other overt forms of middle-class ideology, and the insistence on the labor theory of value, Owenism gave space and nourishment to a wide variety of radical concerns with religion, education, technology, medicine, philosophy, democracy, self-help, trade unionism, feminism, millenarianism, utilitarianism, and even mysticism. It was thus possible for radicals often with very different interests to enter into "the movement," if only sometimes peripherally or only temporarily.

In the light of this diversity, it is not so surprising that phrenology should have come within the Owenite venue. Indeed, given that "Owenism" (not unlike "Puritanism" in the seventeenth century) was in many respects a "generalized response to the experience of social change," having "numerous points of affinity" with early Victorian culture as a whole, it would have been extraordinary had the knowledge not come within the Owenite venue.[2] What *is* surprising, and has never been fully realized by historians nor accounted for in view of the considerable use of phrenology to attack Owenite socialism, is the scale of its cultivation among Owenites.[3] Far more extensive than Carlile's, this cultivation also ran more deeply, insofar as at one level it was part of a rejection of natural knowledge that was "divested of the principle of vitality" and that presented real phenomena as a part of an individualizing "nature of things" rather than in terms of social relations. In considering the various roles of science within early-nineteenth-century radical culture, therefore, one can hardly do better than to explore the nature of what critics – including, eventually, some Owenites themselves – deplored as the "abominable alliance" between Owenism and phrenology.

THE BASES OF RAPPORT

The key to the intellectual rapport between phrenology and Owenism largely lies in the fact that Gall, though an untypical child of the Enlightenment in some respects, was as optimistic as his contemporaries about humanity's potential for improvement. His nonlearning theory had been a reaction to Locke's sensationalism, but he nevertheless used social arguments based on biology in a reformist way.[4] Having postulated biological inequality between people at birth (and assumed the inferiority of females), he looked to the environment, socialization, and striving as leading to the improvement of the human race (though he categorically rejected Lamarck's doctrine of the inheritance of acquired characteristics). He intended, too, that his cerebral theory could be directly applied to the reform of character and thence to the reform of society: By withholding or providing stimuli to particular mental organs, he believed, specific forms of behavior could be encouraged or discouraged. This formed the basis of his hope for the doctrine in the reformation of lunatics and criminals – a hope for phrenology shared incidentally by Lamarck.[5] Gall's belief in biological inequality, moreover, did not necessarily run counter to the psychological principle of other eighteenth-century theorists that all people were equal in their natural faculties. As we saw in Chapter 6, Gall's theory could be taken as proving that all people were indeed equally endowed at birth (with respect to the number of their mental faculties) and hence equal in their *potential* for improvement. Thus even though for Gall the issue was with the *limits* of nature and nurture upon the ideal development of the individual (whereas for the Owenite followers of Locke, Condillac, and Helvetius, the issue was with *altering* nurture so as to mold an ideal nature to be shared equally by all), there was a wide area of overlap between these two different starting points in mental philosophy.[6]

In Britain the basis for their mutual support was enhanced by Spurzheim who, in the course of his extensive tours of the country after 1814, laid stress on the meliorist implications of the doctrine while playing down the fatalistic preformationsist aspects. He emphasized the point that "all organized beings are modified by external influences" and, though primitive nature is never changed, even small influences acting constantly "will necessarily produce, in time, conspicuous changes in mankind." Otherwise, he confessed, man would be "less perfectible than we may wish for."[7] Since it was to the leading reformers of the day that Spurzheim introduced himself and sought to make his mark, such an emphasis was clearly appropriate. Robert Owen, whom Spurzheim met in New Lanark, later recorded with satisfaction that he knew Spurzheim "from his first arrival in this country" and, indeed, had "reason to know that [Spurzheim's] very useful little treatise on education [1821] ... was much influenced by the circumstances of [our] conversations."[8]

George Combe, who in fact did the final editing for the English publication of Spurzheim's treatise on education, was even more cognizant than Spurzheim of the rationales for social reform in Britain. Moreover, as the brother of the Owenite communitarian Abram Combe, George Combe was not only intimately acquainted with Owen's theory and practice, but also was fully alert to the response to Owen's ideas in reformist circles. Aware of how Spurzheim had reoriented Gall's doctrine, Combe anxiously carried the revisions further – to the point of suggesting the possibility through education of quite radical alterations to the primitive nature or original powers of manifestation and the inheritance of acquired characteristics.[9] Since the whole of Combe's phrenological consideration of the constitution of man was in relation to *external* objects, it is hardly to be wondered at that by the 1830s in Britain phrenology was popularly believed to have "left the discoveries of its original expounders at a great distance behind."[10]

As much to the point, however, Owen's "science of society" no less than Gall's "science of mind" was in a state of continual revision in the early nineteenth century as it sought for an ever more coherent philosophical basis upon which to draw for action. In his first publication, *A New View of Society; or, Essays on the Principle of the Formation of the Human Character* (1813), Owen had argued that all the world's evils could be attributed to bad environment and that by changing children's environment in their earliest years a better character could be molded. For the elimination of vice and crime (for which purpose the *Essays* were written) there could be optimism, for "human nature," Owen proclaimed, "is without exception universally plastic."[11] The two main points of Owen's dogma were not, strictly speaking, contrary to anything held by phrenologists. Phrenologists could no more object to the first of these points, that "the old system of the world is founded on the belief that the character of man is formed by himself," than they could possibly disagree with the second – that "the new rational system of society is founded on the knowledge that the character of man is formed for him."[12] Additionally, however, Owen's argument left room for the influence of inborn peculiarities, and to this influence he came to attach increasing importance largely in response to the preaching of phrenology. The finalized form of Owen's psychological propositions that emerged in the early 1830s as the "Five Fundamental Facts" upon which the new society was to be founded contained nothing to which the phrenologists (or almost anyone else) could take exception. Condensed by Owen in the *Book of the New Moral World* (1836–44), the single cardinal "Fact" was a doctrinal compromise: "Man is a compound being, whose character is formed of his constitution or organization at birth, and of the effects of external circumstances upon it from birth to death; such an original organization and external influences continually acting and reacting upon each other."[13] In effect this commonsensical compromise between the secular ideas of Helvetius and Gall (which, as early 1828, was elaborated in an "Address to Phrenologists by an Advocate for the Principle of the Formation of Human Character by the Influence of Circumstances")[14] was a recapitulation of Bentham's belief that the tendencies with which a man is born inclines him to certain types of pleasures, while environment strengthens and weakens or even produces and eliminates such tendencies.[15]

To some, the accommodation of "the absurdities of craniology" by those who believed in the "flattening machine of the original sameness" (as Hazlitt scorned both doctrines, respectively) was the result of both doctrines being utterly deterministic.[16] The feminist and communist Catherine Barmby, for instance, in her article on phrenology in the *Co-operative Magazine* in 1826, showed how readily phrenological conclusions conformed with those of Owen. Like Owenism, she wrote, phrenology illustrates

that the human being is not, in any view, whether of his nature, or of his condition in the universe, free to choose, but that he is *necessarily, what he is*; that his character is created for him by his conformation, as much, or more than by the condition in which he is placed; that he has no self-directing power vested in himself to choose what he would be, or how he would act; that he is impelled to act by the force of those organs which nature has created and combined to form his brain.[17]

In 1840 the Birmingham secretary of Owen's Association of All Classes of All Nations, the Unitarian Hawkes Smith, announced enthusiastically in the *Phrenological Journal* that as far as he was concerned the phrenological doctrine testified to the most important and steadfast of Owen's incantations, that "The Character of

Man is Created For Him and Not By Him." "Phrenology and Owenism," he asserted, "equally involve the doctrine of philosophical necessity, as it is taught by Calvin, President Edwards, Crombie, Priestley, and Southwood Smith; and this is the 'nonresponsibility of man.' "[18]

But, in fact, a truer basis of accord between the doctrines was in the mutual effort of their exponents to *rid* them of gloomy associations with determinism.[19] What Owen and Combe both required, though for different reasons and extending from different determinisms, was to show that in spite of basic nonresponsibility, people were morally accountable. Without some degree of "selfdirecting power" there would be no reason for people to strive for new moral codes. It took Combe eight years to realize that the only way he could justify individual responsibility within phrenological theory was to introduce the doctrine of the effect of external circumstances. With Spurzheim's help he came to see that it was the external factors that influenced the "natural activity of the faculties" producing desire that, "when sanctioned by intellect, constitute Will."[20] Owen required an equivalent balancing from the opposite pole to allow for the effects of a better environment on the mental faculties. "To believe that the character is formed for the individual," he wrote, "does not by any means prevent us from estimating the quality of his action; it only gives us a clue to their origins, and directs us to the means by which to render them such as we desire they should be." The child was thus neither accountable for his organization at birth nor for the circumstances after birth, but the reformer was perfectly justified, he said, "in expressing to him our opinion of his actions, that we might thereby give a motive either to repeat or to alter them according as they are good or bad."[21]

The most complete fusion of Owenism and phrenology along these lines was provided by the mentor of George Eliot, the former Coventry ribbon manufacturer Charles Bray.[‡22] An "honest doubter" who had passed through his crisis of faith by finding new secular moorings in phrenology, Bray was troubled by the need both to have men follow moral injunctions in a secular industrial society and to bring to an end the grosser aspects of the industrial exploitation of labor without interrupting the progress of industrial society. Discovering Owenism in the late 1830s, he felt that through its marriage with phrenology a solution to his problem was to be found and a program for human progress devised. In his most significant work, *The Philosophy of Necessity* (1841), he grafted onto the biological determinism of phrenology Owen's doctrine of circumstances to arrive at a definition of necessity that depended equally upon both. It is unnecessary here to rehearse Bray's argument; at the time it received praise from Owenites and Combeans alike more because of its clarity of exposition than because of its novelty.[23] It should be noted, though, that in terms of its practical implication, Bray's filtering of Combe's philosophy through Owenism resulted in Bray's extolling the view of coordinated individual capital accumulation for the benefit of the community as a whole. The Coventry Labourers' and Artisans' Co-operative Society, which Bray established in 1840, was the implementation of the ethics of cooperative individualism (as distinct from the ethics of labor's struggle against capital for social justice.)[24] Like Herbert Spencer's model industrialism, which made the same ethical plea,[25] the ideal industrial society for which Bray's philosophy and example argued paralleled the ideal physiological structure and function of brain as depicted by phrenology, with mental, and hence human, progress depending on the cooperative interdependence of the parts (within the given structure). Like Combe, Bray asked that restraint be placed on the "natural" Acquisitiveness of people (especially capitalists) in order to eradicate the "unnatural" functional imbalance in the system – in order, that is, to make the capitalist system operate more humanly. Pure reason alone was thus to bring the injustices of class inequality to an end.[26]

We will see that there were specific historical reasons why Bray's marriage of phrenology and Owenism should have been well received by certain Owenites in the early 1840s. For the present it is sufficient to note that Bray's writings were a further manifestation of the accord between phrenology and Owenism that Owenites had long recognized and respected. The *British Co-operator*, for instance, in 1829 considered that phrenologists, had they "rendered no other service to mental science, than that of exactly discriminating each separate state of feeling, they would have done enough to entitle them to the thanks of all succeeding investigations." But, it was added, they had done more: In the face of the political economists' concern with wealth accumulation, and the concern of authority with keeping the emiserated in their place, the phrenologists had gathered together the knowledge that showed the "BEST means of attaining HAPPINESS."[27] Not all Owenites would have gone so far but most appreciated the knowledge as more than merely a helpmate in the creation of a better society. Replacing the view that "some passions and propensities ... [are] innately evil in themselves" with the view that all the mental faculties were in themselves good, some Owenites held phrenology to "prove" (by the presence of "bad" conduct) that faulty mental organization could only be the result of the faulty organization of society.[28] Phrenology was therefore "a test of socialism's practicality," a doctrine flowing from "the same fountain of truth" and streaming in the same egalitarian direction.[29] Thus a contributor to Owen's *New Moral World* in 1835 (shortly after the 1828 "Address" on phrenology's and Owenism's harmony had been reprinted) proposed that phrenology's corroborative proof of materialism and the doctrine of necessity, together with its object of universal happiness, constituted nothing less than a "glorious trinity."[30]

That the glorious trinity was tested in the same fire of religious and social opposition only strengthened Owenite faith in the science. Persons such as the correspondent to the *Morning Chronicle* in 1839 who defined socialists as "a set of mature philosophers whose faith is phrenology, and whose theory (if not practice) is the promiscuous intercourse of the sexes"[31] reinforced the alliance among Owenites by making it seem that the same age-old repression of rational scientific and social truth was at work on both these attempts to discuss openly the functions of the mind and body and to question social organization and orthodox religious control. To the youthful Owenite "social missionaries" Robert Cooper, Frederick Hollick, Holyoake, Charles Southwell, and J. G. Clarke, who were all out to teach that the secular was sacred, this rendered phrenology (in the tradition of the early Carlile) the clinching factor in an advocacy of anticlericalism and materialism.[32] Hence phrenologists such as the Swedenborgian D. G. Goyder, the antimaterialist and antimesmerist J. Q. Rumball, the Low Churchman Charles Cowan, and the Catholic H. W. Dewhurst were led to complain in their phrenology lectures, as the Methodist W. Lowe did in his, of "silly socialists" dragging the science "an unwilling captive, into [their] ... service" in attempts "to prove man's irresponsibility."[33] The Christianizing phreno-mesmerist from Sheffield Spencer T. Hall was another who believed that the socialists had "unhesitatingly received the new theory among them and cherished it with all imaginable fondness" because they took it for granted that "whatever militated against the opinions of mankind at large, must of necessity, help to substantiate theirs."[34] There was a large grain of truth in the charge, yet so long as peripatetic Christian zealots such as the Reverends John Brindley and Brewin Grant toured the country with handbills and diatribes against a phrenology that was "evidently one and the same with the infamous founder of Socialism," it was far more expedient to exploit the abominable alliance than to deny it.[35] At the same time, however, Owenites openly challenged the Christian phrenologists, making it clear that their support – like Carlile's – was for a science that was entirely infidel and undivorced from political struggle.

Beyond these religious, philosophical, and social reasons for Owenite interest in phrenology, there was, finally, the allure of craniology. Given that most Owenites were every bit as intoxicated by the marvels and miracles of science as Zetetics were, the attraction to the craniological mapping of mental faculties is readily understandable. "Only a few years ago we had but four elementary substances in nature," declared a cooperator in 1826,

Now there are proved to be compounds; and we have almost *sixty* elementary substances. So also, by the new and interesting science of phrenology, instead of about four original powers, as perception, memory, judgement, and volition, we have no less than thirty-five powers or faculties, that is distinct organs, clearly marked out in every commonly well organized human brain.

. . . here is work enough, here is abundant scope here is a field of operation sufficiently extensive. Here are thirty-five powers to be developed, to be duly exercised and properly directed, in every human infant. Here are no prejudices to encounter, no errors to root out, no ill-habits to overcome.[36]

Owen himself responded enthusiastically to Spurzheim's and Combe's bump-reading visits to New Lanark between 1820 and 1823. In spite, or perhaps because, of the fact that Combe, during his 1820 visit, managed to upstage Owen by delineating the heads of some of the schoolchildren and thereby converted fellow visitors from the *London Magazine* to a belief in phrenology, Owen was excited enough immediately to purchase books and busts with which to study the science further.[37] It was partly out of this early study that his "psychography" emerged: an attempt to simplify the "recondite speculations" of the Common Sense philosophers with his own phrenological-like list of reified human faculties. He also designed a "psychograph" with which "to exhibit the subject of human nature in a tangible shape" through measuring "the faculties at birth and then determin[ing] how they were altered by circumstances."[38]

Similarly inspired after coming under Combe's influence in Edinburgh in 1821 was A. J. Hamilton of Dalzell, the collaborator with Abram Combe in the first Owenite community in Britain, at Orbiston. Hamilton's initial response was the familiar one of new awareness and rationalization: Feeling that the deep mysteries of life had now been simply solved, he expressed the wish that he had earlier known the true philosophy of mind and knowledge of self so that he might not have "missed that success in life to which he thought he was entitled."[39]

Though Hamilton and Owen subsequently rejected Combeanism as an invidious ideology responsible for leading Owenites away from the pursuit of Owen's social views, neither lost his early enthusiasm for the craniological aspects of the science.[40] Owen and his son Robert Dale typified many Owenites in casting aside their reservations on the science whenever an eminent phrenological delineator presented himself,[41] while the *New Moral World* gave such encouragement to craniology that it twice provided favorable reviews of a *Phrenological Chart* (sixpence colored, ninepence varnished) produced by the former Manchester fustian cutter E. T. Craig.[42] Although Owenites recognized that the exterior reading of the internal faculties was the least defensible aspect of phrenology, they almost gave craniology its final seal of approval when, at the 1843 Congress of Delegates from the Branches of the Rational Society, Walter Newall, the delegate from the London A1 Branch (the John Street Institute) proposed that "a committee be appointed to consider the expediency of applying the principles of phrenology, as a test to ascertain the tendency of character, in Harmony Hall, as well as in any future selection of residency."[43] William Devonshire Saull, the radical London wine merchant and member of the London Phrenological Society who contributed extensively to the erection of both the Hall of Science, City Road, and the John Street Institute, proposed to bequeath his private phrenology museum to Harmony Hall, doubtless believing like the French socialist Etienne Cabet that such communities required *musée de cranologie* for educational purposes.[44] Being surrounded by the hostile, as well as by the freeloading, the offbeat, and the lazy, Owenite communitarians were keenly aware of the need for an easy and rapid means of estimating character. Moreover, there was reason to believe that the only really successful Owenites experiment – the Ralahine Community in County Clare, Ireland, organized by E. T. Craig[‡] between 1831 and 1833 – owed its success entirely to Craig's ability to practically apply phrenology in the screening of candidates and in the assigning of their places in the community's rigid division of labor.[45] It is worth adding that Craig's applications of phrenology at Ralahine were not intended to support the "communistic notions" of Owen, which Craig believed were regrettable "afterthoughts, founded on [Owen's] erroneous ideas of 'Human Nature.' "[46] Ralahine, which the John Street Owenite A. R. Wallace was to praise as the shining example of "pure socialism," was in fact a successful instance of the type of cooperative individualism endorsed by Bray.[47] In effect, it was an agricultual New Lanark that depended for its "success" on phrenological gimmicks such as a "charactograph" (a near-imitation of Owen's "Psychograph" intended to encourage self-discipline and industry by having workers compete against their past performances).[48] To the extent that Owen phrenologically erred by subsequently rejecting the socioeconomic principle underlying such gimmickry, it was perhaps appropriate that upon his death in 1858 a vigil was kept over his coffin and furze bushes scattered over his grave to ward off phrenological headhunters.[49]

COMBE AND OWEN: HARMONY, SHIFT, AND SCHISM

As a rationalist philosophy of character and social reformation, phrenology was to Owenite socialists a harmonizing doctrine – radically expressive, utopian, antitraditionalist, and physiognomically convenient. Paradoxically, Combe's hostility to Owenism in the early 1820s confirms much of this doctrinal harmony and the tandem interests of the respective proponents. At that time Owen, "the Prince of Cotton Spinners," was still the philanthropist and friend of nobles, engaged, as suggested above, in an effort to find the most successful anodynes against social disruption and to instill factory discipline in a laboring population notoriously fractious. Yet while conducting at New Lanark one of the most celebrated experiments in industrial scientific management, Owen was wavering between "an intense desire for the total reorganization of society and a conviction that change needed to be gradual." Having just relinquished a pyramidal view of the "aristocracy resting on the broad base of 'the working and pauper classes,' " he was thinking not of abolishing economic and social inequalities but of the utopian future in which such inequalities would be submerged.[50] To this Owen, concerned with "rules, laws, and what is called order," Combe could only respond with envy. Like others he was "exceedingly delighted" by New Lanark; was as intrigued with it as Lord Brougham, whom he encountered there on his second visit in October 1822.[51] After visiting New Lanark for the third time in 1823, Combe wrote privately, "In Owenism there is a good deal of truth which might be most beneficially applied to the old society,"[52] It was immediately thereafter that he decided to extend his views on phrenology by writing "lectures showing its application to morals, criticism, and political economy."[53]

From the start, Combe's envy of Owen's fame encouraged him to deploy phrenology in a competitive manner. Spurring him on was the disaffection to Owenism in 1821 of his elder brother Abram. Far more spirited and adventurous than his lawyer brother, though no less religiously motivated, Abram turned to Owenism after visiting New Lanark with George in 1820 and after reading Owen's *Report to the County of Lanark* (1821).[54] The Practical Society in Edinburgh, a working-class organization born out of the slump of the early 1820s, provided him with a testing ground for some of the "New Views"; while the Orbiston community (1826–7) was to be a total commitment to their application. In George's view such commitment was excessive and irresponsible; but more irritating personally was Abram's neglect of, if not disdain for, phrenology.[55] Thus in 1823, when Combe first engaged in battle with Owen in the second volume of the *Phrenological Journal*, his writing was characterized by a petty and vindictive spirit. Stressing the importance of innate qualities over the effect of circumstances only so far as a British reformer could dare, and having, as Owen acknowledged, only this "one difference between us," Combe based the greater part of his argument on an appeal to conventional sexual and religious prejudices – views of Owen's "*folly, absurdity* and *immorality*" that Combe knew were wholly untrue from previous conversations and correspondence with Owen.[56] While Owen in his published reply soundly refuted the allegations and redeemed his character, Combe's reputation was permanently blackened among leading Owenites and his popular phrenology made suspect. As A. J. Hamilton pointed out to Combe in a letter written on the back of an article from the *Newcastle Magazine* on the effects of environment on character,

It would have been all very well if you had not said what you have done, respecting Amativeness and a first cause . . . from having *little* (if any) *amativeness yourself*, you are not qualified to write upon the subject *at* all, far less to found objections upon it, to a system of which, you have evidently not made yourself master. . . . You have therefore risked your system by what you have so unnecessarily done![57]

In view of Owen's remarks in the *Report to the County of Lanark* on equality and his expressed desire to put into "immediate practice" the principle "THAT THE NATURAL STANDARD OF VALUE IS, IN PRINCIPLE, HUMAN LABOUR, OR THE COMBINED MANUAL AND MENTAL POWERS OF MEN CALLED INTO ACTION," it is not surprising that Combe should have retaliated with the argument that if Nature had intended "community of property and equality of rank," then the mental faculties for self-preservation would have have been implanted in the brain.[58] Missing from Combe's argument at this point, however, was any underlying sense of urgency; essentially he was attempting only to take the sarcasm out of the critics' snipe: "Why should the public be at the expense of parallelograms, and producing the disorganization of society" when a science of mind exists that if adhered to could, without causing any social upheaval, annihilate every baneful passion obstructing the perfection of human happiness?[59] But it was only a matter of time before the real ideological differences between Owen and himself opened up. The watershed was Abram's death in 1827 and the financial ruin of Abram's family over the Orbiston community. Although at the meeting of the proprietors of Orbiston in 1826 Combe conceded (perhaps only out of politeness) that the "general principles seemed correct," he added that "the tenants would, most assuredly, do best under their own management, as it would be much to their own interest to exert themselves."[60] Three years later he had succeeded in convincing the manager at Orbiston, Alexander Paul, that "from the way that we have all been brought up, and from the differences in our desires and feelings, it will be scarcely possible, under any circumstances, to find an equal number of individuals ... who could go hand in hand with one another in such an experiment."[61] By 1831 Combe was capitalizing on Abram's career and death for convincing-sounding personal insights on human nature in relation to communitarian living.[62] When, in 1837, Hawkes Smith told him that "*your* claims for man ... can never be realized while competition drives us all in its present wild goose chase – Competition can never be destroyed, or checked while the system of individual accumulation exists," Combe thus defended himself:

My opinions are perhaps rendered strong on this point, by having witnessed the mental condition of the Orbiston population. They were totally unprepared for co-operation, and they only consumed the substance of the proprietors. My brother's family were ruined by the experiment and still suffer severely from it.[63]

Meanwhile working-class disaffection in response to the economic crisis of the mid-1820s and in response to the influence of the writings of William Thompson, John Gray, J. F. Bray, James Morrison, and Thomas Hodgskin (who amplified within Owenism the labor theory of value and arguments for economic equality) rallied support to an Owen now to be seen as a radical communitarian and advocate of mutual aid. After 1826 Owen reversed his previous view of the social pyramid to expose "what a powerful burden rested on the labouring class, and how desirable an equal division of property would be."[64] Owen the philanthropist, educator, and factory reformer now became Owen the dreaded "socialist" leading the class-conscious cooperative and trade union movement of the early 1830s and attacking the three most sacred institutions of bourgeois society: private property, religion, and marriage. Though this phase of Owenism withered with the collapse of the National Labour Exchange and the Grand National Consolidated Trades Union in August 1834, and most of those who clung to Owen's doctrine thereafter returned to ideas less concerned with directly attacking capitalist economics, the public impression of Owen and socialism after 1830 was fixed.[65] Nor was this ossification of the image entirely unfounded, for even as Owen turned to paternalistic advocacy of the millennium and claimed to be the exponent of order and harmony between "All Classes of All Nations," he was still able to assert that no principle has ever "produced so much evil as the principle of individualism" and continued to attack the mechanics' institutes, for instance, as supporting the "existing anomalies" and as serving as "instruments for continuing social inequality."[66] Though with his unfailing optimism Owen continued to hope that between phrenologists and the followers of his own views there would be "no necessity for contests of opinion" (thus confirming that there was), phrenologists had good reason to think otherwise and to protect their resource accordingly.[67] Insofar as the only real difference between them and the Owenites in the 1820s had been the matter of the pace of social revolution, in the 1830s the philosophical differences between them over the matter of character formation came to signify ideological positions clearly opposed.[68]

Combe above all was adamant that "Socialism, Fourierism, [and] Owenism" were contrary to human nature. At his most unequivocal – in a letter to William Ellis written on the very day in 1848 when twenty thousand Chartists were marching on Kennington Common – he asserted that whereas "Charles Bray ..., who goes far with us, and ... Robert Chambers, are in favour of an 'organization of labour,' by which they mean some kind of arrangement by which the operatives shall share in the profits produced by the joint action of labour and capital ..., [t]o me it appears that this is impossible." "Brute labour," he added, ought not to reap "the reward which Providence has allotted only to intelligent labour, or labour enlightened, directed and controuled by a cultivated intellect and trained moral sentiments." Lest Ellis should be in any doubt about what was meant by "enlightened labour," Combe explained that he referred to those with the ethics or "mental condition of those in the middle ranks who combine capital and labour."[69] Later that same year, in a letter to Bray, he argued against the importance of the circumstances as in any way assisting the condition of the working class. Their real elevation, he insisted, would consist of "intelligently and perseveringly" training and teaching them "to comply with the natural laws which govern the production and distribution of wealth." Until this was done, no external applications such as land schemes could "rescue them as a class from the natural consequences of infringing these laws." So long as the laborer remained "deficient in morality, industry, intelligence, and self-restraint," neither universal suffrage, good land, the best laws, nor religion would ever save him from"beggary."[70]

So far as is known, Combe never expressed an opinion either way on the uses to which phrenology was put by Owenites. Likely he realized that to have done so would have landed him in same camp as religious reactionaries railing against the "horrible misapplication" of phrenology to the "doctrine and practice of socialism ... that uproot every social and domestic tie ..., destroy all moral accountability ..., overturn the most dearly-cherished institutions, and declare that man is responsible only to himself."[71] To have identified himself with sentiments such as these would not only have been personally reprehensible, but would also have been strategically foolish, for so long as Owenites expressed an interest in phrenology and maintained (as Owen's close colleague George Fleming told Combe in 1837) that "Mr Owen and yourself are preaching exactly the same doctrine,"[72] Combe could hope, not unreasonably, that phrenological truth might succeed in transforming the minds of those persisting in the belief that civilization was still radically imperfect. By not responding to such addresses, Combe could hope to prevent phrenology from being more clearly recognized than it already was as a symbol of bourgeois ideology over which socialist controversy and consciousness might be raised. In part his hopes were founded, as we shall see; but his tactic of silence (if tactic it was) was insufficient to prevent Owenites from attacking his particular phrenological views as a "nauseating mass of cant and humbug."[73]

Before we turn to that, however, it is worth remarking briefly on the strength of other factors that prevented the rise of an ideologically symbolic antiphrenology among Owenites and that, among Owenite rank and file at least, served to efface the reality of the contest between Combeans and Owenites over the control of the legitimating resource of brain physiology. Perhaps most important was the fact that other phrenologists were usually much less explicit and overt than Combe about their politicoeconomic views. Though many of them, as we noted in Chapter 5, similarly buffeted their liberalism against Owenism and came in the 1830s and 1840s similarly to lay new emphasis on the importance of

nature over nurture as a part of a process of blocking out contradictions in their theory, by retaining a low public profile on these
issues they inadvertently ensured that the outspoken Combe would
be singled out as exceptional. Some phrenologists, such as the
Woods, Joshua and Hawkes Smith, and Bray openly asserted that
phrenology "demonstrates the erroneousness of most of the principles of [bourgeois] political economy."[74] Thereby, they helped
to affirm the utility of neutral phrenological "facts" distinct from
the"values" attached to the science by Combe. Certainly, Combe
was isolated in his hostility to cooperatives. As men like Smiles,
Bray, and Chambers were aware, cooperatives were a means of
having workers look to themselves in times of need instead of
becoming a burden on society.[75] The reviewer of Bray's *Philosophical Necessity* in the *Phrenological Journal*, oblivious to the so-
lidaristic significance of cooperatives to workers, desired only that
"for the deep-seated disease that threatens [society's] dissolution"
slightly *more* weight be attached to remedies other than the "natural
union of labour and labour's fruit, capital, in the same individuals,
in an enlightened system of cooperation" – remedies such as political reform, free trade, education, religion, and emigration.[76]

Further blurring the differences between Owenite and phrenological reform was the fact that at appropriate moments Combean
phrenologists were not adverse to lauding Owen as a great educationalist and reformer. No less a promoter of an iron clad bourgeois rule than James Simpson, for example, singled out Owen
in a speech on secular education in 1837 as "the most eminent
illustration of benevolence which this or any former age has produced."[77] That such cordiality was worth the effort is attested to
in the fact that no less a hard-nosed Owenite than Isaac Ironside
was so pleased with Simpson's performance that he immediately
took up the study of phrenology.[78]

It was by no means clear, therefore, where phrenologists stood
in relation to specific social and political philosophies. If, in looking
for the answer, one searched the phrenological literature too
broadly, they appeared, indeed,to stand everywhere. Such was the
realization of a dazed reviewer in 1841 who, like others before
him, could only conclude that

the theory of mind of one phrenologist may be wide as the poles asunder
from that entertained by another, as long as the fact is acknowledged

that the brain is the most direct organic medium of mental agency. For instance, one phrenologist may conceive the mind of man to be chiefly swayed by events from without, or that he is the creature of external circumstances. Other phrenologists may hold him to be in a greater degree the creature of his own internal organization. Another may conceive him to be predominantly the creature of his own will, whilst others may maintain, that man is most strongly, though secretly, affected by spiritual influences.[79]

Interestingly, this reviewer accused Combe of espousing "an equal distribution of property" and presumed that it was because of that "disorganization of society" that "Mr Combe's book [was] so much in favour with the disciples of Mr Robert Owen."[80]

But if much Owenite interest in phrenology depended on Combe not appearing as the only spokesman for the science, as much depended again on the specious reality of "Owenism." Arthur Bestor's careful observations on the rapidity with which Owen moved from one position to another, E. P. Thompson's distinguishing of Owen from "Owenism," and the reminders by J. F. C. Harrison and others that " 'Owenism' provided a reservoir from which different groups and individuals, including working men, could draw ideas and inspiration which they then applied as they chose" all caution us against supposing "Owenism" to be socially or politically coherent.[81] Typically, at the 1832 Co-operative Congress, William Pare could express his opinion on the "fallacy" of identity of interests between the exploited working class and the exploiting middle-class capitalist, at the same time that the Baptist preacher and future lecturer on phrenology Joseph Marriott[‡] could assert that cooperators were not "levellers," had no desire to deprive others of property, and only wished to "embrace all ranks and conditions of men."[82] The latter, softer position tended to predominate among the Owenite rank and file,[83] but was itself manifested in a wide range of particular interests. This diversity is reflected among the various Owenites who lectured or wrote specifically on phrenology, among them the secularists Holyoake,[‡] J. G. Clarke,[‡] and Robert Cooper, the feminist and Baptist-turned-freethinker Emma Martin,[‡] the former Methodist and future Chartist schoolmaster William Lovett, the Unitarians W. Hawkes Smith[‡] and a Mr. McArthur[‡] of Halifax, the cooperators Craig[‡] and Catherine Barmby, and the democrat and mesmerist J. N. Bailey.[‡] One could add, on the basis of their financial and moral support for Owenite projects, the names of Bray, the aristocrat and temperance advocate Arthur Trevelyan, and even the eccentric Pierre Henri Baume,[‡] who lectured on the science at the Westminster Institution in Milbank in 1835. Different again were the Owenite advocates of phrenology attached to the Ham Common Concordium presided over by the "Sage of Burton Street," the former merchant and Pestalozzian educator James Pierrepont Greaves (1772–1842). Like Flaxman before him, Greaves (who was elected a member of the LPS in May 1826) had waded deep into the spiritualist writings of Jakob Bohme, William Law, and Emanual Swedenborg and had come out with, among other things, a phrenology so intellectually alternative at one level, so absurdly religiosymbolic at another, and so banal at yet another as to make it virtually incomprehensible to the world outside.[84] To the "sacred socialists" of Ham Common, however – among whom were the Owenite missionaries Alexander Campbell, Goodwyn Barmby, and William Galpin – this phrenology was not a part of a muddled enthusiasm, but rather was at one with their vegetarianism, temperance, chastity, mesmerism, hydropathy, and religiocommunism in being a part of a total rejection of conventional social norms and in being a rejection of the reigning positivist metaphysics of capitalism – albeit the latter stemmed almost inadvertently from the loathing of the authority of conventional materialist rationality and experimental science. Although socially and intellectually there were many particular points of difference between this phrenology and that preached within Carlile's Allegorical Christianity, behind both was much the same revulsion at the consigning of man to an inanimate and materialist, impersonal and mechanical nature and the same desire to recover a spiritual wholeness that had somehow been destroyed through the advance of industrial civilization.[85] Significantly, it was among these nineteenth-century equivalents of the seventeenth-century Commonwealthmen that Eliza Sharples found refuge after Carlile's death in 1843.[86]

Though unusually expressed, the interest taken in phrenology by the "First Concordians" was by no means radically at odds with the interest taken in the science by other Owenites (including those who by the late 1830s were acclaiming Comtean positivism specifically in connection with human intelligence).[87] Although for the majority Owenites phrenology was, as Thompson has

observed, "the last and conclusive link" in their chain of argument
for a more rational secular society, historical views drawn from
the late-nineteenth-century milieu of William Morris ought not to
obscure the fact that for socialists in the earlier part of the century,
the imagining of the "rational" always involved to lesser or greater
degrees an adherence to the "irrational" or "nonrational" as a part
of the repudiation of the "rational society" of bourgeois competitive capitalism.[88] Within the "Universal Community of Rational
Religionists," as Owenites styled themselves in the early 1840s,
many had no difficulty in combining an interest in "bread and
cheese reform" with a broader millenarian interest in spiritual
development.[89] The building of the alternative or really rational
society always involved both, the imagined New Moral World
being a harmonious integration of the material and the spiritual,
the rational and the sensual, the scientific and the human. Thus
we cannot simply assume that Owenite praise for phrenology as
a "rational and consistent key" to physical, mental, and moral
reform was necessarily a regard for the science premised upon the
same rationalism as that celebrated by the Combeans or, to the
extent that it was, that it was only that.[90] Indeed, the critique of
Combe's phrenology, to which we can now turn, was in large
part an expression of contempt for a science that had too obviously
become only a manifestation of bourgeois rationality functioning
against "the schemes which we [Owenites] propose for amending
the condition of humanity."[91]

REACTION AND REFRACTION

In her 1830 article on phrenology in the American Owenite journal
The Free Inquirer, the shrewd socialist Fanny Wright saw cause to
protest "against the habit, so current among us, of entering the
paths of science, as we do those of faith, prepared to see more
than can be seen, and to believe in the absence of demonstration."[92]
The analogy with religion may have been only coincidental, but
there was certainly more than a hint of suspicion of "the *nature*"
of phrenology. Though she did not say so explicitly, it is clear
that she perceived a possible threat to socialism from the knowledge. Owen, too, had been aware of this ever since the skirmish
with Combe in the early 1820s. So was his son, Robert Dale –
the coeditor with Fanny Wright of *The Free Inquirer*. Thanking

Combe for a copy of his *Essay on Human Responsibility* in 1827, the younger Owen took the opportunity to criticize as "totally indefensible" what he called Combe's "magnified optimism." In arguing that "all practical evil is universal good and all present suffering the certain and direct cause of future happiness," Combe, according to Robert Dale Owen, merely "affirm[ed] that what is, must be, because it is." To Robert Dale Owen, as to his father, this religious incantation was Combe's great folly. Since they had come to disbelieve in the divine wisdom of competitive industrial capitalism as a basis for social life, they could see no possible foundation for Combe's optimism unless it could be proven that "misery and suffering are in themselves good and desirable."[93] For Combe and other phrenologists to claim that man's nature – his biology – was not adapted for a different state of things was to accept the competitive system and possibly reform its imperfections but not to deal with the economic causes of the social ills. The Owenite formula of changing the social and economic relations so as to change man's nature could, as a corrective means, be the only source of genuine optimism.

But it was not until the 1830s, when the real and the symbolic success of the *Constitution of Man* was becoming manifest, that the Owenite leadership began openly to express serious reservations about Combe's phrenological naturalism. Appearing in the *New Moral World* early in 1835 was a "Dialogue ... between the founder of 'The Association of All Classes of All Nations,' and a stranger desirous of being accurately informed respecting its origin and objects," one of whose primary aims was to draw back into more constructive socialist channels those seen as being led astray by phrenology. Thus the stranger in the dialog is made to ask: "Why have you introduced so much of the subject of phrenology into our present discourse?" Owen's reply could not have been clearer: "Because, as phrenology is now taught by its advocates, it is made to occupy that place in the public mind which belongs to a science that will effect far more for the improvement of the human character than it is possible for so weak and imperfect an instrument as phrenology ever to accomplish." It was a weak and imperfect instrument, he added, because it could "advance no further than to conjecture what are the proportions and powers of the human mind.... And as soon as society shall be put into a healthy and rational state, that state to which the world is slowly approaching, phrenology will be rendered almost useless through the operations of the 'science of the influence of circumstances.' " Implicitly acknowledging the ideological contest between the respective "scientisms," Owen was here, in effect, choosing to undermine the credibility of the competitor's social resource rather than suggesting that it be appropriated and alternatively deployed. As if pronouncing over the science's grave, he acknowledged phrenology's great service in directing attention to the study of the mind and to the "gross errors of the present mode of education," in assisting with the study of the laws of organic life, and in revealing the necessity of changing society in accordance with the "eternal, unchanging laws of nature, instead of the ignorant and ephemeral laws of man." But in the final analysis this was not enough: Phrenology had not advanced beyond being a critique of the old society; its anticlericalism and antiaristocracy had gone nowhere to eradicate the inequalities manifested by the new political economy. It was thus to be condemned because, having captured the attention of the public, it was leading them "to consider the present transitory condition of the human character, and of society, as their fixed state ['the natural arrangement of human affairs'] when it is extremely probable that man and society are upon the eve of the most extraordinary changes that have ever occurred in the history of both."[94]

Nowhere else in the contemporary literature up to this time had phrenology's ideological function in relation to the social aims of radicals been so precisely described and exposed. Once exposed, however, companion writing followed, though not before the unholiness of the "glorious trinity" of accord between the doctrines had been fully confirmed by Combe himself in his lectures in the Birmingham Mechanics' Institute in June 1838. In these Combe stated unequivocally that it was the "intention of Divine Providence that the present state of society should exist," and added that workers should be content with their lot in the existing social hierarchy:

If all (said Mr Combe) were to try and be Shakespeares, Chantreys, &c., how should we be supplied with ploughmen, weavers, and builders – how would the social machine be kept moving? ... If all became ladies and gentlemen, who will perform the disagreeable duties of society? who will labour in coal mines? &c., &c.[95]

The "faugh" with which the *New Moral World* greeted these remarks on its front page was unequivocal expression of contempt
for a philosophy now recognized as radically at odds with the
"entire change in the character and condition of mankind" and
with the "equitable, and natural system of united property" to
which Owen had become firmly attached.[96] "It seems to us most
unphilosophical to argue, from the experience of a *difference in
capacity*, that therefore an *inequality in social condition* should follow." Having "at no period been highly impressed with Mr
Combe's moral status as a lecturer," they now saw no reason to
heed him at all.

It was following upon Combe's lectures that Owen's *Dialogue*
strategically appeared as a separate pamphlet. Also issued at that
time was a far more trenchant publication by John Lowther Murphy, a Birmingham dentist and member of Owen's Central Board.[97]
Along with Hawkes Smith, Murphy had been on the committee
of the Birmingham Mechanics' Institute when they invited Combe
to lecture, and upon Combe's arrival he had a front-row seat from
which to observe the country's leading phrenologist. What he
observed did not impress him; indeed, it was Murphy who encouraged Holyoake to write to the *Birmingham Journal* when, after
eagerly serving as Combe's demonstrator for fourteen nights, Holyoake had been offered as remuneration only a chipped plaster
cast and a well-thumbed copy of the *Elements of Phrenology*. Insult
was added to injury when Combe further failed to donate anything
to the Institute Fund after having been given the use of the lecture
hall gratuitously and having handsomely profited from the lectures.[98] Not surprisingly, therefore, Murphy in his *An Essay towards a Science of Consciousness* (1838) boldly attacked phrenology,
calling it a mass of untruths, false assumptions, metaphysical nonsense, and idiotic blunders.[99] It irritated Murphy as much as it did
Owen (to whom the *Essay* was dedicated) that in spite of the
audacious exhibitions of phrenological charlatanry – the phrenologist being "generally surrounded by a gaping multitude, of
bump-feeling people" – that yet the system had numerous admirers. That people could be duped by phrenology's naturalistic
and rationalistic extrapolations, Murphy could understand, but it
was almost inconceivable to him how these people could endorse
the "fanaticisms" of phrenologists when there was plenty of evidence to show that their and their children's own livelihoods,

reputations, and futures were often put at stake by phrenological "professors" working in the interests of some master or mistress. Like Godwin before him, Murphy deplored the arrogant presumption of phrenologists to judge and pronounce upon other people's lives, as if they were priests.[100]

At the core of Murphy's attack on phrenology, however, was his concern with the science's perpetration of a supposedly "natural" system of ethics based on rewards and punishments. Reminiscent of Robert Dale Owen's remark to Combe in 1827 that "you seek to vindicate the wages of God to man," Murphy pointed out that phrases such as "obedience to organic law" and "punishment for disobeying physical laws" were merely secularized forms of orthodox theology, the phrenological popularization of which demonstrated "the ignorance of the people, and of the irrationalness of the system that makes them thus ignorant."[101] Anticipating Mill's essay "On Nature" by more than a decade, Murphy went to the heart of the matter to show that the seeming truth of the phrenological philosophy stemmed from a mistaken "metaphorical use of the term laws to signify a general fact." The "distinction between the metaphorical and literal expressions of 'law' not being known to the majority of people," phrenologists had been able to hoodwink the public into a belief that their ethics were based on some objective neutral authority when in fact their use of "nature" was completely subjective.[102] The phrenological insistence on obedience to natural law, Murphy implied, was a means of establishing social control through the same priestly arbitrated system of rewards and punishments as in theology. Alas, Murphy's own faith in a scientific–secular morality did not allow him to call into question the subjective basis of morality itself. Nor was he in any position to demystify the structural mediations in the science or the organismic metaphors it circulated, since he himself anchored his morality in part on phrenological evidence of human nature![103] Moreover, his own place in the Owenite priesthood forbade any condemnation of mediators or mediating structures between one person and another. Nevertheless, his insight was sufficient to further Owen's exposure of the antisocialist function of natural law in phrenological rhetoric and to confirm the suspicions of Fanny Wright that faith in phrenology was making it difficult for people to perceive the existing system as irrational and both in need of and capable of remedy.

Although such preaching may only have been to the converted, evidence from the early 1840s suggests that many Owenites had taken it to heart or had independently arrived at similar conclusions. The Sheffielder and former stove-grate fitter Isaac Ironside, for instance, after zealously taking up phrenology in the late 1830s, abandoned it shortly thereafter on the grounds not only that it was "not capable of rigid demonstration," but that the political and social views of its major advocates were deeply suspect. "The cant which the advocates of the science have employed," he said, "confirmed ... my views."[104] Similarly, the secretary of the Manchester Hall of science wrote in 1842:

Any one who has carefully studied Phrenology, as hitherto propounded, must have been struck with the strange interweaving of many valuable truths with a system filled with inconsistencies, and distinguished by the duplicity and sycophancy of its advocates, in their endeavours to make it acceptable to both orthodox and heterodox.[105]

On the other hand, though, there were those who strongly reacted to any such strictures on phrenology, one writer in the *New Moral World* in 1838 going so far as to say that Murphy had provided nothing but his own dogmatism to overturn "the observations of innumerable facts [of phrenologists] ... who had no motive in their assertions but the development of truth."[106]

Ironically, within a few years, and shortly after Combe had been indicted for preaching "the *irresponsibility* of Socialism,"[107] it was this latter view (though newly qualified) that was to be almost universally held by Owenites. But it was by no act of Combe's that the trick was effected, nor by any sudden change of heart among Owenites. What brought phrenology back into the Owenite fold and caused even men such as Ironside to embrace the science anew was Engledue's address to the Phrenological Association in June 1842 in which (as Ironside put it) "completely severed [was] the connection between cant and phrenology."[108] As the phrenological opposition helped to confirm, "Dr. Engledue's proposition savours much of necessity;... he has broached doctrines untrue, and upon which the whole fabric of Socialism is built."[109] For the rest of the decade radicals were to take Engledue's phrenology as the standard by which to judge all other phrenological production, especially those of Combe and his

Christian apologists. Thereby the sanctity of the resource itself was not only preserved, but reinforced.[110]

It wasn't only Engledue's uncompromising materialism that re-kindled Owenite enthusiams for phrenology: Equally important was the call he made, in the face of the close-mindedness of the scientific, medical, and clerical professions, for instituting free and open inquiry into the mesmeric or "magnetic excitement of cer-ebration." Following upon Ironside's report (in the *New Moral World* in December 1842) on the investigations into phreno-mesmerism that had been conducted by the members of the Shef-field Hall of Science, the "surpassing interest" in the subject that Engledue confessed was matched by Owenites nearly everywhere. Typically, it was reported by the secretary of the Rational Reli-gionists of Sunderland that

> we consider that this [phreno-mesmerism] will be one of the most – if not *the most* – powerful agents in disseminating correct views of human nature, and indirectly, yet surely, destroying those old pernicious doc-trines that have, in all ages, degraded humanity, and spread misery and suffering among the human race.[111]

Phreno-mesmerism clearly delighted Owenites, not only be-cause it was heterodox and drew large crowds to their Halls of Science, but as well because it involved active participation in a process of scientific experimentation and psychological discovery. Moreover, the scientific principles being sought to account for the phenomenon seemed themselves to be of an active, sentient kind.[112] In theory at least, phreno-mesmerism had the potential to obli-terate the distinction between the world of spirit and its priestly overseers, on the one hand, and the human and material order on the other. Thus, possibly as much by its nature as by the demo-cratic manner of its pursuit, phreno-mesmerism was to appear scientifically "alternative" in a way that, thanks to Combe, phren-ology on its own had ceased to be. Reconceived through mes-merism, "Phrenology *can* be rigidly demonstrated," Ironside maintained; "by mesmeric aid, the developments of every indi-vidual *can be correctly* ascertained . . ., [and] a system of education *can* be based upon it." In his opinion, it was "of the highest im-portance that the scientific portion of our Society [of Rational Religionists] should make it a prominent subject of investiga-tion."[113] Thus shorn of Combeanism and religious cant, and turned

around in opposition to them, phrenological truth was rediscovered. Yet for the most part, it was *only* phrenological truth that
was rediscovered; the truth was not reconstituted. By the activity
of Owenite demi-Galls discovering dozens of new mental faculties
through phreno-mesmerism, the metaphorical and metaphysical
basis of phrenology was only reinforced. The belief of some Owenites that through phreno-mesmerism they were determining
psychological reality for themselves was almost wholly illusion-
ary. It is noticeable, too, that none of them raised any objection
to Engledue's insistence on the need to remodel society according
to the laws of hereditary descent, which, "in the course of three
of four generations," he believed, would allow "Nature's aristocracy" to rise to the top and would permit throughout society "high
moral and intellectual preeminence."[114] The objection that came
from the secretary of the Manchester Hall of Science was different
in kind. He was willing to give credence to Engledue's phrenology
over that of other phrenologists, but he felt that the whole business
of phrenology and phreno-mesmerism was a mistake for Owenites, since by pandering to audience excitement it distracted them
from the serious business of preaching socialism and learning how
to construct the new moral world. "In its present stage," he wrote,
"it is to be feared the Rational Society would only encumber itself
by the connexion [with phreno-mesmerism]."[115]

By this date, however, few rank-and-file Owenites were prepared to take much notice of such caution. Whereas when Murphy
and Owen had voiced their similar criticisms only a few years
before there had been enthusiasm for the latest Owenite experiment – the Queenwood community at East Tytherly in Hampshire
– by the early 1840s many Owenites had become disillusioned
with the whole movement. Ostensibly this disillusionment relates
to the increasingly autocratic manner adopted by Owen's Central
Board as it attempted to deal with the financial problems over
Harmony Hall (Queenwood's lavish showpiece). Clearly this
rubbed many Owenites the wrong way. Occurring as it did in
the midst of the socioeconomic disorder that was giving steam to
the Chartist political movement, there is no cause to censure those
radicals such as Lovett and Hetherington who turned away from
Owen at this point on the grounds that he was refusing to face
up to political and social realities.[116] However, in view of negative
comments such as those of Craig's on Owen's "communistic no-

tions," compared to Engel's fond recollection of the "clearcut communism" of Harmony Hall "[that] left nothing to be desired," it would seem that as much historical weight should be placed on the opposition to Owen's primary social objectives as on his "neo-paternalism."[117] In hindsight, at least, this line of argument seems borne out by the many Owenites who at this time came to feel that it would be more "realistic" for the advance of socialism to put greater effort into disseminating materialist phrenology. The reasoning of these Owenites was also pragmatic and justifiable, for in spite of the realities with which Chartists were contending, the early 1840s experienced a new wave of attacks on "socialism" (popularly deplored as infidelism) in which the antagonists often focused on phrenology and phreno-mesmerism.[118] In response to this "irrationality" even the secretary of the Manchester Hall of Science came around to the opinion that phreno-mesmerism was an appropriate subject for Owenites to concern themselves with.[119] Richard Redburn, the secretary of the John Street Institute, could thus report to the *Phrenological Journal* in 1842 that interest in phrenology among radically minded workers was such as to constitute "an undercurrent ... which no one but those who watch the proceedings of the people can have any idea of, and even they not to the full extent." In his own institute a phrenology class had been established shortly after Epps's lectures there in 1840, and it enrolled fifty members, "mostly mechanics," per quarter-term. But it was "not only in this institution," Redburn maintained, "but in some others of the same society, that the study of Phrenology is pursued." Thus it happens, he added, that "many of the admirers of Mr Owen agree with him as far as he had gone; but there are some who, like myself, do not think he has gone far enough, in laying more stress upon the necessity of understanding the nature and functions of the human brain, which, we must agree, is acted upon by education and external circumstances."[120] Unwittingly, perhaps, Redburn, by calling for Owen's "radicalization" as a phrenology-brandishing freethinker, obfuscated the anticapitalist aspect of Owenite socialism, thereby obliterating the ideological distinction between Owenism and Combeanism and assisting the latter's hegemony. Naturally, therefore, Redburn's communication was greeted with open delight by Robert Cox, then the editor of the *Phrenological Journal*. If it were true, as Cox was certain it was, that socialists held doctrines at variance with human nature, then there was "no better means of dispelling their delusions than to encourage among them the study of Phrenology."[121]

It is doubtful, of course, that radical "delusions" were ever dispelled quite as fully as Combeans would have wished, perhaps not even among Owenites of Redburn's sort. The possibilities of artisan culture were always wide, and elements of compliance with naked or mediated forms of the dominant ideology could readily coexist in individuals and groups in ways that transcend their immediate appearance (as we observed in reference to Carlile's interest in phrenology and noted in passing in reference to A. R. Wallace).[122] What is certain, though, is that during the early 1840s, at the same time as Owen's plans for an alternative communistic society were crumbling, Owenite arguments for the socialist tendency of phrenology became as foreign, if not as seemingly absurd, as Carlile's earlier attempt to prove that phrenology was at the root of the science of God. Indeed, Owen's close associate Lloyd Jones, the former critic of Carlile's anti-Owenite phrenology, observed in 1843 that the apathy to social principles in the branches of the Rational Society was increasing, in part, because some had "split up into phrenological committees."[123] Such an observation makes it difficult to dismiss as one-sided Redburn's report on the direction of Owenism in relation to phrenology. Taken with much other evidence, it tends, rather, to confirm the observation of E. P. Thompson that the phrenologizing career of a person such as E. T. Craig is "almost designed to serve as a symbol of the worker's struggle in the nineteenth century."[124] Not only Owenites of greater historical significance than Redburn – men such as Joseph Marriot, Lovett, Holyoake, and Charles Southwell – but also such Chartists as Arthur O'Neill‡ and Thomas Cooper all felt in essence, if not in so many words, that Owen's lamentable shortcoming was (as Craig put it) his failure to apprehend the "practical consequences" of phrenology.[125] Since to them it seemed that the *Constitution of Man* had revealed (as Lovett confessed to Combe) the "first clear ideas of [our] own nature," their reaction to Owen was all too predictable.[126] So, too, it might be said, were the future careers of these men. Lovett's was typical: Believing that Combe's phrenology had rendered education a "science" for "the first time in history," he abandoned political Chartism and in 1842 established the National Hall Holborn, a place for adult education complete with its own phrenology class. In 1848, at the height of Chartist activity, he opened in the National Hall what was regarded as the first Combean secular day school for children. To further "prostitute his great intellect," as some Chartists accused him, he devoted himself to the production of works such *Elementary Anatomy and Physiology* (1851), in which it was emphasized that "all of the diseases which afflict humanity" could be traced *"to the neglect or infringement of some of the great physical and moral laws of the universe."*[127]

None of these radicals (not even Lovett), however, can be said to have simply "surrendered" to middle-class values. Rather, in a social context in which the applications of egalitarian and anti-capitalist logic seemed increasingly impractical, critical evaluations of the structure of society and insistence on social and political transformations were allowed to be submerged in enthusiasm for a materialist phrenological physiology and secular naturalism that mediated a faith in the virtues of competition and hierarchy as spurs to individual self-improvement and achievement.[128] In reality, the Lovetts, Southwells, and Holyoakes of mid-century were heirs to the early Carlile.[129] Like him, their view of social relations, which was rooted in the preindustrial past of independent artisans, was reconfirmed through phrenology. But in virtually closing down the debate over phrenology's veracity in order, as they thought, simply to exploit the science for the ends of secular self-improvement, they diminished the inheritance. On the one hand, they lost sight of the social prerequisites for phrenology in radical culture, allowing the materialism, secularism, and the virtues of "physical puritanism" to become ends in themselves. Lost, on the other hand, largely because of this, was the desire to fit phrenology within a broader, potentially alternative social conception of "rationality." With Combe's or Engledue's phrenology as the pole star of Reason and Truth, radicals of the stamp of Lovett and Holyoake were blinded to the need to seek for spiritual antidotes to the forces of alienation in capitalist society. To them the deployments of phrenology by the later Carlile or by the Concordians became incomprehensible.[130] A dialectical richness in phrenology's meaning and use by radicals was thus transformed one-dimensionally; phrenology reverted to the materialist terrain of Paine, Thelwall, and the early Carlile, but through that backward rotation of phrenology's wheel of fortune more than one of the vital spokes that had distinguished its working-class from its bourgeois deployment and significance had gone missing.[131]

For the most part, only rhetoric remained – rhetoric not of natural rights, nor of social contracts, nor of wars against private property, but (as Craig championed it through phrenology) of struggles against the powers withholding from the many the knowledge that prepares the way "for mental freedom, by breaking the chains and destroying the despotisms that shackled thought and terrified reason."[132] Such rhetoric, indistinguishable from that of the Combes, the Martineaus, and the Broughams, directed aggression into socially harmless channels and masked reconciliation to the prevailing social order. Indeed, through this rhetoric's equating of "socialism" with the "secularism" coined and celebrated by Combe, socialism itself was rendered innocuous. As Holyoake put it in 1844, with less irony that he supposed, "It is a pleasant thing to write on Socialism. There is no fear of offending anyone."[133]

Yet if, in the final analysis, the examination of phrenology among early-nineteenth-century radicals goes further to illustrate than refute the role of bourgeois ideology as mediated through positivist conceptions of human nature, it also reveals that from the point of view of challenging this "metaphysical citadel" of bourgeois hegemony, all was not darkness after Blake's critique of the metaphysics of Newton. Although modern scientistic capitalist culture may well have encountered its first and last great symbolic act of "negation" in the execution of Lavoisier, responses to science thereafter were not passive, nondiscriminating, and deferential. Especially among those most imbued with a vision of social relations and human fulfillment alternative to that conditioned by industrial capitalism, critical flashes of "illiterate inspiration" on positivist science continued to appear.[134] The irony is that the body of natural knowledge that seems most to have elicited these critical responses in the pre-Darwinian period was the same as that which did most, overtly and covertly, to discourage critical reflection on both science and society. In being so compelling for use in the attack on traditional religious authority, in contributing to pragmatic interest in science, and in consolidating popular faith in the material and moral certainties of biology, phrenology helped to deflect working people's attention away from material historical forces and onto individual pathology. But more than this, by leading them to share the ruling class's image of the nature of cerebral reality, it led them to give tacit consent to the ruling class's right to judge them. Thereby above all did phrenology tighten the corset on working people's ability collectively to determine their own history and reality.

CONCLUSION

The Physiognomy and Phrenology of today are rash and mechanical systems but they rest on everlasting foundations.
> Ralph Waldo Emerson, October 1839: *Journals*, vol. 6 (1966), 285

Remember, that history may leave an important trace ..., that
conditions change and that the conditions necessary to the initi-
ation of some process may be destroyed by the process itself.
> R. Lewotin and R. Levins, "The Problem of Lysenkoism," in
> Hilary Rose and Steven Rose, eds., *The Radicalisation of Science:*
> *Ideology of/in the Natural Sciences* (1976), 60

It is possible ... that man may find an additional magic that will
bring back under his control the vast forces he has unleashed upon
reality. This power, though, is not identical with the one that
first set these forces in motion. And, of course, it can also happen
that man drowns in the floods that he himself has produced.
> Peter Berger, *The Social Reality of Religion* (1969), p. 10

From the perspective of the first half of the nineteenth century,
nothing appears more certain than that during the second half of
the century phrenology entered a precipitous decline. From the
aspiration to science the whole of it slipped into an easily ridiculed
art of character analysis. "At this moment the so-called sciences
of psychology and phrenology stand before the world as hopeless
failures," wrote the anthropologist James Hunt in 1867, adding
that "this is felt, not only by independent thinkers, but even by
the general public, and in many cases by psychologists and phrenologists themselves."[1] Among the "independent thinkers" were
G. H. Lewes and Herbert Spencer. Though Lewes, from a positivist perspective, regarded Gall as revolutionary in assigning the
study of mental functions to biology and in posing the problem of
cerebral localization, he regarded phrenology as a radically imperfect
science promoted by bigots. Likewise Spencer: Although, as Hunt

noted, "there is, perhaps, no modern writer on psychology who has so blindly accepted the fundamental principles of phrenology as he has done," in his *Psychology* (1855) Spencer spoke out strongly against "the unscientific reasonings of the phrenologists" and, like Lewes, condemned its advocates as simple-minded dogmatists.[2]

Among the many phrenologists confirming Hunt's verdict was Charles Bray. As he saw it, in 1885,

phrenology has now fallen into disrepute, first because the clergy have given it a bad name as leading to materialism; and secondly, it has been followed for gain by incompetent "Professors," who profess to reveal a great deal more than phrenology in its present state is able to tell even were such men its competent exponents.[3]

Others sought to cast the blame for phrenology's "failure" squarely onto "materialists, free-thinkers, and infidels" (and onto Engledue in particular); still others attributed it wholly or in large part to the science becoming mixed up with mesmerism (again indicting Engledue as a chief culprit).[4] By no means everyone felt, as many in the medical profession did, that it had been Gall's "sad misfortune" to have had his doctrine made popular; and seemingly unique was the opinion of J. M. Robertson, the historian of freethought, member of Parliament, and vice-president of the British Phrenological Association in the 1890s: Asking himself why phrenology had "so completely lost its status," he had

no hesitation in saying that the process was practically an economic one. That is to say, phrenology was gradually cold-shouldered by the scientific classes, especially the medical, when it was found that in itself it did not "pay," and that to profess it was to be clerically ostracised. . . . in France, as in Britain, the main cause of the decline of phrenology was clearly the religio–economic pressure.[5]

Unanimous, however, were both supporters and opponents of phrenology in their denunciation of the "peripatetic charactervendors," the "head manipulators on the sands," the "phrenomesmerists and fortune-tellers" who were held to have vulgarized the knowledge beyond all former recognition.[6]

But if after mid-century phrenology was no longer intellectually and socially robust in the ways that it once had been, it cannot on that account be dismissed historically. No less than early-nineteenth-century expressions of antiphrenology, late-nineteenth century expressions of contempt for the "humbug" of phrenology are cultural signals, the dismissal of which on that basis would be no less intellectually arrogant than the dismissal of phrenology from the earlier part of the century.

Like Paracelsianism in the seventeenth century and astrology in the eighteenth century, after the major scientific, social, and theological battles over them had been fought in the centuries preceding, phrenology in the second half of the nineteenth century became in many ways more deeply entrenched than ever in everyday thought and expression.[7] As many observed at the time, while the nomenclature and basic cerebral principles of phrenology permeated Western language, the naturalism celebrated by Combean phrenology insinuated itself unobtrusively into the public mind, becoming, not unlike Newtonianism in the eighteenth century or structuralism in the twentieth, one of those powerful but largely "unseen influences on modern thought."[8] More quantifiable was the continued growth in the second half of the century of the imaginative and practical appeals of the knowledge. Even before Lorenzo Fowler[‡] and his brother-in-law Sam Wells (1820-75) stepped off the boat from New York in Liverpool in 1860 and set about bringing to an end the brief hiatus in phrenology's popularization in Britain, Alexander Bain could write in *Fraser's Magazine* that the "phrenological partition of mind" was so well known to the general public that all attempts "either to confirm or impugn it, have a chance of being readily understood."[9] In the aftermath of the revival staged by Fowler and Wells, public awareness and enthusiasm for phrenology was that much higher. Indeed, "so popular became this supposed scientific standard of individuality," reflected a writer in 1907, "that I once heard a prominent clergyman remark that before he addressed a young man about his soul he wished he could be allowed to feel his bumps."[10]

As earlier in the century, the appeals of phrenology were multifaceted and spanned the social classes. Although by 1858 Lord Palmerston may have been exceptional in seeking phrenological counsel (from the phrenologist Frederick Bridges for fifty pounds), among the middle classes, of the sort who encouraged their sons to read Smiles's *Self-Help, Thrift, Duty,* and *Character,* phrenological delineations continued to be seen as useful prerequisites for deciding on education and careers, as well as for the hiring of servants.[11] Nor were bourgeois professionals wholly estranged from the science: Although there was far less explicit countenance of it in the fields of penal reform, psychiatry, and education than previously (its direct fructifying role having been fulfilled), related craniometric and physiognomical pursuits continued to seem relevant. This was especially so in the developing field of racial anthropology, where "anthropometry" came into its own.[12] Mr. James Mortimer, M.R.C.S., the self-confessed "dabbler in science" in the *Hound of the Baskervilles* (1902), was by no means unique in his favorite hobby of collecting and measuring skulls and talking craniology incessantly. Holmes himself, of course, like the young William Osler, was inclined to the phrenological scrutiny of the criminal head – a pursuit that gained credibility through the influence of the late-nineteenth-century Italian criminologist – physiognomist Cesare Lombroso (1835–1909).[13] Also directly and indirectly stemming from phrenology was the work, as well as the interest in the work, on eugenics and psychometrics of Francis Galton, Karl Pearson, and Darwin's son Leonard. The last, who was the president of the Eugenics Society, between 1911 and 1928, invented the anthropometric calipers that between the wars came to be routinely applied to the heads of schoolchildren.[14] Obviously extending from the earlier phrenology, as noted in Chapter 1, was the work on cerebral localization by David Ferrier and others.

But it was above all in popular working-class culture that phrenology was most faithfully preserved and pursued in the second half of the century. Increasingly, as it became one of the "characteristics of the age," as Brewster tagged it in 1863, it adjusted to the practical needs, amusements, aspirations, and comprehensions of ordinary working people. Already, by the 1850s, works such as that by "Gall the Younger" on *The Practical Uses of Phrenology Exemplified in the Application of the Science to Everyday Life* (Glasgow, 1856) or John Mill's *A Catechism of Practical Phrenology* (Leeds, 1851) were becoming more available and sought after than the older high-minded tracts extolling natural law or those instructing on the anatomy of the brain. It is noticeable, too, that more often than not the place of publication was one or other of the big industrial towns of the North. The new consumers of phrenology, while not wholly given over to the lighthearted and the entertaining, as some suggested, had neither the money, the patience, nor the stomach for the reform-vaunted productions of their "social betters."[15]

Reflecting, assisting, and catering to the new market after 1860 were over 150 practical "professors" of phrenology.[16] Most, but not all, were drawn from the same humble backgrounds as the majority of their clientele. For some, like the ungainly "poor Bill S." of the Potteries, recalled by Charles Shaw at the end of the century, becoming a "professor" of phrenology was a way of struggling out of a cruel life of poverty, abuse, and indignity.[17] The path out tended to be either through an apprenticeship, such as that received by J. D. Burns (1835–94) after he joined Fowler's entourage in 1863, or, more commonly, through taking a course of lessons, such as those available from the itinerant Professor Wright (who also taught animal magnetism and taxidermy at ten shillings a lesson!), or from Frederick Bridges's Institute of Mental Geometry in Liverpool, or John Taylor's Phrenological Academy in Morecambe (three guineas for eleven lessons), or at the Phrenological Institute in London run by Deville's successor, Cornelius Donovan.‡ Establishments like these, which were also devoted to private consultation, proliferated in the 1870s and 1880s.[18] But for every one of them there were at least a dozen poor Bill S.'s operating by winter in small shops and front parlors and by summer on the piers and sands of Blackpool, Morecambe, Brighton, Bournemouth, and elsewhere. Considering themselves lucky to get a chance to lecture at a YMCA, such practitioners, one suspects, were *not* like Mr. Mark Moores of the Phrenological Museum of Morecambe (est. 1872) who "never calls at people's houses, or places of business, to seek examinations, and never has done."[19]

If a career in phrenology was largely a way of survival for some, for others it served, additionally perhaps, as a kind of fallback for radical politics in the post-Chartist period of defeat and relative quiesence. The fictional Mr. Wilks depicted by James Ashcroft Noble in 1873 was true to life (and may well have been based on Joseph Barker):

He began his career as a shoemaker and a local preacher among the Methodists. At the time of the Chartist agitation he rushed into politics, became one of its most notorious supporters in his own part of the country, and very narrowly escaped imprisonment. When Chartism collapsed, he took to lecturing on theology, phrenology, and the literature of labour; and is now established in some town of the north of England, where he keeps a bookseller's shop, and examines people's heads – phrenologically, of course. He is, at present, a sceptic of the most advanced type.[20]

By the time Noble wrote, however, the likes of Mr. Wilks or Kingsley's near-identical Sandy Mackaye in *Alton Locke* (1849) were becoming figures of the past. Though as we shall see, phrenology continued to be a shibboleth of antiauthoritarianism for a minority of independently minded plebeian autodidacts, the particular type of hard edge that had been honed by the old guard of radical artisans earlier in the century had become dulled. Whether the science was pursued in the dissenting milieu of the provincial chapel or in the anticlerical milieu of metropolitan clubland, the old inflections of social rebellion were, in mid-Victorian Britain, much less heard than the ethics of improvement and the themes of self-help and the achieving of a "proper understanding of ourselves and our surroundings."[21] As if writing in 1834, William Mattieu Williams,‡ a graduate of the phrenology class in the London Mechanics' Institute in the 1840s, asserted in his *A Vindication of Phrenology* (1894) what was by then entirely platitudinous – that the "highest and incomparably the most important practical usefulness of Phrenology is its application to the business of self-culture as the necessary means of elevating the whole human race."[22] Equally reminiscent and socially innocuous, though no less meaningful to a younger generation, was the reassertion of the theme of secular liberation from the social strictures of old theology. "The lectures of Messrs Fowler and Wells have given phrenology a different position in this country to what it had before they came to our shores," it seemed to a Glaswegian workingman in his valedictory address to Fowler in 1863:

Mr Fowler gives us higher and more ennobling views of the mission and destiny of the human race than we had. His teaching is somewhat different from what we were accustomed to. We are no longer told we are poor, depraved, miserable, evil-disposed wretches, and that, if we get anything better than misery and unhappiness here, and something worse hereafter, we get more than we deserve. Mr Fowler shows us by the light of phrenology that ... not only are we privileged, but it is our duty, so to use them [mental faculties] for the purpose of raising ourselves mentally and morally, and that it is no blasphemy to aspire to as near to the perfection of our Creator as an earthly nature will admit.[23]

Since the phrenology of Fowler and Wells, like that of Williams, had been fashioned in the heyday of bourgeois phrenology in the

1830s and 1840s, and within that mold, it is unsurprising that there should have been this continuity in the rhetoric. The continuity might also be seen to testify to the lack of alteration in the social forces, not to say the basic social structures and relations, that initially had popularly called forth the knowledge.

And yet, though elderly patients of John Epps in Manchester were "forcibly reminded ... of old times" upon hearing the lectures on phrenology and physiology by Fowler and Wells in the 1860s, there were also subtle and significant differences between the old and the new articulations of the knowledge as well as in the nature of its appeal.[24] One partial change was the greater emphasis on hereditarianism, and on race and racial degeneration in particular. Charles Rosenberg observes that in the United States it was in the 1840s that "the exhortatory literature of phrenological improvement became ... increasingly involved with explicit discussions of heredity."[25] In Britain this change was in part directly the result of the American influence of the Fowlers. Joseph Barker, impressed during his tours of the United States by the more earthy frontier frankness of the Fowlers, began publishing cheap editions of their works in Leeds in 1851. Among those works was Orson Fowler's best-selling *Hereditary Descent: Its Laws and Facts Applied to Human Improvement* (1844), along with various other of his tracts on "Amativeness," "Love and Parentage," and "Matrimony." Through the "Yankee courseness" and "painful rudeness" of these works (as Holyoake regarded them), the Fowlers cast, into a language more amenable to the less educated, ideas that Spurzheim and Combe had already made popular and that in the 1850s, were being looked upon as at the center of the phrenological achievement.[26] In 1857, several years before the works of the Fowlers became widely available, and decades of course before Darwinism was to have any popular impact, Hugh Miller noted that

never, perhaps, was the phrenological belief more general than now, that the human race, like some of the inferior races, is greatly dependent for the development of what is best in it, on what I shall venture to term purity of breed. It has become a sort of axiom, that well-dispositioned intellectual parents produce a well-dispositioned intellectual offspring.[27]

Part and parcel of this shift in emphasis and appreciation of phrenology was the increasing bourgeois fear of social degeneration, especially as occasioned through a supposed unleashing of the sensuality attributed to the working class. To teach control of procreation was not only "the most intimate and telling way of inculcating in the lower classes the belief that power over life itself lay in science and nature forces," as F. B. Smith has remarked;[28] it was also, through the deification of that science and those natural forces, potentially the most effective way of inculcating among working people the same bourgeois values that Combe had dispensed through the *Constitution of Man*. Middle and late Victorian phrenological literature abounded in discussion of the evils of sexual indulgence, and it was not uncommon to attribute to phrenologists a certain omniscience in these matters. As an antimasturbation author warned in the 1870s,

The solitary libertine can ... be detected by a multiplicity of signs ... in spite of all concealment; and phrenologists can decypher every line on the map of sensuality, and explain the secret workings and language of the heart. If a lewd woman can select her partner even in the midst of a large assemblage, by the marks of libertinism which he bears about him, the physiologist and phrenologist will certainly have little difficulty in tracing sensuality by similar signs.[29]

But though protoeugenic ideas and notions of race (not radicalism) and sexual purity were to figure more prominently in later Victorian phrenology, it would be a misrepresentation to characterize it wholly in that light. In terms of its prevailing mood, as distinct from its contents (which remained largely descriptive and explanatory), the most distinguishing feature is the greater tendency to antielitist antiintellectualism. The nature of this antiintellectualism was different from that of the status-seeking professionals involved with the science earlier in the century. Although there continued the celebration of practicality, experience, and antiintrospection over abstract philosophizing, the literature became at the same time more than ever opposed to professional intellectuals as a social group arbitrating power. Combe and company had of course previously directed populist democratic rhetoric against the academic intellectual elite, but, as epitomized through Combe's candidacy for the Edinburgh chair of logic in 1836, they also had been openly covetous of the social–academic status they purported to scorn. Phrenologists in the second half of the century were far less ambivalent and much more adamant, perhaps because of the virtual impossibility of their usurping academic positions, but seemingly more out of genuine disapproval of the autocratic behavior of those who would maintain privilege and power by purporting to know better than others. "The intolerable humbug of our public writers as to all matters concerning the Philosophy of Nature, founded on observed facts shall be unflinchingly exposed," declared the editor of a proposed new magazine devoted to popular phrenology and astrology; "the *niaseries* and noodleisms of many so-called philosophers shall be held up to the world for its scorn, contempt, or ridicule, as they may severally deserve."[30]

W. Mattieu Williams, though never a self-conscious spokesman for the rights of the people – despite, or perhaps because of, the fact that he was the son of a fishmonger – and though very much opposed to the vulgarization of "the old phrenology of Gall," nevertheless supported the popularizers of phrenology in order to rebuke the intellectuals. For phrenology to fulfill its "special function" of elevating the human race, he argued, it

must be a popular science, *the* popular science, the science of the vulgar multitude, the common property of all, down to the poorest of the poor. This will be prevented if it first becomes accepted by the aristocrats of learning, or patronised by those who regard our Board schools, etc., as dangerous institutions calculated to render the "common people" discontented with their condition.

In order that its future progress may be wholesome and fruitful, it is desirable that it may continue for some time longer in a state of invigorating adversity, sheltered, sustained and advocated by the radical democracy of the intellectual world, by those who think for themselves and dare to carry out their convictions, even though they are not in accordance with prevailing conventional fashions.[31]

Such rhetoric was partly derived from that of the bourgeois ideologues of the 1830s and 1840s, which itself partly derived from an older (and in radical culture, continuing) Jacobin demand for knowledge that could be understood and shared in by all. Yet it was also more than that: Explicitly, it was an expression of resentment by working people at their social and intellectual exclusion and cultural dispossession, and implicitly it was a part of a new and relevant social critique. In a context in which legitimations of bourgeois "distinction" based on natural rights and ascetic virtues were giving way to those based on intellectual superiority (and academic certification), the assertion of phrenology's place among the "vulgar multitude" was not simply an asocial challenge to an arrogant use of antiphrenology as a resource for intellectual elitism.[32] However inadvertently, it was also a challenge to what was becoming the main rationale for the maintenance of bourgeois social and political power. In effect, late Victorian do-it-yourself phrenology with its deliberate emphasis on the "plain and practical" (bordering at times on antiscience) was the plebeian response to the cultural imperialism of those erecting the myth that a society governed over by intellectuals and scientists was necessarily a better and freer place to live.[33]

In this respect as in others self-help phrenology was at one with, and gave as much to as it got from, the growth of medical dissent and self-healing in the second half of the century, as well as the growth of interest in spiritualism. Both of these phenomena have now begun to attract the attention of historians, and it is clear that however tenuous may have been some of the practical and theoretical links with phrenology, at psychological, social, and rhetorical levels the basis of faith in them and in phrenology was mutually reinforcing.[34] Many of the same individuals were involved; indeed, it seemed to the renegade phrenologist Daniel Noble in 1853, a

striking fact that the ranks of almost every philosophical folly of the present era ... have been recruited from the expiring phrenological school – teachers and disciples alike. Some have become apostles or partisans of the water cure; others of clairvoyance and mesmeric prevision; and some, again, of homoeopathy; whilst a few, I believe, have gone over to the spiritual rappers![35]

Noble's belief that these new phrenologically related interests were merely manifestations of "excessive credulity" is belied, of course, by his own former enthusiasm for phrenology. Nor were these alliances with phrenology so new. In plebeian culture the rapport with heterodox and self-help medicine was longstanding and deep-rooted. As observed in Chapter 6, the desire to understand and control one's own brain was integral to the recognized importance of understanding and controlling one's body, which in turn was part and parcel of the desire not to be ruled over by religious authority. Thus, phrenology had marched hand in hand with temperance, vegetarianism, mesmeric healing, physiology and popular hygiene, self-education, and secularism. After mid-century this rhetorical rapport was strengthened upon the medical profession's closing of ranks and its assertion of authority over popular medical practices such as homoeopathy, hydropathy, medical botany, and various other forms of lay and professional medical dissent. In this new context phrenology became more than ever a comrade-in-arms with heterodox medicine on the countercultural front. The fact that, curatively speaking, orthodox medicine was recognized as being in no better a position than previously to deliver the goods only strengthened both the actual and the rhetorical appeal of heterodox medical ideas and practices. Thus the standard historical emphasis on the medical faculty's abandonment of phrenology in the second half of half of the nineteenth century is misplaced.[36] More correctly, it was the public who in large part abandoned the faculty after the passage of the Medical Act in August 1858. (Appositely, it was in that same month that George Combe died in a hydropathic establishment in Surrey.[37])

Although spiritualism, both as a form of lay healing and as a faith, was a cultural and countercultural phenomenon that reached a crescendo closer to the end of the century, it was intimately bound to phrenology and the other heterodox ideas and practices. Into the twentieth century within middle-class theosophical societies as within the plebeian spiritual lyceums, phrenology remained a favorite topic.[38] Thus continued the direct connections between the subjects that, if historically less pervasive than those with medical dissent, were no less long-standing. When the phrenologist Thomas Timson of the Leicester "Midland Institute of Phrenology, Psychology, Hygiene, Hydropathy, etc." (est. 1882) spoke in the 1890s of "man's magnetic constitution" being "the superfine grade between matter and spirit" and of the soul as consisting of "magnetic poles ... the largest, most brilliant, and most powerful being in the centre and top of the head, in the locality or convolution and phrenological organ of firmness," he was extending a linkage of the science with occult, romantic and Neoplatonic traditions that differed little from that pursued by Greaves and the Concordians in the 1840s.[39] Less garbled, the association with phrenology could be traced at least as far back as Goethe. As we saw in the previous chapter, the popularization and strengthening of these links through the agency of phreno-mesmerism rendered more apparent than real the paradox of a materialist theory of brain contributing to interests in the "irrational" and immaterial. Both phrenological materialism and phreno-mesmerically suggested materialism could contribute to the opposition to priestly authority and interventions. Perceived to a large extent as a means of naturalizing the supernatural, spiritualism was, like phrenology, a contribution to secularism. More problematic is the extent to which late Victorian spiritualism was implicitly a Bergson-like vitalist critique of a social order based on positivist scientific rationality,[40] since spiritualism itself was often investigated according to that rationality. Spiritualism was quintessentially antiintellectualist, however, and hence, like late Victorian phrenology, was implicitly critical of intellectual rationalizations of the existing social structure and relations. It is no accident that bookshops such as that run by the mediums Mr. and Mrs. E. W. Wallis of Manchester advertised, along with their works on spiritualism and theosophy, "Progressive Literature of all kinds" on freethought, palmistry, religion, physiology, medicine and phrenology. Vis-à-vis the productions of late Victorian bourgeois intellectual functionaries, the phrenological works of Fowler, R. B. D. Wells, James Coates, Henry S. Drayton, and others had a natural place beside those of the spokesmen for labor and freethought, Charles Bradlaugh, G. W. Foote, H. M. Hyndman, Robert Blatchford, and J. M. Robertson.[41]

Freed from its former bourgeois moorings and turned around in opposition to the privilege of bourgeois professionals, phrenology in the late Victorian culture of plebeian autodidacts was to a considerable extent an expression of self-determination with collectivist overtones. By the 1890s, when Williams wrote, the "vulgar multitude" had indeed made the knowledge their own, and high-minded intellectuals had reason to express their disapprobation. It is worth noting, too, that the phrenological head now lost the image of scientificity strived for in the 1820s – the mental faculties coming to be filled in pictorially with recognizably human activities (see Figure 8).

Yet, no less than earlier in the century, the radical rhetorical use of the knowledge and the clamor raised against it tended to mask the freedoms that the knowledge itself continued to delegitimize and the repression and submission that it continued covertly to instill. However agressively poised by some plebeians, phrenology remained what it had always been: a representation and naturalization in human nature of hierarchical order. To its functionalist

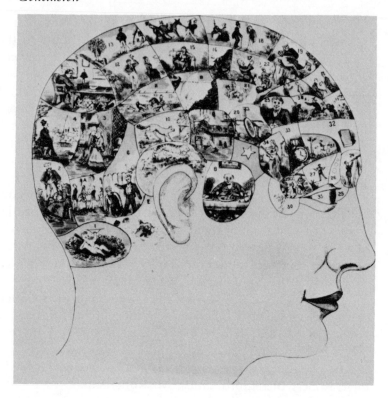

Figure 8. R. B. D. Wells's *Phrenological Chart and Symbolical Head* [1878].

presuppositions, its validation of mental over manual, its pathological orientation to and definition of deviance, and its metaphors
of fragmentation and specialization there came no cultural exor-
cists. If, by the study of the science people continued to feel themselves liberated from enslaving religious dogmas, such as that of
predestination, there did not necessarily follow from this any man-
date freely to explore personhood or to effect participatory social
action. Rather, as before, phrenology itself encouraged an acceptance of the tyranny of the logic and rationality mediated through
one's own cerebral biology. As before, phrenology mostly encouraged changing oneself to fit the system. If there was any
difference at the end of the century, it was only that in the face
of extended bureaucracy and the spectre of state socialism, on the
one hand, and the impersonal racial reductionism of Darwinian
evolution, on the other hand, the phrenological celebration of

individualism (like the spiritual embodiment of it) could be felt to be emancipating in new ways.

But for most people interest in phrenology was motivated by nothing so lofty as the "right" to find one's own place in the competitive social order. More humbly, if no less actively, phrenology continued to be regarded as simply a means to making the most of one's mental and social lot in life. In the 1870s it seemed to some that more than ever

the fun of the thing ..., the novelty has ... ceased to exist and people consult Phrenology for the benefits which they will derive from its teachings, in the management and training of children, choise of pursuits, self-improvement, marriage, how to make the most of their talents, etc.[42]

Thus to Robert Tressell writing at the end of the century, phrenology seemed at one with savings banks, teetotalism, sexual abstinence, Sunday schools, the polishing of boots, and all the other plain, ordinary, and often altruistic things that allowed working people either religiously or secularly to celebrate individualism and thereby assist politically the class that oppressed them economically. In the midst of appalling class exploitation, Tressell saw the whole business of phrenological consultation as continuing to impose upon working people a false consciousness of self or the illusion of social autonomy. Tressell's failure to confront the science head on, as it were, in his chapter on "The Phrenologist" in *The Ragged Trousered Philanthropists* suggests, perhaps, that he was aware that working people made of sterner stuff than his character Mr. Slyme also took sustenance from the knowledge. But it was the Slymes in particular, it seemed – those seeking to leave their class behind – who most naturally hoarded the knowledge and, through its pseudoprofundities, relished in "astonishing their fellow working men."[43]

But arguably it was *because* of working people's greater sense of being stuck within an oppressed class, their sense of the greater fixity of late Victorian social relations, and the generally more pessimistic outlook on nature of the time that the phrenology that Tressell took to be a sign and symbol of oppression was more than ever required and sought after as a secular religious means to ego satisfaction, consolation, hope, and "indelible [cosmological] evidence of comprehensive design, and constant harmony."[44] Phrenology continued to be, as spiritualism had also become, "cheap, easy and expeditious Revelation."[45] It was hardly credible that the public should abandon phrenology "and get nothing in exchange," remarked a commentator in the *Popular Science Review* in 1869; so long as it continued to furnish meaning and to give order and apparent precision to experience by reducing ambiguities, scientific men arguing against this system of knowledge could only "force their audiences to conclude that it is not possible to argue with 'experts'!"[46] As opposed to the "experts," phrenologists continued to deal with the really important and enduring issues of life and death, sex and family, order and meaning. "The sanctum, or consultation-room, of the phrenologist may well be regarded as a hallowed place," wrote the Bournemouth phrenologist J. J. Spark in 1891.

In the course of his ordinary duties he must, as a priest, listen to confessions and give advice on spiritual subjects, as physician give advice on health, as a judge with acuteness decide between contending parties. Besides regularly acting in this triple capacity, he is often a mesmerist, a medical electrician, an hydropathist, a psychologist, and astrologist.[47]

By this date, few phrenologists were any longer aspiring to be ideologues of social change. In the face of another rush of social, economic, and intellectual changes, and the even greater indifference to humanity in mass society, it was rather wholly as ministers to physical and psychological suffering that they functioned to reaffirm the basis of consent to what were now the "traditional" ways of understanding and evaluating life in the urban industrial context. Subtly, phrenology had shifted from being predominantly an Excalibur for change to being a source of "genesis amnesia" – the illusion that "things have always been as they are."[48]

Popular Darwinism, the eugenics movement, the First World War, the Depression, and popular Freudianism were among the many phenomena that contributed to sap and ultimately extinguish the science, art, and religion of nineteenth-century phrenology. By the Second World War the beaches and piers were clear, Leonard Darwin's anthropometric calipers had been laid to rest, and plaster casts in chemists' windows were seen no more. Never again was there to be anything quite like phrenology – at least not with the same capacity to, at the same time, render the intangible tangible, to explain comprehensively the human mind, and to predictively and optimistically act upon and inform the human condition.

But if phrenology's combined theory of brain and science of character was not to endure, the legacy of its cultural significance was. In spite of all the forms of resistence to Gall's doctrine in the nineteenth century, it, more than any other form of psychology, established in the public mind the notion that human behavior was capable of classification and measure and that social, economic, and intellectual success, on the one hand, and problems of crime, delinquency, and addiction, on the other, could be reduced to organic derangement of brain.[49] Though "the path from phrenology to psychosurgery" delineated by Stephan Chorover was not a direct one, there can be no doubt that the "science of IQ" and applied psychology took up where phrenology left off.[50] Minus phrenology's vivid imagery, the new methods of mental testing continued ever more widely to make the brain, and the intellectual faculties in particular, the celebrated cultural part; to encourage people to attend competitively to the differences between themselves; and to legitimate essentially the same hierarchically organized division of labor that phrenology had naturalized in the early nineteenth century. For the period from the 1930s to the 1950s especially, psychology as a "science" was largely what phrenology in its relation to cerebral localization and neurological biology had been for much of the century before, and what ethology–sociobiology and molecular biology have contended to be from the 1960s to the present: not simply a blunt scientism to enforce commitment to the hierarchical and authoritarian structures and relations of capitalist society, but more, the culturally acceptable naturalistic language or code by which people came to scrutinize and rationalize their sense of the social order.[51] Insofar as phrenology has allowed us to focus on this means of and process for cultural consent during the genesis of industrial capitalism, it might not be inappropriate to conclude with Marx, "So you see, phrenology is not the baseless art which Hegel imagined!"[52]

APPENDIX: PUBLIC LECTURERS ON PHRENOLOGY IN BRITAIN TO CIRCA 1860

This biographical list of 233 lecturers on phrenology (21 of them antiphrenologists) includes only those persons who have been identified as lecturing in some public forum. Excluded are (a) those who read papers on the subject to private bodies, such as phrenological or medical societies; (b) persons such as John Conolly or William Lawrence who, in their public lectures on physiology, laws of health, etc. made only indirect or partial reference to phrenology; and (c) practical manipulating phrenologists for whom evidence of public lecturing or teaching on phrenology has not been found. In most cases it can be assumed that the lecturer also gave further lectures near to the dates and locations given here.

Abbreviations

★	*Denotes authorship of published writings on phrenology*
•	*Lectured against phrenology*
BAAS	*Member of the British Association for the Advancement of Science*
DLB	*Dictionary of Labour Biography*
DNB	*Dictionary of National Biography*
DSB	*Dictionary of Scientific Biography*
Lit & Phil	Literary and Philosophical Society or Institution
LSA	Licentiate of the Society of Apothecaries
MEB	Frederic Boase's *Modern English Biography*
MI	Mechanics' Institute
MPA	Member of the Phrenological Association (established in 1838 but for the most part discontinued in 1842 after ENGLEDUE's address on materialism and mesmerism)
MPS	Member of the Phrenological Society of ...

Major sources

H. C. Watson, *Statistics of Phrenology* (1836); *Phrenological Journal* (1823–47); *Phrenological (Anthropological) Magazine and Christian Physician* (1835–9); *Phrenological Almanac* (1842–5); *Phreno-Magnet* (1843); *People's Phrenological Journal* (1843–4); *Zoist* (1843–56); *Journal of Health and Disease* (1846–51); *Journal of Health and Phrenological Magazine* (1851–60); *Human Nature* (1867–78); *Crisis* (1832–4); *New Moral World* (1834–45); *Analyst* (1834–40); *Penny Mechanic* (1836–7); *Oracle of Reason* (1841–3); *The Movement* (1843–5); *Reasoner* (1846–72); *Cooper's Journal* (1850); Thomas Coates, "Appendix IV: List of Lecturers [1835]," in *Report of the State of Literary, Scientific, and Mechanics' Institutions in England* (London, SDUK, 1841).

Lecturers

Biographical information has been drawn principally from the sources listed in Chapter 2 (note 8), together with local directories and fragments from the person's published works where applicable. Where *DNB* or *MEB* entries are available, information has been weighted to those aspects of biography that have largely been ignored, including, above all, involvement with phrenology.

ABELL, Richard, M.D. Edinburgh 1822, b. Ireland; lectured in Cork Inst. 1825; MPS Edin 11/21.

ADAIR, Thomas, of Sheffield; lectured in the Midlands, the North, and Scotland 1843–6; reputed to be the first to introduce phreno-mesmerism into Scotland; his course of lectures on phreno-mesmerism in Newcastle in 1843 was attended by over 1,000 persons.

• AITKEN, ———, M.D.; lectured in Blandford Lit & Phil, Dorset, 1839.

AITKEN, Mrs. William C., lectured in Dundee 1835 with husband as demonstrator.

AITKEN, William C., MPS Dumfries (sometime sec.); sec. for the organization of the Phrenological Exhibition in the Dumfries MI, which was attended by 5,000 persons in 1842; lectured in Scotland 1835–8.

* ALEXANDER, Disney, apothecary of Hull and medical author; an apostate of the Church, he became a Methodist lay preacher in the 1790s; med. supt. of the Wakefield Pauper Lunatic Asylum 1831–6 (succeeding Sir William Ellis); elected corresp. MPS London 12/26; lectured in Wakefield in the 1830s as well as in Leeds and elsewhere; also lectured on health at Sowerby Bridge MI 1839; provided a testimonial on phrenology to Sir George MACKENZIE in 1836.

* ALLEN, Matthew (1783–1845), M.D. Aberdeen 1821; youngest of ten children of a dissenting preacher of York; a spendthrift, inveterate liar, and persuasive personality; apothecary of York Lunatic Asylum 1819–24, having previously run a shop in Edinburgh and been imprisoned for debt; established a model asylum in Epping Forest in 1825, which his third wife continued to run after his death; friend of Tennyson and EPPS; elected a corresp. MPS Edinburgh 11/21 and MPS London 11/24; took to lecturing on phrenology for pecuniary reasons in 1816, being the first after SPURZHEIM to establish himself as an itinerant on the science in Britain; his lectures in the Leeds Lit & Phil in 1825 were reported as the best attended to date; lectured less frequently on the science in the 1830s, during which time he was also a member of the London Anthropol. (Phren.) Soc. (M. C. Barnet, biog. *Med. Hist.*, 9 [1965], 16–28)

ANDERSON, J., surgeon of Richmond; lectured there 1835; also lectured on anatomy, physiology, and zoology.

BAILEY, James Napier, author and Owenite social missionary; lectured on phreno-mesmerism in the Rotunda (5/43) and on a semipermanent basis at the (Owenite) John St. Inst. 1843.

• BAKER, W., debated phrenology with Peter JONES at Finsbury Hall 4/48; lectured at London Inst. on Evidences of Christianity etc.

★ BALLY, William, modeler and delineator; b. Switzerland; while in Birmingham in the 1830s he employed HOLYOAKE for a while to bring him customers; traveled with SPURZHEIM 1829–31 and then with BARBER on phrenological tours; ran the Phrenological Gallery on King's St., Manchester, and served as curator of the Manchester Phren. Soc. 1838; MPA, signing the declaration of expediency 1842; contributed to *Phren. J.*; regarded by Mancunians as the best practical phrenologist in England; taught plaster casting in Manchester MI and lectured on this craft in other Midland towns in the 1830s; lectured on phrenology (chiefly to mothers and guardians) in the Manchester Athenaeum 1842; retired to Switzerland 1848, donating his collection of over 1,000 casts to the Manchester MI.

★ BARBER, Jonathan (1784–1864), M.R.C.S.; practiced medicine in Scarborough and London before emigrating to America in 1820 and becoming the most distinguished teacher on elocution in Yale and Harvard; V.P. Boston Phren. Soc.; friend and pupil of SPURZHEIM; lectured and manipulated in U.S. and Canada in 1836, and on the continent and in Britain 1838–42; debated with BRINDLEY in Bristol in 1842; also lectured on elocution in London; returned to medical practice in Canada in the mid-1840s as a homoeopath; professor of oratory at McGill University until 1862. (*MEB*)

BARKER, Edward (1798–1832), Sheffield pen knife manufacturer and operator of the Sheffield Lead Works; Unitarian; notable chemist; active radical in the 1820s; curator of mineralogy department of the Sheffield Lit & Phil; lectured regularly on phrenology at the Sheffield Medical Inst.; BAAS.

BARLAS, Rev. George, Christian phrenologist; lectured in Scotland c. 1835.

★ BAUME, Pierre Henri J. (1797–1875), b. Naples; eccentric wealthy supporter of radical causes; former spy in the employ of the King Ferdinand of Sicily; friend of CARLILE; established the Experimental Gardens, Islington; lectured on phrenology in the Westminster Inst., Millbank, 1835. (*DNB*)

★ BEAMISH, Richard (1798–1873), civil engineer, F.R.S. 1836; M.I.C.E. 1829; assistant engineer on the Thames Tunnel 1826 and resident engineer of Gloucester and Forest of Dean Railway to 1850; brother of Francis Beamish (M.P. for Cork 1837–41 and MPA) and North Ludlow Beamish (Sheriff of York and F.R.S.); resided at Prestbury, near Cheltenham; MPA 7/40, signing the declaration of expediency 1842; contributed to *Phren. J.*; lectured in Cheltenham and in the Midlands 1839–42 and in Cork 1844; also devoted to hydropathy and elocution. (*MEB*)

★ BEDFORD, Rev. John G. (1810–79), Wesleyan preacher in Glasgow and Manchester; trained as a solicitor in Wakefield; MPS Bath, read various papers on Christian phrenology and contributed to *Phren. J.*; conducted a discussion with the antiphrenologist Mr. Kenyon of New York 1838. (*MEB*; *DNB*)

★ BEGGS, Thomas (1808–96), b. Edinburgh; apprenticed as a bookbinder in Leeds; engineer and brass founder in London 1848–71; sanitary engineer in Southwark 1871–92; took the temperance pledge in 1838 and became sec. Total Abstinence Society of Nottingham and, in 1846, of the National Temperance

League; sec. of the Complete Suffrage Association 1842 and of the Health of Towns Association 1848; educationalist; wrote on juvenile depravity and on the deterrent effect of capital punishment; MPS Sheffield 1843; chairman of the new London Phren. Soc. 1856; commenced the weekly *Phreno-Magnetic Vindicator* 6 Mar. 1843; lectured in the Midlands 1842–4. (*MEB*)

BIGNELL, J. H., lectured in Portsmouth 1833.

BILTON, ———, MPS Portsmouth, resigned in 1832 after having been accused of mixing politics with phrenology in a lecture on "The Light Which Phrenology Affords toward Ameliorating the Condition of Mankind."

BIRCH, William John (1811–63), barrister; son of a captain in the East Indian commercial service; educated Balliol and New Inn Hall, Oxford (B.A. 1832); leading contributor to freethought funds; supporter of Italy; author of *An Inquiry into the Philosophy and Religion of Shakspere* (1848); delivered seven free lectures on phrenology in Manchester Lyceum 1840; also lectured on popular religious fallacies and on "natural theology deduced from the mind" in Manchester MI and Liverpool MI 1840. (*MEB*)

★ BOYD, John, of Edinburgh; established himself as a practical phrenologist in Aberdeen; claimed to be one-time pres. of Hunterian Med. Soc. and hon. MPS Majorca; regarded by respectable Edinburgh phrenologists as a "person of flaming pretentions"; lectured and manipulated in Scotland 1844–6.

★ BRAY, Charles (1811–84), Coventry ribbon manufacturer 1835–56, freethinker and author, proprietor of *Coventry Herald and Observer* 1846 (later *Herald and Free Press*); friend and tutor of George Eliot 1841–50, interesting her in phrenology; committed to free trade; became interested in Owenism in 1840s; established and presided over the Coventry Labourers' and Artisans' Co-operative Society 1843; established a working men's club 1845; interested in homoeopathy, hydropathy, mesmerism, and spiritualism; BAAS; corresponded with COMBE; MPA 5/40, signing the declaration of expediency 1842; mem. of COX's Psychological Soc.; delivered six lectures to Coventry MI 1836 and also ran a phrenology class there. (*DNB*; *MEB*)

★ BRIDGES, Frederick (d. 1883), practical phrenologist from c. 1832; traveled in U.S. in the 1840s collecting skulls etc.; established the School of Practical Phrenology and Physiology, Mt. Pleasant, Liverpool, before 1850; lectured in the North and Midlands 1840s–60s.

• ★ BRINDLEY, John, dissenting preacher, sometime schoolmaster of March, Cambridgeshire; leading antisocialist agitator often combining the attack on socialism with an attack on phrenology, which he regarded as highly destructive of Christianity; appointed sec. Religious & Useful Knowl. Soc. for his efforts; edited the *Anti-Socialist Gazette* 1842; publicly debated phrenology with RUMBALL in Worcester in 1838, 1839 and again in Liverpool 1842 (passing out handbills – "Anti-Phrenology for the People"); debated with BARBER in Bristol 1842 and with DEVILLE at the Adelphi in London 1842; invited after COMBE's lectures in the Birmingham MI to give a course of six antiphrenology lectures there in 1836 (being paid 18 guineas), which led to W. H. SMITH's two lectures in reply – it was Brindley's reply to Smith (in four lectures delivered at the Birmingham Soc. of Arts) that led him to make the connected attack on socialism; thereafter he devoted more time to attacking socialism than phrenology.

• ★ BROMLEY, Rev. J., Wesleyan minister 1811–50; mem. Portsmouth and Portsea Phil. Soc. 1/22 when his lectured there against GALL and SPURZHEIM's doctrine as fatalistic and materialistic; lectured against the doctrine in Doncaster Lyceum 1836, leading to the debate with LEVISON.

BROOKES, H. (or Brooks), lectured mainly on mesmerism, but sometimes demonstrated phreno-magnetism; began lecturing in Kent 1842 and toured the southern counties 1843; a conservative style.

BROWN, James, surgeon in Glasgow; lectured in Glasgow MI 1825.

★ BROWNE, William Alexander Francis (1805–85), L.R.C.S. 1826, M.D. Heidelberg, F.R.S.E. 1861; pres. Royal Med. Soc. Edinburgh; physician in Sterling 1830; supt. Montrose Royal Asylum 1834–8 and Crichton Royal Inst. 1838–57; med. commissioner in lunacy for Scotland 1857–70; pres. Medico-Psychological Assoc. 1866; MPS Edinburgh 4/24, MPA 5/40, and on the council of the Edinburgh Ethical Soc. for the Practical Application of Phrenology; intimate of Combe family; highly popular as a lecturer on phrenology (attracting 1,000 listeners in Dunfermline in 1838); attended last meeting of Edin Phren. Soc. 12/70; contributed to *Phren. J.* (MEB)

BUIK, James, MPS Dundee; lectured in Forfar 1833.

★ BUNNEY, Lieut. Joseph, practical phrenologist "of Christian principles"; office at 62 Regent's Quadrant, London; claimed to have begun lecturing on phrenology c. 1830 and to have "examined one-half the members of our leading universities, Oxford and Cambridge"; appears lecturing [as J. Benny?] at the Surrey Educational Inst. 1848 and on the "Pleasures of Scientific Research and Sensual Gratification, Contrasted" at the Soho Mutual Instruction Soc. 6/50.

★ BURKE, Luke (d. 1885), MPS London; theist and prolific writer; member of HOLYOAKE's Utilitarian Soc. 1847; launched the *Ethnological Journal; or, Magazine of Ethnology, Phrenology, and Archeology* 1848–9, n.s. 1854 (referred to by the *Derbyshire Advertiser* as "a daring infidel publication"), *The Future* 1860–2; edited *People's Phren. J.* 1843–4; lectured at the London MI 1843 (on one occasion with EPPS); also lectured on ethnology and the chronology of the Old Testament.

BUSHEA, Henri (or Bu Shea, or Beau Sheau), "professor," "Dr.," and "L.L.D."; itinerant manipulator; present at the antiphrenological lectures of BRINDLEY in London 1842 and had to be carried off the stage; regular itinerant in the Midlands 1842–6 (see Fig. 7); in Sheffield 3/41–3/42, where he established a museum and lectured at the MI and elsewhere in an effort to prove the harmony of phrenology with Scripture; announced the formation of the Sheffield Phren. Inst. and Anti-Socialist Soc. 8/41.

BUSHELL, Josiah, hon. sec. Pershore MI, Worcester, where he lectured on phrenology in 1850; also lectured on the Mosaic account of creation.

• BUTLER, Rev. William Joseph (d. 1869), rector of St. Nicholas's Church, Nottingham, 1825–66; delivered an anti-*Constitution of Man* lecture in the Nottingham Assembly Rooms (to 70) 5/40, replied to by DOW.

BUTTERWORTH, J. S., lectured on phrenology and mesmerism at Marsden MI 1852–3 and at Lockwood MI 1860–1, both near Huddersfield.

★ CAMERON, George Douglas (d. c. 1845), b. Scotland; M.D. Edinburgh 1820; practiced in Liverpool; introduced H. C. WATSON to phrenology c. 1823; contributed to *Phren. J.*; delivered course of 12 lectures in the Paris Rooms, Liverpool, 1824 and lectured to small audiences there 1825, 1827; rebuffed by Liverpool Roy. Inst. when he offered to lecture on phrenology 1828; MPS Edinburgh 12/24.

CANTOR, Dr., lectured successfully in Leeds, Bradford, Wakefield, and Sheffield MIs 1842.

★ CARGILL, William, East India Co. merchant; testimonial to MacKENZIE 1836; sec. Newcastle Phren. Soc.; brother of Dr. J. Cargill (who was also MPS Newcastle); contributed to *Phren. J.*; lectured in Newcastle 1838, leading to dispute with Dr. Samuel Knott.

CARLILE, Eliza (née Sharples) (d. 1852), feminist; lecturer at the Rotunda; common law wife of Richard CARLILE; penniless upon his death in 1843, she was taken in by the Ham Common Commune; interested in mesmerism and subjects occult; lectured in Carlisle, Gravesend, London mid-1830s and on "the philosophy and theology of Phrenology" at the London Hall of Science 1839.

★ CARLILE, Richard (1790–1843), radical publisher and leading British atheist and materialist after the Napoleonic Wars; imprisoned for his seditious publications; lectured on phrenology in Manchester and the North 1829 and, after his conversion to allegorical Christianity, on phrenology as affording an aid to prayer, repentance, and salvation, in Brighton 1836. (*DLB*; *DNB*)

★ CARSON, James C. L. (1815–86), Irish; M.D. Glasgow 1837; med. advisor to over 30 assurance companies; wrote against capital punishment and the Plymouth Brethren; evangelical Christian phrenologist; did delineations; contributed to *Phren. Almanac*; gave three courses of lectures at Coleraine MI 1842, 1850, and courses in Dublin 1851. (*MEB*)

CARSTAIRS, ———, surgeon of Sheffield; lectured on phreno-mesmerism at Wakefield and Leeds 1843 and at Sheffield Phren. Soc. 1842; MPS Sheffield.

• ★ CATLOW, Joseph Peel (d. 1867), lectured in Nottingham and Manchester 1843 on the delusion of phreno-mesmerism.

★ CHURCH, Richard, hon. sec. Yorkshire Soc. for Promoting National Education 1850s; lectured at Chichester Lit & Phil 1833.

★ CLARKE, Rev. Henry, of Chorley, Lancs.; interested in phrenology from c. 1825; Christian phrenologist; contributed to *Phren. J.*; lectured in Dundee Mechanics' Phren. Soc. 1835, and with AITKEN in various Scottish towns 1835–6.

★ CLARKE, J. G., Owenite socialist and freethinker; lectured on phrenology as buttress to Owen's Rational Religion in and around Manchester c. 1838.

COLEMAN, ———, lectured in Wolverhampton Lit. & Sci. Soc. 1837.

COLLYERS, Robert H., author of American phrenological works and scientific inventor; English student of SPURZHEIM, whom he claimed to have met in Paris; went to U.S. 1836 and set up as a lecturer in New York on the "Wonders of the Microscopic World"; graduate of Berkshire Medical College, Pittsfield, Mass., 1839; converted to mesmerism; lectured to large audiences in New England 1841–3, competing with COMBE in Hartford in 1839; lectured in Liverpool on phreno-mesmerism 1843, returning to Boston 1845; returned to England in the 1860s and was present at the meetings of the Ethnol. Soc. of London in 1863; sentenced to three months in prison for fraud in 1876. (T. Stoehr, "Physiognomy and Phrenology in Hawthorne," *Huntington Lib. Q.*, 37 [1974], 399–400)

★ COMBE, George (1788–1858), leading popularizer of phrenology in Britain; author of the *Constitution of Man*; involved in BAAS but opposed its exclusiveness and its exclusion of phrenology; promoter, leading contributor to, and sometime proprietor of *Phren. J.*; founder of the Edinburgh Phren. Soc. 1820; between 1822 and 1840 lectured in Edinburgh, Glasgow, Birmingham, Bath, Newcastle, Aberdeen, and in U.S. and Germany; first began teaching and lecturing on phrenology in Edinburgh 5/22; first lectures to working-class audiences in 1832. (*DNB*; *MEB*; C. Gibbon, *Life* [1878])

★ CONNON, John, editor of *Tyne Pilot*; graduate of Aberdeen Univ.; author of prize-winning essay on the application of phrenology to the choice of parliamentary candidates 1840; MPA 5/40; contributed to *Phren. J.*; lectured in South Shields MI 1842.

COOK, _____, lectured in Leeds Lit. Inst. 1842.

• ★ COVEY, Charles (1795–1834), M.R.C.S., surgeon to Birmingham Dispensary; lectured against phrenology in Phil. Inst., Birmingham, 1831. (*Aris's Birm. Gaz*, 6 October 1834)

★ COWAN, Charles (1806–68), M.D. Edinburgh 1833 and Paris 1834; M.R.C.S. Edinburgh; son of the Rev. Thomas C. Cowan of Reading (d. 1856); lecturer on anatomy in Bath, where he practiced medicine 1835–9; hon. phys. Reading Dispensary and sen. phys. to Roy. Berks. Hospital 1839 to death; an early exponent of auscultation; early and energetic member of the BMA; anti-homoeopath in the 1850s; author of several medical works; regarded as one of the best speakers in the medical profession; active in Low Church politics in Reading and author of various works on Church association, modern spiritualism, and biblical literalism; contributor to *Phren. J*; provided COMBE with a testimonial in 1836; Christian phrenologist; lectured 1836–43 in Reading (in 1836 to over 800 persons in a benefit for the Royal Wiltshire Hospital) and Bath; MPA 9/40; rejected phrenology in the 1840s after encountering the criticisms of M. P. J. Flourens. (*MEB*; obit., *Br. Med. J.*, 1868, p. 650)

★ COX, Edward William (1809–79), eldest son of William C. Cox, a manufacturer of Taunton; educated in that place and lectured there on phrenology in the MI in 1834; called to the bar 1843; sergeant-at-law 1868; proprietor and conductor of the *Law Times* 1843–79 and various other legal journals; Conservative M.P. for Taunton 1868–9; wrote on politics and on spiritualism; life-long interest in phrenology and psychology; established and presided over the Psychological Society 1875 to death. (*DNB*; *MEB*)

* COX, Robert (1810–72), third son of Robert Cox, leather dresser of Geordie Mill, Edinburgh; nephew of COMBE; coeditor of *Phren. J.* 1830–7, 1841–7; intimate of Robert Chambers; Writer to the Signet, but did not practice and declined Combe's offer of his business when Combe retired in 1836; antisabbatarian writer; sec. Liverpool Lit., Sci., & Commer. Inst. 1836–40; lectured in Liverpool Lit & Phil 1837; defended phrenology against attack by A. HIGGINSON in Liverpool Lit & Phil 1838; MPA 9/40, resigned 1842; MPS Edinburgh and present at its last meeting 12/70. (*DNB*; *MEB*)

* CRAIG, Edward Thomas (1804–94), Manchester fustian cutter; Owenite cooperator and organizer of the Ralahine Commune, Co. Clare, Ireland; assistant editor of *Star in the East* after 1836; lectured occasionally on phrenology before 1836 and constantly thereafter to become one of the most active itinerants in Britain in the 1840s, when he was for a time employed as a peripatetic lecturer for the Yorkshire Union of MIs; in 1843 he added mesmerism to his lectures and edited the weekly *Mesmerist*; manipulated on stage and privately; used a cast of Rowland Detrosier as a model of perfect organization; became MPA 8/40 while living in Nottingham; pres. Br. Phren. Soc. 1888; continued to work in education, social reform, journalism, and ventilation. (*MEB*; *DLB*)

* CROOK, William Henry, itinerant science lecturer; involved with BAAS, strongly opposing the proposals for its autocratic organization in 1831; MPS London 1825; claimed to have discovered the faculty of Alimentiveness (hunger); lectured in most British towns c. 1825–35, mainly in Lit & Phils; also wrote and lectured on mnemonics; believed by GOYDER to have been responsible for introducing phrenology into Bristol.

* CRYER, William, M.D., M.R.C.S.; of Bradford; included phrenology in his lectures to the Bradford MI 1843; advocated mesmerism; later pres. Hunterian Soc. (Edinburgh), hon. mem. Verulam Phil. Soc., London.

CUBI, Madam, described herself as the "Spanish martyr of phrenology" (cashing in on the reputation of the Spanish phrenologist Mariano Cubi y Soler [1801–75]); manipulated and lectured in London in the 1840s.

* CULL, Richard, Bedford Sq., London; lectured to Staines Lit & Phil 1838, London MI 1837; contributor to *Phren. J.*; MPA 8/40, resigning 1842; BAAS; sec. Ethnol. Soc., 1855; wrote on medical and quasi-medical subjects.

* DAVEY, William (d. 1858), lectured in Edinburgh and Dublin and elsewhere 1848–58 with his coadjutor for 10 years, J. W. JACKSON; turned from lecturing and demonstrating phrenology and phreno-mesmerism to mesmerism.

* DEVILLE, James (1777–1846), leading phrenological manipulator and cast maker in London in the 1820s and 1830s, among whose customers were Harriet Martineau, Charles BRAY, George Eliot, R. D. Owen, Richard CARLILE, the duke of Wellington, and Prince Albert; from humble origins, he became in the 1810s a lampmaker with a profitable business in lighthouse fittings and a plaster caster; Fellow of the Zoological Soc.; mem. (subsequently chairman) of the Society of Arts, and mem. Inst. Civil Eng.; fellow engineer Bryan Donkin encouraged him in the early 1820s to branch into phrenological casting, whence arose his interest in phrenology; organized SPURZHEIM's lectures at the Crown and Anchor Tavern 1825; though regarded as an illiterate by some phrenologists, he contributed to the *Phren. J.* and wrote various guides to accompany the phrenological heads he produced; MPS London and sometimes treasurer; MPA 9/40, resigned 1842; lectured at MIs and Lit. Inst. throughout Britain in the 1830s and gave private lectures in his museum-shop in the Strand; left a collection of over 5,000 skulls and casts (Obit., *Phren. J.*, 19 [1846], 329–44)

★ DEWHURST, Henry William, surgeon, fellow Roy. Jennerian Soc.; mem. London Vet. Med. Soc.; mem. Plinian Soc., and mem. West Med. Soc.; associate of EPPS, pres. and founder of the Verulam Phil. Soc. of London, 1834–7; delivered lectures on phrenology, natural history, astronomy, etc. ("at a day's notice") in London and in the provinces 1820s–1830s; a Catholic, he was sometimes accompanied at his lectures by an Irish priest, the Rev. D. Delaney; had some kind of controlling interest in the *Parthenon*.

DOBSON, _____, lectured on phrenology with GAINSBY in Sunderland Athenaeum to a large audience 1843.

DODD, W. J., surgeon, Monkwearmouth; lectured in Sunderland 1836 and South Shields MI 1841.

★ DONOVAN, Cornelius (c. 1820–72), "professor" of phrenology 1840s–1870s; lectured in nearly every town in England (esp. in the South East and the south Midlands) with some lecturing in Scotland and Ireland, largely in MIs; gave special instruction to the phrenology class at the West. Lit. Inst. (Leicester Sq.) 1842; succeeded DEVILLE as London's leading practical phrenologist and head caster; established London School of Phrenology, Strand (later Trafalgar Sq.); maintained orthodox political and religious views; MPA 5/40; contributed to *Phren. J.*; mem. Ethnol. Soc.

D'ORSAY, Alexander James D. (1812–94), teacher of English in Glasgow High School 1834–50; maintained a ruthless control over Glasgow Phren. Soc. until forced to withdraw; MPA 9/40; lectured in Glasgow MI, where he also taught grammar; lectured in Forfar 1836 at the invitation of the town magistrates; ordained 1847 and graduated from Corpus Christi College Cambridge 1859 where he was appointed chaplain 1860–4; first lecturer of English history at Cambridge 1860–4; appointed professor at King's College, London, 1864. (*MEB*)

DOVE, _____, itinerant lecturer on phrenology and mesmerism in Scotland, based in Glasgow 1843 (?Patrick Edward Dove, 1815–73, editor of the *Commonwealth* published in Glasgow 1858, the first 20 numbers of the *Imperial Dictionary of Biography*, and, with M. Rankin, *Imperial Journal of the Arts and Sciences: MEB*).

DOW, James K, Lancastrian schoolmaster of Nottingham; lectured c. 1838–41; replied to BUTLER's attack in eight lectures 1840–1; MPA.

DUFF, Rev. Henry, of Leith; two popular lectures in Leith and Glasgow 1835.

★ DUNN, Robert (1799–1877), L.S.A. 1825, M.R.C.S. 1828, F.R.C.S. 1852; mem. Med.-Chirug. Soc. of London and the Westminster Med. Soc.; fellow of Ethnol. Soc.; educated at Guy's and St. Thomas' Hospitals; taught at Andersonian Univ.; correspondent of COMBE; author of psychological and medical works; lectured in Scotland 1842; MPS London 12/26. (*DNB; MEB*)

★ EADON, Samuel (1809–91), b. Sheffield; master of an academy in Beef St., Sheffield, then schoolmaster of Pisgah Vale before commencing studies in Edinburgh (M.A. 1834); attracted to hydropathy and homoeopathy in the early 1840s and became a homoeopathic physician in Banbury in the 1850s; joint editor with Charles Pearce of the *Homoeopathic Record*; studied medicine in Aberdeen and received his M.D. in 1861; prolific pamphleteer on alternative medicine, grammar, the land question, and phrenology; interested in the last since mid-1830s; V.P. Sheffield Phren. Soc. 1844–7; MPA 8/40, signing the declaration of expediency 1842; lectured on the harmony between phrenology and scripture in the 1840s; interested in mesmerism and phreno-mesmerism after witnessing La Fontaine's demonstrations in 1842; friend of CRAIG. (*Phren. Record*, 1892, pp. 7–8)

EDEN, Rev. "Dr.," of 70 Regent St., London; "Professor of Moral Philosophy and Cerebral Physiology"; lectured on phrenology and mesmerism Banbury MI 1847 (see Fig. 6).

ELLIS, John, frequent lecturer on phreno-mesmerism at Owenite Halls of Science and workingmen's clubs in the 1840s, especially in London and in Stockport. (Possibly the same who was an Owenite social missionary and author of a radical attack on marriage 1845; possibly also the John Ellis of the Sheffield Phren. Soc., 1846.)

★ ENGLEDUE, William Collins (1813–58), M.D. Edinburgh, L.R.C.S.E. 1835, LSA 1836; student of the Edinburgh medical lecturer and supporter of phrenology John Mackintosh and student pres. Roy. Med. Soc.; provided MACKENZIE with a testimonial 1836; practiced in Portsmouth 1835 to death; founded Royal Portsmouth, Portsea, and Gosport Hospital 1846 as well as various public baths and washhouses; coedited the *Zoist* with John Elliotson; promoter of mesmerism and materialism; leading figure in both the Portsmouth and the London Phren. Socs.; lectured at Portsmouth Lit & Phil 1834–5, Hampshire Phil. Soc. 1836, and eight lectures at the Darwen MI 1840; MPA and largely responsible for its dissolution. (*MEB*)

★ EPPS, John (1805–69), M.D. Edinburgh 1826; Calvinist background; committed Nonconformist; ubiquitous London radical (free trade, anti–Church State, republicanism, etc.); mem. Westm. Med. Soc.; pres. Jennerian Inst., pres. Anthrop. Soc. of London 1845; author of numerous works on medicine, botany, grammar, and religion; early leader of British Homoeopathic Movement and a lecturer on materia medica at the London Homoeopathic Hospital 1851; joint editor of *Lon. Med. & Surg. J.* 1828–9; editor of *J. of Health and Disease* 1845–52 and *Notes on a New Truth* 1856–69; stood unsuccessfully for M.P. for Northampton in 1847 with Chartist backing; MPS Edinburgh 4/26; MPS London; MPA; began lecturing on phrenology the same year he took up private medical practice in London, 1827, and became one of the most familiar figures in the educational institutions in London and the provinces; contributed to *Phren. J.* and edited the *Phrenological (Anthropological) Mag. & Christian Physician* 1835–9. (*DNB; MEB*)

EVE, Ebenezer, practical phrenologist; pupil of DONOVAN; delivered a course of lectures to the Notting Hill and Kensington Co-operative Soc. 1862.

★ FALKNER, Alexander, cashier at Commercial Bank, Newcastle; contributed to *Phren. J.* and *Phren. Almanac*; MPA 9/40, signing the declaration of expediency 1842; lectured in Newcastle to large audiences 1841–2; operated private phrenology museum.

• FIELDING, ———, a "young surgeon" who lectured against phrenology in Hull in 1827. (?Robert S. Fielding [1806–55], LSA 1833, practiced in Riccol, near York: *Med. Dir.*, 1856, p. 733)

FIFE, Sir John (1795–1871), M.R.C.S. 1814, F.R.C.S. 1843; sen. surgeon Newcastle Infirmary; founded Newcastle Medical School and Eye Infirmary; mayor of Newcastle 1838, 1843; J.P.; chairman and sponsor of Newcastle MI; involved with most local social reform movements; knighted in 1840 for his part in suppressing Chartism in Newcastle; key figure in Newcastle Phren. Soc.; provided MACKENZIE with testimonial in 1836; lectured to a crowded audience in Newcastle Lit & Phil 1836 and in Carlisle MI 1836. (*DNB*; *MEB*)

★ FORSTER, Thomas I. M. (1789–1860), F.L.S. 1811, M.B. Cambridge 1819, fellow Roy. Astron. Soc.; naturalist, astronomer, meteorologist, author; eldest son of Thomas Furley Forster, Russian merchant and naturalist (1761–1825); converted to Catholicism 1824; friend of Sir Joseph Banks, John Herschel, and William Whewell; credited with 35 papers in the Roy. Soc. Cat.; founded, with the mathematician B. Gompertz, the Animals' Friend Soc., of which he became hon. for. sec. when he retired to Bruges in the late 1820s; BAAS; attracted to GALL's doctrine in 1806 and coined the word *phrenology* in 1815; acquainted with SPURZHEIM from 1815; first person to lecture on phrenology in Edinburgh (Wernerian Soc., 1816); MPS London 3/25. (*DNB*; *MEB*; *Recueil de ma vie* [1837])

★ FOWLER, Jessie A. (1856–1932), the last of the American "phrenological Fowlers"; daughter of Lorenzo Niles and Lydia FOWLER; lectured, wrote, and delineated with her father in Britain from 1870s; editor of *Phren. Mag* to 1889; mem. Br. Phren. Assoc.; returned to U.S. after the death of her father. (M. B. Stern, *Phrenological Fowlers* [1971])

★ FOWLER, Lorenzo Niles (1811–96), younger brother of the New York phrenologist Orson Squire Fowler (1809–87); emigrated to England in 1860 with his wife Lydia (1823–63), daughter Jessie FOWLER, and partner Samuel Wells (1820–75) and conducted a very successful lecture tour, in the wake of which sprang up many new phrenological societies; his lectures on phrenology, sex, marriage, physiology, heredity, etc. were delivered to working-class audiences at special reduced rates; established the Fowler Inst. in Ludgate Circus as a place for courses of instruction and practical phrenology and as a depot for hundreds of cheap Fowler publications issued from New York; returned to the English lecture circuit in the 1870s, being particularly popular with audiences in the Midlands; established, in 1886, and presided over the Br. Phren. Assoc. (*MEB*; Stern, *Phrenological Fowlers* [1971])

FOX, J. J., delivered three lectures to Devizes Lit. & Sci. Inst., Wilts., 1841.

FROST, J. H., lectured to Spilsby Lit. Inst. 1852.

GAINSBY, ———, lectured on phreno-mesmerism with DOBSON at the Athenaeum in Sunderland 1843.

★ GALL, Franz Joseph (1757–1828), the "inventor" of phrenology; born in Tiefenbronn near Pforzheim, Germany, of Roman Catholic parents; studied medicine in Strasbourg 1777; moved to Vienna 1781, where he received his M.D. 1785; his lectures on the new theory of the brain being proscribed by Emperor Francis I in 1801, he conducted a lecture tour (accompanied by his assistant SPURZHEIM) of the principal towns in Europe, arriving in Paris 1807 where he remained writing, lecturing, and carrying on a highly respectable medical practice until his death. In the spring of 1823 he made a brief visit to London where he lectured on phrenology (in French) at Bossange & Co., Great Marlborough St., to a numerous and fashionable audience; hon. MPS Edinburgh 3/20. (*DSB*)

• ★ GLOVER, Robert Mortimer (1816–59), M.D., medical author and historian of Newcastle Lit & Phil; included phrenology in his lectures on quackery in Newcastle Lit & Phil 1841.

GOULD, Frederick (1817–1900), chemist of Kingston, Surrey; F.L.S. 1849; apprenticed to a chemist in Bath before moving to Kingston, Surrey, 1839; mayor of Kingston 1880; founded and served as first pres. Kingston Lit. & Sci. Inst., where he lectured on phrenology 1841, 1853; MPA. (*MEB*)

★ GOYDER, David George (1796–1878), practical phrenologist of Glasgow; educationalist, sometime apothecary and Swedenborgian preacher; Church background; apprenticed to a brush maker 1810 and a printer 1814; Swedenborgian schoolmaster in Bristol in early 1820s; became inspector of Pestalozzian schools and traveled widely; settled briefly in Hull and Newcastle before moving to Glasgow where he became the resident practical phrenologist; attracted to phrenology in 1822 after CROOK's lectures in Bristol, but did not begin lecturing until 1839; traveled extensively in England and Scotland and lectured in every village within a 40-mile radius of Glasgow; edited the *Phren. Almanac*; MPS Glasgow, MPA 9/40; operated a private phrenology museum in Glasgow; died in Bradford. (*MEB*; *Autobio.* [1857])

GRAHAM, ———, MPS Glasgow; lectured in Kirkcowan 1841.

• ★ GRANT, Rev. Brewin (1821–92), son of a Leicestershire wool comber; evangelical opponent of "Rationalism, Romanism and Radicalism," including phrenology; active 1840s and 1850s; engaged with DONOVAN in a public debate in Birmingham 1849 and lectured against the science in Sheffield 1858; described by HOLYOAKE as "rabbit-minded, with a scavenger's eye for the refuse of old theological controversy"; became a Congregationalist minister in Birmingham 1848–53, Sheffield 1856–68; became an Anglican priest 1871. (*MEB*)

GREEN, John, Owenite social missionary, appointed to Liverpool 1838, at other times in Manchester and Stockport; lectured on phrenology in Blackburn 1837, Wigan 1838, and probably elsewhere; emigrated to U.S. where (according to HOLYOAKE) he was killed by a train.

★ GREGORY, William (1803–58), M.D. Edinburgh 1828, F.R.S.E. 1832; fourth son of James Gregory, professor of medicine in Edin; studied chemistry under Liebig in Giessen 1835; accepted a lectureship at the Andersonian Univ. 1837, at Dublin Univ. 1838, at King's College, Aberdeen, 1839, and then the professorship of chemistry at Edinburgh 1844 (his competitor, Lyon Playfair, being his successor in 1858); author of various works on chemistry and on mesmerism; pres. Scottish Curative Mesmeric Assoc. 1856; BAAS; active MPS Edinburgh in the 1830s and 1840s and the leading figure in the Aberdeen Phren. Soc.; MPA 9/40, signing the declaration of expediency 1842; contributed to *Phren. J.*; delivered a course of popular lectures at the Andersonian Univ. 1839 (*DNB; DSB; MEB*)

GULLAN, John G., teacher in Glasgow; delivered course of lectures in the Andersonian Univ. 1835; MPA.

★ HADDOCK, Joseph Wilcox (1800–61) of Bolton; LSA 1834, M.D. St. Andrews 1850; med. referee for Waterloo and Provincial Assurance Co.; his *Somnolism and Psycheism* (1849), which supported phreno-mesmerism, was delivered as two lectures in the Temperance Hall, Bolton, 1848.

★ HALL, Spencer Timothy (1812–85), son of a Nottinghamshire Quaker cobbler; worked as a stockinger and a printer before aspiring to poetry, essays, and journalism; known as the "Sherwood Forester"; took up hydropathy and homoeopathy in the 1850s and practiced in Derby, Kendal, Burnley, and elsewhere before settling in Blackpool 1881; interested in spiritualism; took up the cause of phreno-mesmerism 1843, lecturing and demonstrating in most towns in England and Scotland; edited the *Phreno-Magnet* (1843); sec. Sheffield Phren. Soc. 1843; died a pauper. (*DNB; MEB*)

HAMILTON, Mr., unidentified popular "mountebank" active in the 1840s; appeared in Newcastle and Carlisle 1841, in Sheffield on phreno-mesmerism 12/45.

HAMILTON, Mrs., of Paisley, practical phrenologist and lecturer; regarded by respectability-seeking phrenologists as a quack but by Owenites as a popular defender of women's rights on the basis of equal mental endowment in both women and men; highly successful at drawing large audiences; appears to have remained largely in Scotland before the 1840s, subsequently in London and elsewhere, lecturing mostly in Halls of Science and MIs on "The Course of Women's Freedom" and "The New Age of Harmony," usually also giving delineations; last appears lecturing on phrenology to a Public Discussion Class in the Council Chambers, Oxford, 1856.

• ★ HAMILTON, Rev. Richard Winter (1794–1848), L.L.D. Glasgow 1844; D.D.; author, minister of the Albion Independent Chapel, Leeds, and pres. Leeds Lit & Phil 1836–8; delivered his *Essay on Craniology* (1826) to the Leeds Lit & Phil, referring to phrenology as "a mischievous fable to posterity," replied to by H. D. INGLIS. (*DNB*)

• * HAMILTON, Sir William (1788–1856), F.R.S.E. 1818, last major exponent of Scottish Common Sense philosophy; elected to chair of logic, Edinburgh, 1836 after competing with COMBE; lectured against phrenology in Edinburgh Assembly Rooms 1827 in a fundraising campaign for the Committee for the Relief of Distressed Operatives; also lectured against the science in the Roy. Soc. of Edinburgh 1825, 1826. (*DNB*; *MEB*)

* HANCOCK, William, solicitor of Wiveliscombe, Somerset; sec. Exeter Phren. Soc., 1841; contributor to *Phren. J.*; MPA 8/40, signing the declaration of expediency 1842; three lectures to Taunton MI 1838; also lectured on physiology c. 1835.

HARRIS, _____, itinerant phreno-mesmerism in Hawick, Galashiels, Melrose, 1843.

HART, _____, lectured on phreno-mesmerism with BAILEY at South London Hall of Science 5/43 (?William Benedict Hart [1813–58] M.R.C.S. 1827, LSA 1837, of Spitalfields: *Med. Dir.*, 1859, p. 973).

* HAWKINS, John Isaac (1772–1855), civil engineer; son of Isaac Hawkins of Taunton; lived for many years in Bordentown, N.J., where in 1852 he started the *J. of Human Nature and Human Progress*; mem. Inst. Civ. Eng. 1824 and a consulting engineer in London 1816–49 before returning to New York; invented, among other curiosities, the ever-pointed pencil; Swedenborgian; BAAS; established in 1835 the Common Good Society along with his friend EPPS (who described him as more enthusiastic than intelligent); pres. Kentish Town Mechanics' Lit. & Sci. Inst. 1836; became interested in phrenology in 1815; treasurer of London Phren. Soc. until 1842 when he established and presided over the Christian Phren. Soc., of which Epps was V.P. [in 1844 this society was superseded by the London Anthropol. (Phren.) Soc.]; MPA 8/39; contributed to *Phren. J.* and *Phren. Almanac*; lectured to many London institutes in the 1830s and 1840s. (*MEB*)

HENDERSON, William Ramsay (1810–32), of Warriston, near Edinburgh; son of a wealthy Edinburgh banker; amateur landscape painter and dilettante; became deeply interested in phrenology in the early 1820s; MPS Edinburgh 3/24; left over £5,000 for the advancement of phrenology, to include publication of a cheap edition of the *Constitution of Man* for "intelligent individuals of the poorer classes and Mechanics' Institutions, etc" – the funds were also used to float *Phren. J* during lean years; attempted to lecture to the working classes of Leith but abandoned lecturing due to his embarrassing stutter.

HICKS, Edwin Thomas, in the same league as DONOVAN, CRAIG, GOYDER, and LEVISON as a popular itinerant lecturer in the 1840s; for a time he was based in Bristol where he delineated and spoke in defence of BARBER's phrenology against BRINDLEY's attack in 1842; lectured mainly in the south of England; also dipped into electrical psychology and mesmerism, the latter leading to a public debate with fellow itinerant, but antimesmerist, J. Q. RUMBALL in Gloucester 1845.

• ★ HIGGINSON, Alfred (1808–84), LSA 1832, M.R.C.S. 1832; brother-in-law of Harriet Martineau; hon. surg. Liverpool South Dispensary; demonstrator of anatomy at Liverpool Med. School 1840–4; contributor to *Cyclopedia of Anatomy and Physiology*; inventor of Higginson's syringe; lectured on anatomical and physiological aspects of phrenology relative to existing knowledge of the structure and functions of the brain, Liverpool Lit & Phil 1838; debated with R. COX. (*Proc. Roy. Soc. Med.*, 25 [1932], 635–8)

★ HODGSON, William Ballantyne (1815–80), educationalist, political economist, reformer, and phrenologist; born in Edinburgh of Calvinist parents, his father being a working printer; intimate of COMBE, William Ellis, BRAY, Cobden, Bright, and EPPS; MPS Edinburgh, mem. Edinburgh Ethical Soc. for the Practical Application of Phrenology, and MPA 8/40; sec. Liverpool MI 1839, becoming its principal 1844–7 at £400 per annum; elected by the Merchant Co. of Edinburgh in 1871 to occupy their newly endowed chair of political economy in the University; prominent in nearly every liberal reform movement in the 1840s and 1850s; coedited works of the Unitarian reformer W. J. Fox; contributed to *Phren. J.*; began lecturing on phrenology at age 22 in various Scottish towns to large audiences of operatives; delivered courses of lectures in Liverpool 1840–7, Sheffield 1847; in response to his lectures in Edinburgh in 1855 the Edinburgh Working Men's Phren. Soc. was established (it survived past 1864); also taught physiology and laws of health. (*DNB*; *MEB*)

HOLDENNESS, J. F., lectured in London 1837–8 to MIs in New Road and Islington.

★ HOLLAND, George Calvert (1801–65), M.D. Edinburgh 1827; son of a Sheffield artisan; apprenticed to a hairdresser before being befriended and educated by Unitarians; began medical practice in Manchester but was forced to remove to Sheffield 1829 because of his public advocacy of phrenology; appointed hon. phys. Sheffield General Infirmary; established Sheffield Physiol. Soc. 1837 and was an active supporter of the Lit & Phil; in 1840 his exposure of the fallacies of Corn Law repeal cost him his former friends and his medical practice; became involved in railway projects and acted as the director of two banks; upon the collapse of the latter, he moved to London; returned to Sheffield in 1851 as a homoeopathic physician and established the Sheffield Homoeopathic Hospital 1853–4; also attracted to mesmerism; alderman of Sheffield 1862 to death; wrote several medical works and edited the *Sheffield Homoeopathic Lancet*, 1853; V.P. Sheffield Phren. Soc.; lectured on phrenology in Halifax 1827–8 and Chesterfield 1831. (*DNB*; *MEB*)

HOLM, Henry Haley (1806–46), M.R.C.S. 1828; son of J. D. HOLM; an inheritance allowed him to devote all his time to phrenology and comparative zoology; lived with SPURZHEIM Paris and at his father's home in Bedford Sq , and with his father inherited Spurzheim's London collection of skulls and paraphernalia; first to give a course of lectures on phrenology in a recognized British medical school (London Hospital, 1832–3); arrested in 1828 and fined £50 for disinterring the bodies of his mother, brother, and sister and severing their heads for phrenological study; MPS London 12/25 until 1832 when he and a few others (including Sir James Clark) formed a more exclusive group to discuss phrenology;

MPA; delivered a course of lectures at the Western Inst. 1838. (Obit., *Phren. J.*, 19 [1846], 286–9; *Hendon & Finchley Times & Guardian*, 28 Mar. 1958)

★ HOLM, John Diderick (1772–1856), grandson of John Haley Holm (d. 1763), a moneyer of the Royal Mint. Sweden; b. Sweden; moved to London 1805 as a foreign merchant, from which occupation he retired in 1817 to commence an amateur career in phrenology, having much earlier met GALL in Paris; friend and executor of SPURZHEIM; MPA; lectured every Thursday at his home in Gower St. 1828–32 and in Bedford Sq. 1832 to his death; also lectured 1832–6 at Grainger's Theatre of Anatomy, Southwark Inst., London and Baltic Tavern, North London Inst., Eastern Athenaeum, Gothic Hall, Inst. of Useful Knowledge, and Milltown Inst.; lectured at the South London Owenite Hall of Science 1843. (*MEB*)

★ HOLYOAKE, George Jacob (1817–1906), Birmingham whitesmith, educated at the MI where he became interested in phrenology as well as Owenism, freethought and Chartism; became an Owenite missionary but eventually rejected Owenism and devoted all his attention to the propagation of rational secular religious views, preceding Charles Bradlaugh as the leading secularist in Britain; unfortunate encounters with BALLY and COMBE made him suspicious of some of the motives of phrenologists but he lectured on the science in the Sheffield Hall of Science 8/41 to a large audience (and presumably at other Halls of Science at this time); in 2/46 he delivered a lecture at the Rationalist Inst., London, on "The Phrenological Philosophy of George Combe and Dr Engledue, Including Our Unsettled Personal Reminiscences"; in the John St. Inst. 12/48 he lectured on "Other Ways of Telling Character Than by Palmistry and Phrenology." (*DNB*; *DLB*)

HUGHES, C. G., (sometimes spelled Hughs), delivered a lecture on "The Phrenological Character of Jesus Christ" to the Owenite John St. Inst. 1843; also on mesmerism to Southampton MI 1843 and on phreno-mesmerism to various London institutes c. 1843.

★ HUNTER, Robert (1795–1864), M.D. Glasgow 1828; lecturer on anatomy and surgery, Portland St. School of Med. 1826; at the Westminster Hospital, London, 1841–50, and at Andersonian Univ. 1850–60; pres. Faculty of Phys. & Surg., Glasgow, 1855–7; surg. Glasgow Roy. Infirmary 1857; lectured on phrenology at Glasgow MI 1833 and with J. R. WOOD at Greenock 1834–6; testimonial to COMBE 1836; MPS Glasgow and MPA; wrote popular manuals on phrenology.

HUNTER, William, professor of logic at Andersonian Univ.; delivered a course of lectures on phrenology at the Andersonian; testimonial to COMBE 1836.

HUSPAND, ———, gave a free lecture on phrenology at York MI 1839; also lectured on the philosophy of sleep and on civilization in Africa.

★ HYTCH, E. J., law stationer of Islington; organized and tutored the Saturday evening phrenology class at the London MI 1839–44; gave courses of lectures at the MI 1841, 1846 to large audiences; noted as a Christian phrenologist; contributed to *Phren. J, Phren. Almanac, People's Phren. J.,* and *Christian Physician*; also contributed to the *Lancet* and wrote a volume of poetry; MPA 5/40, resigning 1842.

★ INGLIS, Henry David (1795–1835), traveler and miscellaneous writer; son of a Scottish advocate; editor of the *Chesterfield Gazette* prior to 1830 and of the Jersey *British Critic* 1832–4; settled in London and contributed to *Colburn's New Monthly Mag*; one of the V.P.'s of the Leeds Lit & Phil 1826 when he replied to the Rev. R. W. HAMILTON's animadversions on phrenology. (*DNB*)

★ INGLIS, James (1813–51), M.D. Edinburgh 1834, M.R.C.S. 1834, F.G.S.; b. Glasgow; distinguished himself in medicine while a student; hon. phys. Ripon Dispensary 1837, thereafter practicing in Halifax; largely involved in the organization and proceedings of the Halifax Lit & Phil and was curator of its geological department; author of various medical essays, including essays against homoeopathy; contributed to *Phren. J.*; MPA 8/39, signing the declaration of expediency 1842; testimonial to MACKENZIE in 1836; lectured in Halifax Lit & Phil 1843. (Obit., *Med. Dir.*, 1852, pp. 647–8; *MEB*)

★ INWARDS, Jabez (1817–80), practical phrenologist and advocate of temperance, life insurance, and self-help; associate of TOWGOOD and the Quaker hydropath and temperance advocate William Horsell in the Phrenological Depot and Museum, 492 Oxford St., London; lectured 1843–c. 1860 in London workingmen's institutes, Notting Hill, Holborn, and in the provinces (also on other scientific and literary subjects); helped form with BEGGS and others the new London Phren. Soc. 1856. (*MEB*)

★ JACKSON, John Williams (1809–71), b. Somerset of Wesleyan family, lamed at 13; moved from Bristol to London 1832 where he attempted to launch himself as a writer, spending an unsuccessful 7 years in the British Museum in this pursuit; turned to lecturing and in Bridgeport met William DAVEY with whom he lectured for 10 years until Davey's death in 1858; settled in Edinburgh 1855 and lectured on phrenology and mesmerism and ran a phreno-mesmeric clinic; supplemented his income with newspaper and periodical journalism; moved to Glasgow after Davey's death and presided over the Curative Mesmeric Assoc. and became a leading figure in the Glasgow Assoc. of Spiritualists; mem. (new) Phren. Assoc. of Edinburgh 1864; after marrying in 1866 he returned to London; contributed to the *Zoist, Anthropol. J.*, and *Human Nature*. (Memoir by his wife in his *Man Contemplated* [1875])

★ JENNINGS, James, wealthy patron of adult education and Owenite cooperative efforts; editor of the *Family Cyclopedia*; lectured on phrenology to London MI 1828.

• JEVONS, William, Jr. (1794–1873), Liverpool Unitarian; uncle of the better-known political economist W. S. Jevons (1835–82); first son of Thomas Jevons who married into the Liverpool political and banking family of Roscoe; wrote on *Moral Philosophy* (1827) and astronomy (1828); educator, ran a day school in Liverpool that included a class on mental and moral philosophy (from 1822); lectured on phrenology in Liverpool Lit & Phil 1828 and again 11/34 on "Functions of the Brain with Strictures on Phrenology."

JOHNSON, _____, Owenite; lectured on phreno-mesmerism in Newcastle 1843.

JONES, Edward, of Holywell, Wales; lectured on phrenology and mesmerism in Wales in the 1840s with his brother.

JONES, Peter, connected with the phrenology class in the London MI (possibly succeeding HYTCH), then organized the Sunday afternoon phrenology class in the John St. Inst. 1846–8; lectured at most of the radical institutions in London, occasionally found on the debating platforms defending the science; gave address 1847 as Goldsmith's Row, Fleet St.; debated phrenology with BAKER 1847.

KEIR, _____, gave popular lectures on astronomy, geology, natural history and phrenology c. 1836–7 in Ireland, Scotland, and the Midlands.

★ KIRTLEY, Martin, surgeon, Barnard Castle; lectured in the Barnard Castle MI 1836; contributed to *Phren. J.*

KISTE, Adolphus, itinerant lecturer on phrenology and phreno-mesmerism; MPS Liverpool, MPA 8/40; with VERNON in Liverpool, Exeter, Torquay, and elsewhere 1840–1.

LACON, Joseph, solicitor and general literary author; pres. Liverpool Philomathic Soc.; early promoter of Liverpool MI and gave the first lectures on phrenology there 1832–3.

LEE, A., lectured on the formation of the skull and the structure of the brain in London MI 1837. (Likely Alexander Cooper Lee [d. 1850?], M.D. Erlangen 1831, London practitioner and editor of medical texts by Astley Cooper and John Elliotson.)

LEGER, Théodore (1799–1853), b. and educated Paris; resided in Mexico where he acquired and spent two fortunes; medical mesmerist 1850; lectured on phrenology at Hungerford Hall, London, 1851; gave seances and examined heads at 20 Gerrard St., Soho, 1852. (*MEB*)

★ LEIGHTON, Andrew, Liverpool manufacturer; contributed to *Phren. J.*; 7/40, signing the declaration of expediency 1842; MPA later involved with spiritualism; lectured to Liverpool Hope St. Mutual Improvement Soc. c. 1862.

★ LEVISON, John L., itinerant phrenologist, lecturing throughout England mainly at MIs 1828–43; delivered a course of lectures at the London Inst. 1832 to an audience of 800; leading phrenologist of Hull before moving to Doncaster where he opened a phrenological museum and became V.P. of the Lyceum; subsequently moved to London; lectured on dentistry and "dental quackery" in Birmingham 1842 and was involved there with phreno-mesmeric experiments; in 1849 he was established as a dentist in Brighton; contributed to *Phren. J.* and wrote on mental culture and temperance; MPA, signing the declaration of expediency 1842.

LOGAN, Simon, artist; of Walworth, Surrey; MPS London and MPA 8/39; highly popular lecturer in Scotland, the east of England, and London 1836–41; also lectured for Popular Education Assoc. in London 1836 at the Southampton Coffee House.

★ LOWE, Hudson, of Chelsea; contributed to *Phren. J.*; MPS London and MPA; lectured in Lit. & Sci. Inst.'s in 1840s.

★ LOWE, William Robinson (1820–56), wholesale chemist and town councillor of Wolverhampton; zealous sanitary improver and working-class educationalist; nominally of the Church of England and highly Christian phrenologist; life cut short by an embarrassing bankruptcy; BAAS; contributed to *Phren. J.*; MPA 8/39, signing the declaration of expediency, 1842; lectured at Wolverhampton MI 1840–2 and Ironbridge 1841; also lectured on geology, education, and literature. (Memoir in *Lectures* [1857])

LUNDIE, H., lectured on phreno-mesmerism in Devizes, Scotland, 1844 (possibly the same who appeared in English towns in the early 1840s and was regarded by the Sheffield Phren. Soc. as an itinerant quack).

MCARTHUR, ———, (1813–49), stationer of Halifax; b. Inverness and worked for a time in Edinburgh as a printer; educated at MIs; became a Unitarian; moved to London and then to Halifax where he heard Lloyd Jones lecture on Owenite cooperation and became a convert and subsequently sec. Preston Social Soc.; devoted himself to working-class education and improvement in Halifax and lectured there on phrenology; upon his death HOLYOAKE noted in the *Reasoner* that McArthur "taught and lectured with a zeal and activity almost above his strength. His lectures on Phrenology will not soon be forgotten by those who heard them."

★ M'BEAN, G. N. B., "professor" of phrenology in Newcastle-under-Lyme 1844; in Ulster 1850s, also lecturing on medical galvanism and "man's formation"; mem. (new) Phren. Assoc. Edinburgh 1864.

M'DOUGAL, ———, surgeon, of Galashiels, attempted to lecture in Galashiels 1835 but "overruled by the general clamour of its dangerous tendency."

M'GIBBON, ———, itinerant lecturer on phreno-mesmerism in Scotland 1843, from Greenock to Aberdeen.

MACGLASHAN, William, "a lank bare-boned tailor"; otherwise described as a teacher and librarian of the Dundee Phren. Soc.; did delineations and lectured to working-class audiences in Inverarity, Monifeith, Glammis, and Dundee 1835–6.

★ MACKENZIE, Sir George Steuart, 7th baronet (1780–1848), F.R.S. 1815, F.R.S.E. 1799, mineralogist and geologist, pres. Astron. Inst. Edinburgh; BAAS; early member of the Edinburgh Phren. Soc.; sponsor and contributor to *Phren. J.*; close friend of COMBE; turned to mesmerism 1843; proposed the Phren. Assoc. in 1835 and resigned from it in 1842; lectured on phrenology to his tenants at Dingwall 1822, on phrenology and education in Jersey MI 1839, and in Royal Yacht Club 1840. (*DNB*)

MACKENZIE, William (1791–1868), surgeon, of Glasgow; b. Glasgow, son of a muslin manufacturer; studied in London and Vienna, returned to Glasgow 1819; abandoned divinity in 1810 for medicine; appointed to University of Glasgow in 1828 and surgeon-oculist for the queen in Scotland 1838; became a famous eye specialist and professor of anatomy at Andersonian Univ.; early advocate of phrenology; lectured in Glasgow 1822–5 and included phrenology among lecture topics in his anatomy course. (J. Marshall, *Glas. Med. J*, 35 [1954], 258–70)

M'TAGGART, David, surgeon, of Halifax; delivered two public lectures for the Sheffield Phren. Soc. 1845.

MARRIOTT, Rev. Joseph (b. 1794), of a wealthy London family; destined for a legal career, which he abandoned to become a dissenting preacher in Lancashire; attracted to Owenite socialism and became a committee member for Warrington 1831 and wrote Owenite tracts; turned to public lecturing on phrenology in the 1840s; for some time based at Bristol where he lectured and delineated, later lecturing at the Royal Adelaide Gallery, London, and various workingmen's institutes in the 1840s; also lectured on social and domestic economy in the North and Midlands; made proposals to establish Ragged Scientific Institutes and spoke on phrenology at Goswell St. Inst. 1848 after HOLYOAKES's lecture on "Logic of Death."

MARTIN, Mrs. Emma (1812–51), b. Bristol; brought up a strict Baptist, she doubted orthodox Christianity after hearing Alexander Campbell 1839; left her husband and became a freethought lecturer, mainly in socialist halls in London and in the provinces; gave private lectures to women on physiology in London 1840s; debated "marriage and divorce" with the Rev. R. S. Bayley in London Hall of Science 1840; prevented from defending socialism, infidelity, and phrenology against BRINDLEY in Leicester in 1840; supposed to have made a deathbed repentance, but HOLYOAKE nevertheless spoke at her graveside; wrote on infidelity; gave course of five lectures on phrenology at the Sheffield Hall of Science 1839. (*MEB*; *DLB*)

MATHEO, _____, Italian immigrant resident in Exeter 1838; lectured in Exeter, Plymouth, and Tavistock MIs 1838–40; in Sheffield 1841.

MAYNOTT, _____, defended phrenology against O'CALLAGHAN in a lecture in Dover 1839.

MILLER, George (d. 1879), G.P. of Emsworth, Hants., LSA 1831, M.R.C.S. 1833; educated at University College; surgeon to Havant Poor Law Union, later of Sidmouth, Devon, where he was also consulting surgeon to the dispensary; contributed to *Lancet* and other medical journals; pres. Emsworth Lit. Soc., where he lectured on phrenology 1835, 1842; MPA.

MILNE, D., lectured on "The Logic of Phrenology," Finsbury Hall, 1849; normally lectured on cooperation and secular rationalist subjects.

MOIR, Andrew, surgeon, Aberdeen; lectured in Aberdeen 1838, also giving lectures on anatomy and physiology to Aberdeen Phren. Soc.

* MONTGOMERY, James (1771–1854), poet and editor of the *Sheffield Register*; imprisoned for libel 1795; became increasingly conservative in the 1830s; lectured on phrenology in Sheffield Lit & Phil 1826, defending the doctrine against Sir William HAMILTON's attack, but wrote against phrenology's tendency to fatalism 1829. (*DNB*; *MEB*)

NEWMAN, W. H., lecturer at various London mutual improvement and workingmen's institutes 1843–8; conducted an evening phrenology class at the City of London Mutual Improvement Soc. (est. 1836) in 1843, where he also frequently lectured along with EPPS and HOLYOAKE.

★ NICHOL, David (d. 1865), M.R.C.S. 1816 and ext. L.R.C.P.; practiced in Swansea, where he was hon. phys. to the Infirmary (retiring 1846) and hon. sec. Roy. Inst. of South Wales; contributed to *Phren. J.*; MPA 5/40; delivered two courses of lectures in institutes in Swansea 1836–41.

★ NOBLE, Daniel (1810–85), M.R.C.S. 1833, F.R.C.S. 1852, F.R.C.P. 1859; b. Preston; educated at Guy's Hospital; settled in Manchester 1834 and lectured on psychological medicine at Chatham St. School of Medicine before establishing himself as a leading physician and consultant; author of numerous works on physiology and psychological medicine; pres. Lancashire and Cheshire branch of the Br. Med. Assoc.; visiting physician of Clifton Hall Retreat and Why House Asylum, Buxton; declined a county magistracy; active in local sanitary reform; MPA 6/40 and MPS Manchester being the pres. 1835–8; contributed to *Phren. J.*; friend of COMBE and DUNN; lectured in Manchester Lit & Phil 1837; renounced phrenology 1846 after William Carpenter attacked his views. (*MEB*)

NYMAN, _____, lectured on phreno-mesmerism in London 1843; claimed to have had lecturing experience in U.S.

• O'CALLAGHAN, _____, antiphrenology lecture in Dover Phil. Inst. 1839.

O'NEILL, Arthur (1819–96), popular Birmingham Chartist and founder of the Christian Chartist Church; son of a coachmaker; studied medicine in Glasgow 1835 before turning to theology 1837; earned his living by lecturing on science and theology, including physiology and physics among his topics; signed the teetotal pledge 1837; attracted to Chartism 1838 and elected to the executive committee of the Glasgow Chartist 1839, aged 20; founded the Zion Baptist Chapel in Birmingham 1840 and ran a large Sunday school; joined middle-class Radical Reform League 1840; lectured on phrenology in his chapel 1841; imprisoned 1842. (*MEB; DLB*)

OVEREND, Hall (d. 1831), surgeon to Sheffield Infirmary; son of a Sheffield clerk; local science activist with a natural history museum in Church St.; Quaker, but later announced himself a convert to freethought; involved in local reform movement; brother of John (1769–1832) of the Lombard St. banking firm of Overend, Gurney, & Co.; claimed to be the first to introduce phrenology into Sheffield; delivered four lectures in the Lit & Phil 1830; lectured in Nottingham 1824; his son Wilson (1806–65) became a leading surgeon and medical lecturer in Sheffield; his eldest son, John (1802–32) M.D. Edinburgh 1824, of Doncaster became a MPS Edinburgh 2/24; obit., *Gents. Mag.*, 1832, p. 187.

OWENS, _____, initially a member of VERNON's entourage, assisting him in demonstrating and lecturing on phreno-mesmerism in Staffordshire and Bristol MI 1844; by 1850s he was lecturing on his own in London; claimed to be a M.R.C.S. 1839.

PASQUALL, _____, lectured at Almondbury MI, near Huddersfield, 1862.

• ★ PRICHARD, James Cowles (1786–1848), M.D. Edinburgh 1808, diploma Oxford 1835, F.R.S. 1827; attended Dugald Stewart's lectures while in Edinburgh, later studied at Cambridge and Oxford; appointed hon. phys. St. Peter's Hospital, Bristol, 1811 and hon. phys. Bristol Infirmary 1814; published on ethnology 1813 and was pres. London Ethnol. Soc. 1847–8; commissioner of lunacy 1844–8; identified himself completely with conservative activities in science and social life; a Quaker, he joined the Church before leaving Oxford; a member of the Bristol Inst. and a leading figure in the Bristol Lit & Phil where he lectured on phrenology and mesmerism 1/35, concurrent with the writing of his criticisms on phrenology in the *Cyclopedia of Practical Medicine* and in his *Treatise on Insanity*. (*DNB*; *DSB*)

★ PRIDEAUX, T. Symes, b. Southampton c. 1790; friend of ENGLEDUE; contributed to *Phren. J., Zoist,* and the *Anthropol. Rev.* 1860s; mem. Ethnol. Soc.; argued against phreno-mesmeric fallacies (indeed, argued over points of doctrine with most of his colleagues); attracted to phrenology 1806 upon reading the account of the science in the *Lon. Med. & Phys. J.* lectured in Blandford Town Hall, Dorset, and in Guernsey 1838–40; also wrote on the economy of fuels and on grammar.

• PROUDFOOT, Thomas (1791–1859), M.D. Edinburgh 1819, formerly an army surgeon; physician to Kendal Dispensary; magistrate; lectured against phrenology to the Kendal Natural History Soc. 1842.

R____D, _____, lectured in Portsmouth 1834–5.

RAINE, William Tanner, teacher; began lecturing on phrenology 1842 with penny lectures at the Dockhead MI and in Bermondsey (he believed these were the first penny lectures on phrenology given in the metropolis); mem. HAWKINS' Christian Phren. Soc.; contributed to *Christian Physician* 1836.

RICHARDSON, William, itinerant phrenologist and manipulator in Durham and Northumberland; self-taught; also lectured on electricity, pneumatics, chemistry, etc.

• RIGG, J, of Birmingham; commenced antiphrenology lectures in Birmingham 1843 and in Halifax (?John Clulow Rigg, d. 1868, son of the Rev. John Rigg; asst. to a physician of Barton-on-Humber; clerk to Mr. Kell, stockbroker; editor of *The Watchman* 1848–64).

ROBERTSON, James (d. c. 1890), L.R.C.S.E. 1832; surgeon of Johnstone, Renfrewshire; mem. Med.–Chir., Phil., and Geol. Soc.'s, Glasgow; MPA 5/40; delivered a course of 10 lectures in Johnstone in support of a public reading room 1838. (Not to be confused with the James Robertson who died in 1840, who was pres. Paris Anthropol. Soc. founded by SPURZHEIM, who corresponded with COMBE and MACKENZIE, and who left to the EPS £15,000 that, due to foreign legal disputes, was never received.)

ROBINSON, _____, lecturer on scientific subjects; lectured on phrenology to Great Tower St. MI 1837.

ROOTES, William Symonds (d. 1876), M.D. Edinburgh 1839, M.R.C.S. 1845; son of George Rootes, M.D.; trained at St. George's Hospital; med. officer Ross Union, Herefordshire, and hon. phys. Ross Dispensary; lectured to Hereford Lit & Phil 1841.

ROPE, Robert, of Sheffield; professional chemist and medicine manufacturer; included a lecture on phrenology in his lectures (12/40–5/41) to Sheffield MI; also lectured on physiology, chemistry, electricity, and philosophy.

* RUMBALL, James Quilter (1795–1872), M.R.C.S. 1817, LSA 1822; son of John Rumball, surgeon of Abington; itinerant phrenologist; claimed to have studied under Monro at Bethlem Asylum and to have become a pupil of SPURZHEIM's c. 1820; wrote several med. works of dubious value and, in 1844, on the need for the BAAS to recognize phrenology; proprietor of the unlicensed Harpenden Hall Asylum for the Insane at St. Albans, Herts.; contributed to *J. Psychol. Med.* and to *Phren. J.*; established a phrenology shop at 3 King William St., the Strand, 1840 to compete with DONOVAN's establishment; MPA; proposed 1/44 to establish a new Br. Phren. Soc. and a new phren. mag., neither of which projects materialized; lectured in London and the provinces 1830s, 1840s, and to large audiences at the Adelaide Gallery 1843; conducted a strenuous campaign against materialism and mesmerism (especially phreno-mesmerism) 1843, pursuing VERNON around England; debated with BRINDLEY in Worcester 1839–40 and in Liverpool 1842; read Herbert Spencer's head. (*MEB*)

RYDING, _____, lectured in Limerick Phil. Inst. 1830s.

RYLEY, _____, lectured on phreno-mesmerism in Sheffield 1843.

* SAMPSON, Marmaduke Blake (d. 1876), City correspondent or financial editor of *The Times* 1846–79; formerly for many years sec. to the Treasury Committee of the Bank of England; wrote for the *Economist* and the *Spectator* and edited the *Popular Record*; an accomplished classical scholar; met COMBE in New York 1838 and maintained a long correspondence with him on phrenology, currency, and stocks and shares; a founding member of EPPS's Brit. Homoeopathic Assoc. and on its committee 1840s; established himself as an authority on the phrenological treatment of criminals, criminal jurisprudence, and reform; contributed to *Phren. J.*; MPA 9/40, putting forward with SIMPSON the declaration of expediency 1842; lectured to large audiences in various London institutes late 1830s and early 1840s. (*MEB*)

* SANDWITH, Thomas (1793–1867), trained at St. Bartholomew's Hospital; practitioner in Beverley from c. 1815; M.D. Erlangen 1843; surgeon to House of Correction for the East Riding of Yorkshire and Poor Law union med. officer; author of several medical works; contributed to *Phren. J.*; lectured in the Hull and Beverley MI 1835.

* SCOTT, James, M.D. Edinburgh; med. supt. Royal Navy Lunatic Asylum at Haslar, Gosport, from 1822; MPS Edinburgh 1/24 and MPA 9/40; pres. Portsmouth Phren. Soc. 1830s; testimonial to COMBE 1836; lectured in Gosport and Portsmouth 1834–5.

★ SCOTT, John, science lecturer including phrenology in his list of subjects; mem. National Assoc. Promotion of Social Sciences; active c. 1850.

SHARPLES, Eliza – see CARLILE, Mrs.

SHUTTLEWORTH, T. B., of Sheffield; MPS Sheffield 1844; lectured on phreno-mesmerism 1843.

★ SIMPSON, James (1781–1853), Scottish advocate and secular educationalist; close friend of COMBE (provided testimonial 1836), Richard Cobden and Thomas Wyse; MPS Edinburgh 4/23 and MPA 8/39, putting forward with SAMPSON the declaration of expediency 1842; sponsor of and contributor to *Phren. J.*; lectured on phrenology and education 1836–44 in Edinburgh, Newcastle, Birmingham, Bath, Manchester, Aberdeen, and elsewhere; as interested in the cleanliness of the bodies of the working class as in their morality, he was much involved in the campaign for public baths in Edinburgh; subsequently interested in mesmerism. (*DNB; MEB*)

SLEEP, _____, three lectures on phreno-mesmerism in Ross 1847.

★ SMART, Alexander, sec. Dundee Mechanics' Phren. Soc.; lectured in Dundee 1833.

SMITH, John, of Tetley Row; lectured on phreno-mesmerism in Bradford MI 1843.

★ SMITH, Joshua Toulmin (1816–69), eldest son of W. Hawkes SMITH; articled to a Birmingham solicitor 1832; student at Lincoln's Inn 1835, called to the bar 1849; a student of literature and philosophy with an interest in economics and educational reform, he taught with his father in the Birmingham MI, lecturing there on phrenology 1835; influenced by Harriet Martineau's account of U.S., he emigrated to Michigan 1835 where he attempted, but failed, to earn a living by writing and lecturing on phrenology; returned to England 1842 and continued his legal studies; became a noted constitutional lawyer opposing government centralization and founded the weekly *Parliamentary Remembrancer* (1857–65); first pres. Geologists' Assoc. 1859; MPS London and MPA 8/39, being one of the sec.'s of latter 1840; corresponded with COMBE 1836–50 and contributed to *Phren. J.* (*DNB; MEB; J. in America*, 1837–8, ed. F. B. Streeter [1925])

★ SMITH, Sidney, itinerant phrenologist; of Edinburgh; contributed to *Phren. J.*; MPS Edinburgh and on council of Ethical Soc. for the Practical Application of Phrenology; turned more to politics and social reform in the 1840s; lectured in major Scottish centers, North of England, and Manchester 1836–8; also lectured on repeal of Corn Laws and on temperance, often incorporating such items as "improvements in agriculture" into his phrenology lectures to draw larger crowds.

SMITH, T. W., student in the medical department of St. Peter's hospital, Bristol; lectured 2/38 Bristol MI (?Thomas Wade Smith [d. 1857], M.R.C.S. 1843: *Med. Dir.* [1858], p. 874).

* SMITH, William Hawkes (1786–1840), Birmingham radical and Unitarian; at various times author, shopkeeper, printer, engraver, stationer, notary public, editor of *Birmingham Inspector* (1817) and *Midland Chronicle*; V.P. Birmingham MI; attracted to Owenism and Combean phrenology 1830s; arranged the Phren. Assoc. meeting in Birmingham 1839; Christian socialist; contributed to *Phren. J.*; corresponded with COMBE; a friend of BRAY; taught phrenology in the Birmingham MI and publicly vindicated Combe's phrenology in two lectures 1838 after a course of antiphrenological lectures by BRINDLEY; also gave free lectures on geology in other midland towns 1830s; MPA 8/39. (Obit., *Phren. J.*, 13 [1840], 284; *New Moral World*, 7, 8 [1840], 1260–1, 59).

SNAPE, _____, dentist, student of BRIDGES; lectured to Chester MI 1836 on the practical advantages of phrenology in daily life; gave free lectures on phrenology and on the teeth in the Potteries 1840s.

* SPURR, Mrs. Thomas, of Sheffield; associated with Sheffield phrenologists; lectured on "The Brain as the Organ of Intellect" along with other physiological, religious, and educational topics to Sheffield "ladies" 1836.

* SPURZHEIM, Johann Gaspar (1776–1832), M.D. Vienna 1813, L.R.C.P. 1817; b. near Koblenz, Germany, of Lutheran parents and intended for the clergy; studied divinity and philosophy at the Univ. of Treves; traveled to Vienna c. 1797 and took up medical studies in 1800 first as a pupil and then as an associate of GALL; accompanied Gall on his European tour 1805–6 and settled with him in Paris 1807; separated from Gall 1813 and traveled to England where he lectured at intervals 1814–31, returning frequently to Paris where he lectured publicly before 1824 and privately thereafter; rendered phrenology popular among the British public, both lay and medical, from the early 1820s; based himself in England at the London home of J. D. HOLM; hon. MPS London and Edinburgh; contributed to *Phren. J.*; lectured to audiences ranging from 70 in Sheffield 1829 to over 700 for his course at the London Inst. 1826; died of fever in Boston 1832 while on American lecture tour. (*DSB*; A. Carmichael, *Memoir* [1833])

STALLARD, Joshua Harrison (d. c. 1856), G.P. of Leicester; surgeon to Leicester General Dispensary, Union Workhouse, and regiment of militia; wrote on female labor, health and hygiene, pauper lunatics, economics, Scottish Poor Law, municipal government, and sanitation; opposed homoeopathy and hydropathy 1850s; lectured on phrenology to Leicester Lit & Phil 1/47.

• * STANILAND, S. (d. c. 1851), M.R.C.S. 1828, LSA 1829; G.P. of Farnham; became a demonstrator of anatomy at the Leeds School of Medicine; delivered two lectures against phrenology in Farnham Lit. Inst. 1839 to which ENGLEDUE replied in print; the latter's influence may have caused his removal to Leeds.

STARK, William, of Norwich; F.G.S.; lectured to 300 in Norwich Museum 1840; MPA 6/40.

* STEBBING, J. Rankin, of Southampton; contributed to *Phren. J.*; lectured at Southampton and Winchester MI and Cowes Lit. & Sci. Inst. 1833–44.

STOCKS, (?J. E.), phreno-mesmerist of Sheffield; lectured in Doncaster 1843, at Sheffield Hall of Science 1839.

★ STRATON, James (d. 1856), fishing tackle manufacturer; leading phrenologist of Aberdeen and founder, in 1836, of the Aberdeen Phren. Soc.; MPA, signing the declaration of expediency 1842; preoccupied with classifying heads or "mathematics of phrenology"; contributed to *Phren. J.* and *Zoist*; lectured in Manchester Athenaeum 12/51. (*MEB*)

SWEETLOVE, Ellis (d. c. 1843), LSA 1829, M.R.C.S. 1829; educationalist and medical reformer; patron of Liverpool MI, where he lectured on phrenology 1833; also lectured at the Liverpool Polytech. and at the Liverpool Lit., Sci., & Commerc. Inst., 1833–5; also lectured locally on the philosophy of atmosphere and other scientific subjects.

★ TAIT, William (d. 1870), licentiate of the Faculty of Physicians and Surgeons of Glasgow 1833; house surgeon and apothecary of Paisley Dispensary and House of Recovery and one of the district surgeons of the City Parish before taking up practice in Lauder; mem. Med. Soc. and Med.-Chirg. Soc. of Glasgow; author of medical essays; contributed to *Phren. J.*; MPA 7/40, signing the declaration of expediency 1842; lectured in Galashiels and Lauder MIs 1835–6.

TAYLDER, T., lectured in St. Austell Lit. Inst., Cornwall, 1839.

• THOMAS, Rev. J. N. H., sermonized against Combe's *Constitution of Man* 11/36 in St. James Chapel, Edinburgh (see Fig. 5).

• THORPE, _____, M.D. (?Edinburgh 1810); practiced in Leeds; antiphrenology lecture to Leeds Lit. Inst. 1838.

★ TICHBORNE, Thomas, MPS Hampshire; employed in the Stamps and Taxes Office, Somerset House, 1840s; correspondent of EPPS; lectured in Hampshire and Portsmouth and at London Inst. 1832–5, 1839.

TOOMBES, _____, lectured in Tower St. Mutual Improvement Soc. 1837.

TORBET, John, surgeon of Paisley; MPS Edinburgh 11/21; lectured to 70 in Paisley Phil. Inst. 1824–5.

★ TOWGOOD, Frederick (d. 1860), temperance and antitobacco advocate; coeditor of *J. of Health* 1850; treasurer of the new London Phren. Soc. 1856; lectured at Camden Hall 1855.

TOWNSEND, _____, of Haworth, two lectures on phreno-mesmerism in Huddersfield 1843.

★ TURLEY, Edward Astbury, educationalist of Worcester; MPS London 3/25 and MPA; very successful lectures in Worcester Athenaeum and Guildhall 1839 and 1834–6, respectively.

★ TURNER, Henry, Sheffield warehouseman; leading West Riding secularist from c. 1857; follower of Joseph Barker; learned his phrenology at a Sunday school in Sheffield; sec. Sheffield Phren. Soc. 1840s; taught phrenology at the Sheffield MI, illustrating the science with the heads of Richard Oastler, Isaac Ironside, HOLYOAKE, and Owen.

TURNER, Thomas (1793–1873), F.R.C.S. 1843; house surgeon of Manchester Infirmary 1817–20; surgeon to Manchester Royal Infirmary 1830; instrumental in establishing schools of medicine and surgery in Manchester; professor of philosophy at Manchester Roy. Inst. 1843; mem. Prov. Med. & Surg. Assoc. and contributed to their *Transactions* 1835; leading figure in the Manchester and Salford Sanitary Assoc. (est. 1852); BAAS; lectured at Manchester Roy. Inst. on education illustrated by phrenology and utilizing casts provided by BALLY 1844. (*DNB*)

* VERNON, W. John (d. 1850), scientific evangelist with theatrical inclinations; lectured with KISTE in the South of England 1840–3, specializing after 1843 in phreno-mesmerism; MPA 8/40, and delivered a paper at the 1841 meeting; preceded BURKE as editor of the *People's Phren. J*; contributed to *Phren. J.*; his lectures in Exeter sparked the formation of the Exeter Phren. Soc.; in 1845 he advertised himself as a "consultant on mesmerism and phrenology" at a Regent St. address; involved with Chartism, he was imprisoned for 18 months for sedition 1848 and died shortly after his release. (*Reynolds Political Instructor*, 26 Jan. 1850, pp. 89–90)

* WATSON, Hewett Cottrell (1804–81) botanist; editor of the *Phren. J.* 1837–41; one of the 10 children of the Cheshire County magistrate Holland Watson; destined for a military career but due to a knee injury, which left him with a limp, he turned to law (articling in Manchester) and then to medicine (studying in Edinburgh 1828–32); a small inheritance freed him from the need to earn a living; first became acquainted with phrenology through CAMERON in Liverpool c. 1823 and became an ardent advocate after meeting COMBE and other leading exponents in Edinburgh; reacted against his father's Toryism and his Church of England upbringing; confessed himself a democrat and wrote on self-government 1848; BAAS; MPS Edinburgh and MPA 8/39; lectured in Warrington 1839 and Manchester Athenaeum 1839, 1843; turned away from phrenology 1840 and devoted himself to botany and evolution. (*DNB*; *MEB*; *DSB*)

WATTS, _____, lectured on physiology, phrenology, and phreno-mesmerism in Birmingham MI 1836 and Manchester 1843 (likely John Watts [1818–87], son of Coventry ribbon weaver; Owenite and sec. Coventry MI who conducted a boys' school in Manchester Hall of Science 1841–4: *MEB*).

* WEIR, William (1794–1876), M.D. Glasgow 1829; licentiate of the Faculty of Physicians and Surgeons, Glasgow, 1814, and fellow 1816; pres. Faculty, 1847–9; surgeon to Roy. Infirmary, Glasgow, 1829, and physician there from 1840; lectured on physiology and was sec. to the Portland St. Med. School 1830–42; involved in BAAS negotiations 1839; the son of a music teacher who was also sometime precentor in St. George's Church, Glasgow; original promoter of and coeditor with A. Buchanan of the *Glas. Med. J.* 1830–2; contributed to *Phren. J.*; MPS Glasgow and MPA 7/40, signing the declaration of expediency 1842; held chair of phrenology in Andersonian Univ. 1846 (£50 per annum); lectured publicly in Glasgow 1831–4 and 1841–2, Greenock 1835; testimonial to COMBE 1836; owned a private phrenology museum. (*MEB*)

WENMAN, _____, MPS London 1826; lectured in London 1820s.

★ WHITE, John (1806–68), LSA 1828, M.R.C.S. 1829; of Finchley, Middlesex; author of *Popular Lectures on Man* (1841) and *Lessons on House-Wifery* (1849); lectured in the Lancasterian Schoolroom, Tottenham, 1837, Tottenham MI 1838, and Highgate Lit. & Sci. Inst. 1841; esoteric Christian phrenologist; appears as a manipulator (and possibly a lecturer) in Bath 1850s.

★ WHITNEY, William Underwood (1813–95), LSA 1835, M.R.C.S.E. 1835; trained at Bath and at St. Bartholomew's Hospital; G.P. of Westminster; after 1850 surgeon to the Westminster Female Refuge, med. officer Western Dispensary, and surgeon to Emanuel Hospital; sec. Westminster Mechanics' and Lit. Inst. 1837, where he fostered a phrenology class (to which DONOVAN gave special instruction) and where he lectured on phrenology 1830s; contributed to *Phren. J*; lectured on "The Character of Nations – Phrenologically" at the Cadogan Inst. 1840.

WILLIAMS, James (1811–68), Chartist and Owenite of Sunderland; worked in a confectionary shop owned by a Quaker who taught him peace and teetotal principles; subsequently a book and news agent; arrested for Chartist activity 1839, he spent six months in prison; referred to in the Owenite *New Moral World* in 1843 as our "excellent and valued friend"; became a town councillor of Sunderland; lectured on phreno-mesmerism in the North East 1843. (*MEB*)

★ WILLIAMS, William Mattieu (1820–92), son of a London fishmonger; worked with William Ellis in the London MI to establish secular primary schools; studied at the Univ. of Edinburgh 1841–2 and subsequently made a European tour; manufactured electrical instruments; headmaster of COMBE's secular school in Edinburgh 1848–54, then, to 1863, science teacher in the Industrial Department of Birmingham Midland Inst.; manager of the Birmingham Polytechnic 1881–2; contributed science notes to the *Gents. Mag.* 1880–9; an advocate of shorthand; acquired his knowledge of phrenology at the London MI where he also lectured 8/48 and tutored on the subject. (*MEB*; memoir by J. Angell in Williams, *Vindication of Phrenology* [1894])

WILLIS, Robert (1799–1878), M.D. Edinburgh 1819, M.R.C.S. 1823, L.R.C.P. 1837; on Abernethy's suggestion appointed librarian to the Roy. Coll. of Surg. 1827, a post he held until 1845 when he took up practice in Barnes, Surrey; translator of SPURZHEIM and of William Harvey; wrote various medical works as well as a life of Spinoza (1870) and Servetus and Calvin (1877); MPS Edinburgh 6/20 and MPS London 1824; delivered a course of lectures in London early 1824 that were notable for their failure to attract more than seven auditors. (*DNB*; *MEB*)

WILSON, ———, lectured on phreno-mesmerism in Falkirk 1843.

WILSON, Alexander (d. 1846, Co. Wexford), born in Scotland and originally employed as a shopkeeper in Dumbartonshire; worked briefly for the *Scotsman*; an extremely reserved person with literary tastes; apparently driven to phrenology lecturing for pecuniary reasons and itinerating mainly in Ireland 1836–46, also manipulating; gave one lecture in Birmingham Athenaeum 1842. (Obit., *Phren. J.* 20 [1847], 95)

* WILSON, John, of Dalton (in Furness?); "professor" of phrenology; practiced in Cheltenham 1840s; lectured in Ireland and England 1830s; wrote several religious works of a strongly Christian phrenological bent; gave course of six lectures at Birmingham Roy. Med. School at the request of the Phren. Soc. 1842.

WITHAM, Henry T. M. (d. 1844), of Barnard Castle; Roman Catholic and Whig; amateur geologist; resided for eight years in Edinburgh where he joined the Phren. Soc. 4/33; became V.P. of the Wernerian Soc. 1828 and mem. Roy. Soc. Edinburgh; was one of the few Catholics to be involved in the early history of the BAAS and was active in the arrangements in Newcastle 1838; became high sheriff of County Durham 1844; testimonial to MACKENZIE 1836; established and presided over the Barnard Castle MI and lectured on phrenology there 1836. (Obit., *Phren. J.*, 18 [1845], 188)

* WOOD, Charles Thorold, Jr., of Campsall Hall near Doncaster; son of a captain in the Horse Guards and brother of Neville Wood (1818–86; MPA and editor of the *Analyst* and *The Naturalist*); educationalist and ornithologist; established the Campsall Soc. for the Diffusion of Useful Knowledge 1832 and lectured to it on phrenology; contributed to the *Christian Physician*; lectured at Leicester Lit & Phil and in London 1837, at Doncaster Lyceum 1838, and in Sheffield 1839.

* WOOD, Frank, surgeon; wrote for Charles Partington's *Scientific Gazette*; MPS London 4/24; applied to lecture to the London Inst. 1826 (delivery of lecture unconfirmed).

WOOD, John Robertson, M.D. Glasgow 1831; grandson of a Presbyterian minister and brother of a moderator of the Free Church of Scotland in Dumfries; sometime lecturer on anatomy in the Glasgow MI; figured prominently 1828 as a supporter of Thomas Campbell against Sir Walter Scott as rector of the Univ. of Glasgow; moved to London where he died at an early age; lectured in Glasgow MI for six months on physiology and phrenology 1833, in Greenock 1833–6, and on one occasion in the Reformed Presbyterian Church in Glasgow.

WOOD, Willoughby, brother of Charles WOOD; lectured on "music, phrenologically" in Sheffield Lyceum 1838; also lectured in Doncaster where he attacked orthodox political economy.

NOTES

The "Note on sources and abbreviations" at the front of the book explains the organization of the bibliographical material and provides a key to abbreviations other than standard journal abbreviations.

Introduction

1. For bibliographical sources on science, medicine, and technology and its recent reinterpretation, see: Pietro Corsi and Paul Weindling, eds., *Information Sources in the History of Science and Medicine* (1983); P. T. Durbin, ed., *A Guide to the Culture of Science, Technology, and Medicine* (N. Y., 1980); Ina Spiegel-Rosing and Derek de Solla Price, eds., *Science, Technology, and Society: a cross-disciplinary perspective* (Beverly Hills and London, 1977); and G. S. Rousseau and Roy Porter, eds., *The Ferment of Knowledge: studies in the historiography of eighteenth-century science* (Cambridge, 1980). Specifically for the sociology of scientific knowledge, see: Barry Barnes, ed., *Sociology of Science: selected readings* (Harmondsworth, 1972); Michael Mulkay, *Science and the Sociology of Knowledge* (1979); and the journal *Social Studies of Science*. For rejected scientific knowledge, see: Roy Wallis, ed., *On the Margins of Science: the social construction of rejected knowledge*, Sociological Review Monographs 27 (Keele, 1979); for philosophy: Yehuda Elkana, ed., *The Interaction between Science and Philosophy* (Highlands, N. J., 1974). The quotation is from Noam Chomsky, "Objectivity and Liberal Scholarship," in his *American Power and the New Mandarins* (Harmondsworth, 1969), 23–129 at p. 50.
2. This is as true of Susan Cannon's otherwise valuable *Science in Culture: the early Victorian Period* (N.Y., 1978) as it is of Stephen Cotgrove and Steven Box, *Science, Industry and Society* (1970) or Hilary and Steven Rose, *Science and Society* (Harmondsworth, 1969) or Peter Mathias, ed., *Science and Society, 1600–1900* (Cambridge, 1972).
3. L. Pyenson, " 'Who the Guys Were': prosopograhy in the history of science," *Hist. Sci.*, 15 (1977), 155–88 at p. 179. Partial exceptions are Charles Gillispie, *Genesis and Geology: a study in the relations of scientific thought, natural theology, and social opinion in Great Britain, 1790–1850* (1951; N.Y., 1959), esp. chap. 7, pp. 184–216; David Layton, *Science for the People: the origins of the school curriculum in England* (1973); Alfred Kelly, *The Descent of Darwin: the popularization of Darwinism in Germany, 1860–1914* (Chapel Hill, N.C., 1981); and two unpublished theses: D. A. Hinton, "Popular Science in England, 1830–1870," Ph.D. thesis, Bath, 1979; and Susan Sheets Pyenson, "Low Scientific Culture in London and Paris, 1820–1875," Ph.D. thesis, Pennsylvania, 1976.
4. S. Shapin and A. Thackray, "Prosopography as a Research Tool in the History of Science: the British scientific community, 1700–1900," *Hist. Sci.*, 12 (1974), 1–28 at p. 21.
5. Theodore Roszak, *Where the Wasteland Ends: politics and transcendence in postin-

dustrial society (N.Y., 1972), p. xxiv. See also; P. D. Anthony, *The Ideology of Work* (1977), p. 94 et passim.

6. By Paul Feyerabend, *Science in a Free Society* (1978), p. 31.

7. See: Susan Budd, *Varieties of Unbelief: atheists and agnostics in English Society, 1850–1960* (1977), p. 1.

8. Adorno q. in Martin Jay, *The Dialectical Imagination: a history of the Frankfurt School and the Institute of Social Research, 1923–50* (1974), p. 222 (on the need to distinguish carefully between *meaning* and *function* in its quasi-causal sense, see: Peter Winch, *The Idea of a Social Science and Its Relation to Philosophy* [1958], pp. 115–16); Douglas, *Cultural Bias*, Royal Anthropological Institute Occasional Paper no. 35 (1978), p. 1.

9. The best succinct account of Gall and his doctrine is Robert M. Young's entry on "Gall" in the *DSB*, vol. 5 (1972), 250–6. This also contains a useful bibliography and primary and secondary sources.

10. On the origins and antiquity of Gall's ideas, see: M. Bentley, "The Psychological Antecedents of Phrenology," *Psychological Monographs*, 21 (1916), 102–15; Max Neuburger, *The Historical Development of Experimental Brain and Spinal Cord Physiology before Flourens* (1897) trans. E. Clarke (Baltimore, 1981); Edwin Clarke and C. D. O'Malley, *The Human Brain and Spinal Cord: a historical study illustrated by writings from antiquity to the twentieth century* (Berkeley, 1968); E. Lesky, "Structure and Function in Gall," *Bull. Hist. Med.*, 44 (1970), 297–314; H.W. Magoun, "Development of Ideas Relating the Mind with the Brain," in C. Brooks and Paul Cranefield, eds., *The Historical Development of Physiological Thought* (N.Y., 1959), 81–108; N. H. Steneck, "Albert the Great on the Classification and Localization of the Internal Senses," *Isis*, 65 (1974), 193–211; A. E. Walker, "The Development of the Concept of Cerebral Localalization in the Nineteenth Century," *Bull. Hist. Med.*, 31 (1957), 99–121. Opponents of phrenology, taking the doctrine's antiquity to argue against its novelty, and supporters, using it to show the doctrine's "respectable heritage," related Gall's ideas to (among others) Boerhave, Haller, Von Swieten, Schellhammer, Glasser, Jacobi, Vieussens, Monro, Vicq d'Azyr, Reil, John Baptista Porta, Agrippa, Delaporta, Tiedemann, Prochaska, Willis, Swedenborg, Jherome of Bruynswyke, and the C9th John the Irish Scot. See: P. M. Roget, "Cranioscopy," *Encyl.Brit.*, Suppl. 4th–6th ed. (Edin., 1824), vol. 3, 419–37 at p. 420; Thomas Laycock, "Phrenology," ibid. (8th ed., Edin., 1859), vol. 17, 556–67 at p. 557; A. Macalister, "Phrenology," ibid. (9th ed., Edin., 1885), vol. 18, 842–9 at pp. 842–3; John Elliotson, "The Term Organs of the Brain, used before Gall," *Zoist*, 3 (1845), 22–4; J. Eliot Hodgkin, "Phrenology in the Sixteenth Century," *Notes & Queries*, 8th ser., 5 (24 Mar. 1894), 224–5; Terrance O'Toole, "Origin of Phrenology," *Dublin Penny J.*, 1 (18 Aug. 1832), 60–1; "The Phrenology of the Middle Ages," *Gents. Mag.*, 103 (1833), 126–8; "Historical Notice of Early Opinions Regarding the Functions of the Brain," *Phren. J.*, 2 (1824/5), 378–91; "Antiquity of Phrenology," *Lancet*, 5 Aug. 1826, p. 599; "Pnrenology as Old as Creation," *Edin. Mag. & Lit. Misc.*, 93 (Mar. 1824), 268–75; "Swedenborg's Doctrine of Craniology," *Lon. Med. Repository*, 6 (1828), 92–3.

11. Young, "Gall," p. 252; idem, *Mind, Brain, and Adaptation in the Nineteenth Century: cerebral localization and its biological context from Gall to Ferrier* (Oxford, 1970); and K. Dallenbach, "The History and Derivation of the Word 'Function' as a Systematic Term in Psychology," *Amer. J. Psychol.* 26 (1915), 473–84, esp. at p. 484.

12. Macdonald Critchley, *"The Divine Banquet of the Brain": the Harveian Oration* (1966), p. 6.

13. As q. in Louis Chevalier, *Labouring Classes and Dangerous Classes in Paris during the First Half of the Nineteenth Century*, trans. F. Jellinek (1973), p. 411.

14. Lavater, *Essays on Physiognomy: for the promotion of knowledge and the love of mankind*, trans. T. Holcroft (1789), as q. in Willard L. Valentine and D. D. Wickens, *Experimental Foundations of General Psychology* (3rd ed., N.Y., 1949), p. 6. See also: Theodore Poupin, *Caractère phrénologiques et physiognomiques des contemporaines les plus celebres, selon les systemes de Gall, Spurzheim, Lavater, etc.*

(Paris, 1837); A. Ysabeau, *Lavater et Gall* (Paris, n.d.). On Lavater and the many editions of his works in England (20 by 1810) see: J. Graham, "Lavater's Physiognomy in England," *J. Hist. Ideas*, 22 (1961), 561–72.

15. [Richard Chenevix], "Gall and Spurzheim: phrenology," *Foreign Q. Rev.*, 2 (1828), 1–59 at p. 37.

16. See: Brian Easlea, *Witch-hunting, Magic, and the New Philosophy: an introduction to debates of the scientific revolution, 1450–1750* (Brighton, 1980), pp. 111 ff.

17. While Linneaus in the mid-C18 was attempting to identify the races of man in terms of corelated psychological and biological categories, and Battie and the Monros were endeavoring to classify human types by their "nervous" disposition, Emanuel Swedenborg was independently elaborating a theory of cerebral localization very similar to Gall's. See: G. S. Rousseau, "Psychology," in Rousseau and Porter, *Ferment of Knowledge*, 143–210 at p. 172; and K. Akert and M. P. Hammond, "Emanuel Swedenborg (1688–1772) and His Contribution to Neurology," *Med. Hist.*, 6 (1962), 255–66.

18. See: Chevalier, "The Preoccupation with Physical Characteristics and Its Significance," in his *Labouring Classes*, pp. 409–17 at p. 410; and Young, "Gall," pp. 252–3.

19. Stephan L. Chorover, *From Genesis to Genocide: the meaning of human nature and the power of behavior control* (Cambridge, Mass., 1979), p. 143; and see: Erna Lesky, *The Vienna Medical School of the Nineteenth Century* (Baltimore, 1976), chap. 1.

20. Gall, *Anatomie et physiologie du système nerveux en général, et de cerveau en particulier, avec des observations ... de l'homme et des animaux*, 4 vols. and atlas (Paris, 1810–19), which, with J. G. Spurzheim as coauthor of the first two volumes, was revised and published as *Sur les fonctions du cerveau et sur celles de chacune de ces parties*, 6 vols. (Paris, 1822–5), trans. Winslow Lewis, Jr. (Boston, 1835). Another translation was begun in 1844 in London but was never completed; parts of Gall's opus were translated by Ellen Epps into the *J. Health & Dis.* between 1846 and 1852. The complaint of some London phrenologists that "Very few phrenologists have ever seen Gall's works" was well founded. See: *Zoist*, 13 (1856), 441; and John Elliotson, "On the Ignorance of the Discoveries of Gall Evinced by Recent Phrenological Writers," *Lancet*, 25 Nov. 1837, 295–8.

21. *Med. & Phys. J.*, 4 (1800), 50. A Mr. Geisweiler of Parliament St., London, was said to be in possession of a manuscript sent from Gall in Vienna. Fuller reports appeared in *Monthly Rev.*, *Monthly Mag.*, and *Philosophical Mag.* from 1802; in *Edin. Rev.* from 1803; *Literary J.* from 1805; and *Gents. Mag.* from 1806. Two important early English sources on Gall were *Dr. F. J. Gall's System of the Functions of the Brain Extracted from Charles Augustus Blöde's Account of Dr. Gall's Lectures, Held on the Above Subject at Dresden: translated from the German to serve as an explanatory attendant to Dr. Gall's figured plaster-skulls* (n.p., n.d. [c.1805]) – Blöde was secretary of finance in Dresden; and [Henry Crabb Robinson], *Some Account of Dr. Gall's New Theory of Physiognomy ... with the Critical Strictures of C.W. Hufeland, M.D.* (1807), which was based on hearing Gall's lectures in Jena in 1805 and which formed the basis of the first encyclopedia entry on the subject: "Craniology," in *Rees's Cyclopedia* (1807), vol. 10 (rev. ed., 1819), n.p., 15 cols.

22. See, for examples: D. de Giustino, "Reforming the Commonwealth of Theives: British phrenologists and Australia," *Vict. Stud.*, 15 (1972), 439–61; Arthur Fink, "Phrenology," in his *Causes of Crime: biological theories in the United States, 1800–1915* (Phil., 1938), 1–19; David W. Lewis, *From Newgate to Dannemora: the rise of the penitentiary in New York, 1796–1848* (Ithaca, N.Y., 1965), 232–50; A. Price, "A Pioneer of Scientific Education, George Combe (1788–1858)," *Educ. Rev.*, 12 (1959/60), 219–29; and R. J. Cooter, "Phrenology and British Alienists, c. 1825–1845," *Med. Hist.*, 20 (1976), 1–21, 135–51, repr. in Andrew Scull, ed., *Madhouses, Mad-Doctors, and Madmen: the social history of psychiatry in the Victorian era* (Phil., 1981), 58–104. See also; Sir Geoffrey Jefferson, "The Contemporary Reaction to Phrenology," in his *Selected Papers* (1960), 94–112.

23. On those not referred to elsewhere (see index) see: (for James Hunt) R. Rainger,

"Race, Politics, and Science: the Anthropological Society of London in the 1860s," *Vict. Stud.*, 22 (1978), 51–70; W. M. Sensemen, "Charlotte Bronte's Use of Physiognomy and Phrenology," *Trans. Bronte Soc.*, 12 (1957), 286–9; I. Jack, "Physiognomy, Phrenology, and Characterization in the Novels of Charlotte Bronte," ibid., 15 (1970), 377–91; M. B. Stern, "Poe, 'The Temperament' for Phrenologists," *Amer. Lit.*, 40 1968), 155–63; E. Hungerford, "Poe and Phrenology," *Amer. Lit.*, 2 (1930/1), 209–31; idem, "Walt Whitman and His Chart of Bumps," *Amer. Lit.*, 2 (1930/1), 350–84; J.B. Wilson, "Phrenology and the Transcendentalists," *Amer. Lit.*, 28 (1956/7), 220–5; Taylor Stoehr, *Hawthorne's Mad Scientists: pseudoscience and social science in the nineteenth-century life and letters* (Handen,Conn., 1978); T. Hillway, "Melville's Use of Two Pseudo-Sciences," *Mod. Lang. Notes*, 64 (1949), 145–50; and H. Aspiz, "Phrenologizing the Whale," *Nineteenth Century Fiction*, 23 (1968), 18–27. Among French writers reliant on phrenology were Balzac, Baudelaire, Alfred de Vigny, Eugene Sue, and George Sand.

24. In large part this is the perspective of David de Giustino, *Conquest of Mind: phrenology and Victorian social thought* (1975); and John D.Davies, *Phrenology, Fad, and Science: a nineteenth-century crusade* (New Haven, 1955; repr. ed., 1971). See also: O.Temkin, "Gall and the Phrenological Movement," *Bull. Hist. Med.*, 21 (1947), 275–321; T. M. Parssinen, "Popular Science and Society: the phrenology movement in early Victorian Britain," *J. Soc. Hist.*, 7 (1974), 1–20.

25. Shapin, "Phrenological Knowledge and the Social Structure of Early Nineteenth-Century Edinburgh," *Ann. Sci.*, 32 (1975), 219–43; idem, "The Politics of Observation: cerebral anatomy and social interests in Edinburgh phrenology disputes," in Wallis, *Margins of Science*, 139–78; idem, "Homo Phrenologicus: anthropological perspectives on an historical problem," in Barry Barnes and Steven Shapin, eds., *Natural Order: historical studies of scientific culture* (Beverly Hills and London, 1979), 41–71. See also: David Turnbull, ed., *Phrenology: the first science of man* (Deakin University, 1982) and the excellent review of this by R. Yeo in *Proc.Austral. Ass. Hist., Phil., (and) Soc. Stud. Sci.*, no. 13 (1982), 26–9.

26. See: R. M. Young, "The Impact of Darwin on Conventional Thought," in Anthony Symondson, ed., *The Victorian Crisis of Faith* (1970), 13–35 at p. 16.

27. *The Secularization of the European Mind in the Nineteenth Century* (Cambridge, 1975), pp. 170, 183.See also: Budd, *Varieties of Unbelief*, p. 128; F. A. Hayek, *The Counter-Revolution of Science* (Glencoe, Ill., 1955), p. 206; E. P.Thompson, "The Peculiarities of the English," in his *The Poverty of Theory* (1978), 35–91, at pp. 61 ff., but cf. R. M. Young, "The Historiographic and Ideological Contexts of the Nineteenth-Century Debate on Man's Place in Nature," in Mikuláš Teich and Robert M. Young, eds., *Changing Perspectives in the History of Science* (1973), 344–438 at pp. 423 ff.

28. Robert Merton, *Science, Technology, and Society in Seventeenth Century England* (2nd ed., N.Y., 1970), p. 209. See also: Zygmunt Bauman, *Culture as Praxis* (1973); C. Geertz, "Ideology as a Cultural System," in David E.Apter, ed., *Ideology and Discontents* (Glencoe, Ill., 1964), 47–76; H. Marcuse, "Remarks on a Redefinition of Culture," in Gerald Holton, ed., *Science and Culture* (Boston, 1965), 218–35; James P. Spradley, ed., *Culture and Cognition: rules, maps, and plans* (San Francisco, 1972); and Y. Elkana, "Introduction: culture, control system, and science," in R. S. Cohen et al., eds., *Essays in Memory of Imre Lakatos* (Dordrecht, Holland and Boston, 1976), 99–107.

CHAPTER 1: *From out the cerebral well*

1. Morell, *An Historical and Critical View of the Speculative Philosophy of Europe in the Nineteenth Century* (1846), I, pp. 411–26, II, pp. 529 ff.; Lewes, "Phrenology,"in his *Biographical History of Philosophy* (rev. ed., 1857), 655–74; and Lange, *The History of Materialism and Criticism of Its Present Importance* trans. E. C.Thomas (1881), III, pp. 113–25.

2. A. G. W. Whitfield, "Clark and Combe: fact and fantasy," *J. Roy. Coll. Phys.*,

11 (1977), 268–72 at p. 272. For similar references Daniel W. Hering, "Phrenology," in his *Foibles and Fallacies of Science* (1924), 152–57; C. J. Herrick, "Error in Neurophysiology," in Joseph Jastrow, ed., *The Story of Human Error* (N.Y., 1936), 251–67; Joseph Jastrow, "The Skull Science of Dr. Gall," in his *Wish and Wisdom: episodes in the vagaries of belief* (N.Y., 1935), 389–403; Lowell S. Selling, " 'Quack' Number One: Gall," in his *Men against Madness* (N.Y., 1940), 121–72; and Martin Gardner, "From Bumps to Handwriting," in his *Fads and Fallacies in the Name of Science* (2nd ed., N.Y., 1957), 292–8.

3. See R. Wallis, *Margins of Science*, esp. the essay by H. Collins and T. J. Pinch, "The Construction of the Paranormal: nothing unscientific is happening," 237–70; and R. M. Young, "Getting Started on Lysenkoism," *Rad. Sci. J.*, 6/7 (1978), 81–105.

4. Dallenbach, "Phrenology versus Psychoanalysis," *Amer. J. Psychol.*, 68 (1955), 511–25; Medawar, "Further Comments on Psychoanalysis," in his *The Hope of Progress* (1972), 57–68 at p. 68; Rose, "Scientific Racism and Ideology: the I.Q. racket from Galton to Jensen," in Hilary Rose and Steven Rose, eds., *The Political Economy of Science: ideology of/in the natural sciences* (1976), 112–41 at pp. 117, 129; Eysenck, *Fact and Fiction in Psychology* (Harmondsworth, 1965), pp. 130–1, *Sense and Nonsense in Psychology* (Harmondsworth, 1958), p. 61, and *Uses and Abuses of Psychology* (Harmondsworth, 1954), pp. 28–9. See also: L. Mann, "Psychometric Phrenology and the New Faculty Pscychology," *J. Special Educ.*, 5 (1971), 3–14; and S. Waksman, "Psychometric Phrenology Revisited: comments on neuropsychological testing," *J. Consult. & Clin. Psychol.*, 46 (1978), 1489–90.

5. For the critique of positivism and the use–abuse framework, see: L. Levidow, "A Marxist Critique of the IQ Debate," *Rad. Sci. J.*, 6/7 (1978), 13–72; and Thomas McCarthy, *The Critical Theory of Jürgen Habermas* (Cambridge, Mass., 1978), esp. at pp. 5–8, 40–52.

6. Mendelsohn, "The Social Construction of Scientific Knowledge," in Mendelsohn et al., eds., *The Social Production of Scientific Knowledge* (Dordrecht, Holland and Boston, 1977), 3–26. Cf. Joseph Ben-David's idealist account of the origins of C17 science in his *The Scientist's Role in Society* (Englewood Cliffs, N.J., 1971) as criticized in T. Gran, "Elements From the Debate on Science in Society: a study of Joseph Ben-David's theory," in Richard Whitley, ed., *Social Processes of Scientific Development* (1974), 195–209. See also: P. Wright, "On the Boundaries of Science in Seventeenth Century England," in Yehuda Elkana and E. Mendelsohn, eds., *Sciences and Cultures: sociology of the sciences*, vol. 5 (Dordrecht, Holland, 1981), 77–100; and Frank Manuel, *A Portrait of Isaac Newton* (Cambridge, Mass., 1968), p. 119.

7. D. Dickson, "Science and Political Hegemony in the Seventeenth Century," *Rad. Sci. J.*, 8 (1979), 7–37, at p. 10. For the economic background see: Joyce Appleby, *Economic Thought and Ideology in Seventeenth-Century England* (Princeton, 1978), esp, at p. 245.

8. *History and Class Consciousness: studies in Marxist Dialectics* (1923; trans. R. Livingstone, 1971), pp.7–11, 89–98, et passim. The relevant passages are cited in Gareth Stedman Jones, "The Marxism of the Early Lukács," *New Left Rev.*, no. 70 (1971), repr. in Stedman Jones, ed., *Western Marxism: a critical reader* (1977), 11–60 at pp. 13-14. See also: R. M. Young, "Man's Place in Nature," pp. 398–9, 402, 405, 414, 430–4.

9. "Science *Is* Social Relations," *Rad. Sci. J.*, 5 (1977), 65–129.

10. E.g., David de Giustino, *Conquest of Mind*; John D. Davies, *Phrenology: fad and science*; Alastair Cameron Grant, "George Combe and His Circle: with particular reference to his relations with the United States of America," Ph.D. thesis, Edinburgh, 1960; T. M. Parssinen, "Phrenology Movement"; A. McLaren, "Phrenology: medium and message," *J. Mod. Hist.*, 46 (1974), 86–97; O. Temkin, "Gall and the Phrenological Movement"; A. Wrobel, "Orthodoxy and Respectability in Nineteenth-Century Phrenology," *J. Pop. Culture*, 9 (1975), 38–50.

11. Ostensibly a "scientism" is an illegitimate extrapolation from a well-established scientific domain to a social domain. But since science itself is constructed under social conditions and subsumes these conditions, "scientisms" may be said only

to accomplish overtly for social legitimation what sciences do covertly. See: L. Hodgkin, "A Note on Scientism," *Rad. Sci. J.*, 5 (1977), 8; D. Dickson, "Technology and Social Reality," *Dialectical Anthropology*, 1 (1975), 34–37; and Phil Brown, "Scientism of Dialectics?" in his *Toward a Marxist Psychology* (N.Y., 1974), 11–37. Cf. the positivist distinction between science and scientism in F. V. Hayek, "Scientism and the Study of Society," in his *Counter-Revolution of Science*, 129–42; G. Eastman, "Scientism in Science Education," *Science Teacher*, 36 (1969), 19–22; Robert B. Fisher, "Science and/or Scientism," in his *Science, Man, and Society* (Phil., 1971), 43–4; and W. H. White, "Scientism," in his *The Organization Man* (N.Y., 1956), 25–35.

12. E.g., "Phrenology was one of those curious sidetracks of knowledge down which intellectuals in their eagerness to embrace some new thing of great promise wander. It generally takes several years before the true character of these movements appears, at which time, if the promise is shown to be hollow, most will revert to good sense, leaving the field to the charlatans. The twentieth century has shown us the pattern repeated many times." H. Schwartz, "Samuel Gridley Howe as Phrenologist," *Amer. Hist. Rev.*, 57 (1952), 644–51 at p. 651.

13. On Broca and the history of cerebral localization see: Edwin Clarke's entry on Broca in *DSB*; M. Critchley, "The Origins of Aphasiology," *Scot. Med. J.*, 9 (1964), 231–42; K. Goldstein, "Pierre Paul Broca, 1824–1880," in Webb Haymaker and F. Schiller, eds., *The Founders of Neurology* (Springfield, Ill., 1953), 259–63; W. Reise and E. C. Hoff, "A History of the Doctrine of Cerebral Localization," *J. Hist. Med.*, 5 (1950), 51–71 and 6 (1951), 439–70; William Hanna Thomson, *Brain and Personality or the Physical Relations of the Brain to the Mind* (1907), pp. 21 ff.; A. E. Walker, "Concept of Cerebral Localization"; Young, *Mind, Brain, and Adaptation*; and O. L. Zangwill, "The Cerebral Localization of Psychological Functions," *Advancement of Science*, 20 (1963/4), 335–44.

14. *The Story of the Brain*, Henderson Trust Lectures, no. III, University of Edinburgh, 29 Feb. 1924, pp. 15, 4.

15. See: P. Bailey, "Cortex and Mind," in J. M. Scher, ed., *Theories of the Mind* (N.Y., 1962), 3–14; J. McFie, "Recent Advances in Phrenology," *Lancet*, 12 Aug. 1961, 360–3; and S. L. Chorover, "The Pacification of the Brain: from phrenology to psychosurgery," in Thomas P. Morley, ed., *Current Controversies in Neurosurgery* (Phil. 1976), 730–67.

16. See H. Charlton Bastian, "Phrenology: old and new," in his *The Brain as an Organ of the Mind* (1880), 511–47; James George Davey, "The Localization of the Functions of the Brain," *J. Psychol. Med.*, 2 (1876), 252–62; Bernard Hollander, *The Old and the Modern Phrenology: a lecture* (1889); idem, "The Fundamental Principles of Phrenology in the Light of Modern Science," *Phren. Rec.*, 1 (1893), 5–16; idem, *The Revival of Phrenology* (1901); idem, *Scientific Phrenology* (1902); C.W. Saleeby, "The New Phrenology," *The Academy and Literature*, 67 (1904), 510–11; S. Paget, "The Revival of Phrenology, 11"*Fortnightly Rev.*, 78 (1905), 1107–15; M. Allen Starr, "The Old and the New Phrenology," *Pop. Sci. Monthly*, 35 (1889), 730–48; J. Knott, "Franz Josef Gall and the 'Science of Phrenology,' " *Westminister Rev.*, 166 (1906), 150–63; J. M. Robertson, "The Revival of Phrenology," *Free Press*, 5 (1895), 352–72, 616–43, 6 (1896), 246–63.

17. Review of "Lettre de Charles Villers, etc. *i.e.* A letter from Charles Villers to George Cuvier, of the National Institute of France, on a new Theory of the Brain by Dr. Gall, in which that Viscus is considered as the immediate Organ of the Moral Faculties," *Monthly Rev.*, 39 Appendix of Foreign Literature (1802), 487–90. On Yelloly (1774–1842), M.D. Edin. 1796, L.R.C.P. 1800, F.R.S. 1814, F.G.S. 1828, see *DNB*.

18. *Lit. J.*, 5 (1805), 1334.

19. *Recherches sur le système nerveux en général, et sur celui du cerveau en particulier; mémoire presenté à l'Institut de France, le 14 mars 1808; suivi d'observations sur le rapport qui en a été fait à cette compagnie par ses commissaires* (Paris, 1809; published concurrently in Strasbourg). The institute's report on the *Memoir* (which was

conducted by the eminent French scientists J. R. Tenon, Antoine Portal, R. B. Sabatier, Philippe Pinel, and George Cuvier) was printed in "Séance du lundi 25 avril 1808", *Institut de France, Académie des Sciences: procés rebaux des séances de l'académie* ..., and was translated in *Edin. Med. & Surg. J.*, 5 (Jan. 1809), 33–66, which was then reprinted in *Med.& Phys. J.*, (London), 21 (Feb. 1809), 149–61, where it was later noted that the hostility to the theory in the recent numbers was based on opinions "not founded ... on any direct publication of Gall ... but rather on the statements of his pupils and partizans." William Royston, "Sketch of the Progress of Medicine," *Med. & Phys. J.*, 24 (1810), 3–4.

20. The only journals dissenting from this early hostility were *Monthly Mag.*, the London *Med. & Phys. J.* and *Phil. J.* On the last journal see: Chapter 2, esp note 61; *Monthly Mag.* began noticing the doctrine in October 1802 with an "Account of Dr. Gall's Cranioscopical Lectures," 14 (1803), 212–13 and thereafter produced various expository accounts (see: vol. 14 [1802], 379–81, vol. 18 [1805], 492–95, vol. 19[1805], 12–15, and, with a foldout illustration, vol. 21 [1806], 197–203, 290–2); *Med. & Phys. J.* 14 (Oct.1805), 327–36, published "A Concise Account of Dr. Gall's New Doctrine of the Brain, and the Faculties of the Mind," which had been written by Justus Arneman (or Arnamann), M.D., one of the editors of the journal who had heard Gall's lectures in Berlin. By the mid-1820s, however, this journal was largely opposed to phrenology: e.g., vol. 56 (1826), 367–9.

21. *The Works of Jeremy Bentham*, John Bowring, ed. (1843), VII, pp. 433–34 (but cf. Bentham's other, more flattering remarks on Gall's doctrine in 1821 and 1827 in ibid. [N.Y., 1962], VIII, p. 537, VII, p. 433); for a cartoon by Lambert (fl. 1826–43) see: W. F. Bynum, "An Old Maid's Skull Phrenologised," *J. Hist. Med.*, 23 (1968), 386 and plate; Cocking's cartoon prefaces *Three Familiar Lectures on Craniological Physiognomy* (1816).

22. The former was first published in *Whims and Oddities*, 2nd ser. (1827), reprinted in *Comic Poems* (1886), 126–30; the latter appears in *Poems by Two Brothers* (2nd ed., 1893), pp. 200–3.

23. In *Flim-Flams! or, the life and errors of my uncle, and the amours of my aunt! with illustrations and obscurities, by Messieurs Tag, Rag, and Bobtail* (1805), I, pp. 41–53.

24. *Encephalology; or a very brief sketch of Dr. Hirnschadel's ologies of the cranion and phren perfected by the rationals* (1824), reviewed in *Monthly Crit.Gaz.*, 1 (1824), 347–8.

25. John Morley, *The Life of Richard Cobden* (1881), I, p. 26. On Cobden's subsequent endorsement of phrenology see: below Chapter 4, note 99.

26. *Edin. Lit. J.*, 4 (27 Feb. 1830), 149; see also the review of Wade's play in the *Times* q. in *Phren. J.*, 6 (1829/30), 353–4. Phrenology did not make either good poetry or satire: *Edin. Lit. J.* said of the anonymous *Phrenology in Edinburgh* (Edin., 1830 [*sic*]), "We thought Phrenology itself the dullest thing in the universe till we saw this sixpenny poem, which has convinced us that there is one thing still duller – namely, the sixpenny poem." Vol. 2 (19 Dec. 1829), 411.

27. Vol. 76 (June 1806), 502.The lines were from Rochefoucault.

28. "Villers, sur une Nouvelle Theorie de Cerveau," *Edin. Rev.* 2 (1803), 147–60 (Charles de Villers was the educational theorist responsible for introducing the ideas of Gall into France in 1802).

29. Brown, *Observations on the Zoonomia of Erasmus Darwin M.D.* (Edin., 1798); for biographical details on Brown see David Welsh, *Account of the Life and Writings of Thomas Brown* (Edin., 1825).

30. "When I say that the exercise of our moral and intellectual faculties depends upon material conditions," Gall wrote, "I do not mean to imply that our faculties are a product of the organism; this would be confounding *conditions* with *efficient causes*." Q. in J. C. Marshall, "Freud's Psychology of Language," in Richard Wollheim, ed., *Freud: a collection of critical essays* (Garden City, N.Y., 1974), 349–65 at p. 354.

31. Brown is sometimes accredited with being a republican and is generally regarded as the last representative of a vigorous Scottish school that was modified by

French influence but unaffected by German idealism; see: *DNB* and Elie Halevy, *The Growth of Philosophical Radicalism*, trans. M. Morris (1972), p. 435. It is Brown's attachment to these views that explains the paradox of British phrenologists later coming to regard him as their philosophical forerunner. See: Combe, *Elements of Phrenology* (9th ed., Edin., 1862), p. 7; *Diary of the Late John Epps, MD*, ed. Mrs. [Ellen] Epps [1870], p. 388; Daniel Noble, *The Brain and Its Physiology* (1846), pp. 68–70; [R. Chenevix], "Phrenology," p. 15; and David Uwins, *A Treatise on Those Disorders of the Brain and Nervous System Which Are Usually Considered and Called Mental* (1833), p. 22n. But it is doubtful if Edinburgh phrenologists would ever have claimed Brown "a phrenologist in disguise" had not Brown's biographer, David Welsh, been an EPS member (see *Phren. J.*, 2 [1824/5], pp. 98–104, 308–21).

32.   The idea, so opposed by Kierkegaard, that arguments steeped in passion are on that account necessarily less credible was elaborated by Locke in his *Essay on Human Understanding* (1690), bk. IV, chap. 19; see also R. Knox, *Enthusiasm* (Oxford, 1950); and G. Rosen, "Enthusiasm," *Bull. Hist. Med.*, 42 (1968), 393–421.

33.   See: H. D. Spoerl, "Faculties versus Traits: Gall's solution," *Character and Personality*, 4 (1935/6), 216–31; and M. Bentley, "Psychological Antecedents," pp. 102–15.

34.   See: G. N. Cantor, "The Edinburgh Phrenology Debate, 1803–1828," *Ann. Sci.*, 32 (1975), 195–218 at p. 206.

35.   [Gordon], "The Doctrines of Gall and Spurzheim," *Edin. Rev.*, 25 (June 1815), 227–68. He had earlier established his viewpoint in "Functions of the Nervous System," ibid., 24 (Feb. 1815), 439–52, and elaborated on his purely anatomical reasons for dissenting from Gall and Spurzheim's ideas in *A System of Human Anatomy* (Edin., 1815), esp. pp. 79–174, 150. These works were replied to by Spurzheim, *Prospectus of the Anatomical Views of Drs. Gall and Spurzheim on the Brain and Nerves, Confronted with the Edinburgh Review (No. 49, June 1815, Art. X) and Dr. Gordon's Opinions in His System of Human Anatomy and Surgery, Vol. I, Edinburgh, 1815* (Edin., [1815]); and more extensively in idem, *Examination of the Objections Made in Britain against the Doctrines of Gall and Spurzheim* (Edin., 1817). The controversy was examined in different lights in "Retrospect," *Lon. Med. Repository*, 8 (July 1817), 4–9 (which tended to side with Gordon); "Drs. Gall & Spurzheim on the Structure of the Brain," *Medico-Chirurgical Rev.*, 4 (July 1817), 53–63 and (Aug. 1817), 117–34 (which sided with Spurzheim); and "The Craniological Controversy," *Blackwoods*, 1 (April 1817), 35–8 (highly antiphrenological) and (July 1817), 365–7 (pointing out the bigotry). Spurzheim's *Physiognomical System* also received major reviews in the *Eclectic Rev.* [by David Uwins], n.s., 3 (April 1815), 321–35 and (May 1815), 459–69; *Quart. Rev.*, 13 (April 1815), 159–78; *Brit. Critic*, n.s., 3 (May 1815), 468–87; *Lon. Med. & Phys. J.*, 33 (June 1815), 485–505; *Lon. Med.Repository*, 4 (July 1815), 53–63 and (Sept. 1815), 208–29; *Monthly Rev.*, 77 (Oct. 1815), 147–65; and *Augustan Rev.*, 1 (1815), 281–5. On Gordon, see: Daniel Ellis, *Memoir of the Life and Writings of John Gordon, Late Lecturer on Anatomy and Physiology in Edinburgh* (Edin., 1823).

36.   Spurzheim observed this change in the *Physiognomical System*, p. 120. See also: Raymond Williams, *Keywords* (1976), pp. 163–7; Maurice Mandelbaum, "Materialism" in his *History, Man, and Reason* (Baltimore and London, 1971), 20–8; and G. A. Foote, "Mechanism, Materialism, and Science in England, 1800–1850," *Ann. Sci.*, 8 (1952), 152–61.

37.   Gordon, "Doctrines of Gall and Spurzheim," p. 239.

38.   Ibid., p. 268. For Gall and Spurzheim on anatomy see their *Anatomie et physiologie du système nerveux* (Paris, 1812), which was the other work that Gordon was reviewing in 1815 and which subsequently appeared as Spurzheim, *The Anatomy of the Brain, with a General View of the Nervous System*, trans. R. Willis (1826).

39.   It contained an appendix on Gall and Spurzheim's "Crane," pp. 185–207, taken from the *Dictionaire des sciences medicales* (Paris, 1813) vol. 7, 260–66.

40.   Supplement to the 4th, 5th, and 6th editions of the *Ency. Brit.* (Edin., 1824),

vol. 3, 419–37. Replied to by Combe, "Cranioscopy, by Dr. Roget," *Phren. J.*, 1 (1823/4), 165–76. See also: D. L. Emblem, "The Encyclopedia Britannica and Phrenology," in his *Peter Mark Roget: the word and the man* (1970), 132–52. On Roget (1779–1869) M.D. Edin. 1798, F.R.S. 1815, F.G.S. 1828, see: *DNB* and below, Chapter 2. Kidd, *An Introductory Lecture to a Course in Comparative Anatomy, Illustrative of Paley's Natural Theology* (Oxford, 1824), pp. 58–72. On Kidd (1775–1851) M.D. 1804, F.R.C.P. 1818, F.R.S. 1822, F.G.S. 1828, see: *DNB, DSB*, and below. Chapter 2, note 29.

41. *Ency. Brit.* (7th ed., Edin., 1842), vol. 17, 454–73; the last six pages are an afterword explaining why the views had not changed; the whole was published separately as Roget, *Treatise on Physiology and Phrenology from the Seventh Edition of the Encyclopedia Britannica*, 2 vols. (Edin., 1838). Replied to in [Hewett Cottrell Watson], *Strictures on Anti-Phrenology, in Two Letters to Macvey Napier, Esq. and P. M. Roget, M.D.: Being an exposure of the article called "Phrenology," recently published in the Encyclopedia Britannica* ([for private distribution], Oct. 1838); and idem, "Phrenology and the *Encyclopedia Britannica*; or the deliberate obstruction of Truth," *Phren. J.*, 11 (1838), 278–82.

42. Sir George MacKenzie and Dugald Stewart, "Correspondence between Sir G. S. MacKenzie and Dugald Stewart, 1821," *Phren. J.*, 7 (1831/2), 303–9. Barclay, *An Inquiry into the Opinions, Ancient and Modern, concerning Life and Organization* (Edin, 1822), pp. 372–81; replied to in George Combe and Dr. Barclay, "Correspondence betwixt Mr. George Combe and Dr. Barclay," *Phren. J.*, 1 (1823/4), 46–55; Andrew Combe, "Observations on Dr. Barclay's Objections to Phrenology," *Trans. Phren. Soc.* (Edin., 1824), 393–429. On Barclay (1758–1826) M.D. Edin, 1798, F.R.S.E. 1807, see: *DNB, DSB*, and below Chapter 2, note 29.

43. Home, "The Croonian Lecture: microscopical observations on ... the brain and nerves showing that the materials of which they are composed exist in the blood...," *Phil. Trans. Roy. Soc. Lon. for the Year 1821*, pp. 24–46. See also: Spurzheim, "Remarks on Dr. Baillie and Sir E. Home" (q. from the 2nd ed. of Spurzheim's *Physiognomical System*), *Lon. Med. & Phys. J.*, 34 (1815), 309–16. On Home (1756–1832), F.R.S. 1787, see: *DNB, DSB*; on Matthew Baillie (1761–1823) M.D. Oxford 1789, F.R.C.P. 1789, F.R.S. 1790, see: *DNB, DSB*.

Bell, "[On Gall in] Second Part of the Paper on the Nerves of the Orbit, Charles Bell. Communicated by Sir Humphry Davy, Bart., President of the Royal Society. Read June 19, 1823," *Phil. Trans. Roy. Soc. Lon. for 1823*, pt. II, pp. 306–7. Replied to in [Andrew Combe], "Mr. Charles Bell on the Functions of the Nerves," *Phren. J.*, 1 (1823–4), 58–65; [James Simpson], "Additional Evidence of the Existence of a Sense of Equilibrium as a Primitive Mental Power, Derived from the Consistency Which Obtains between Its Supposed Functions and the Recent Physiological Discoveries of Mr. Charles Bell," *Phren. J.*, 4 (1826–7), 266–84; and Spurzheim, *Appendix to the Anatomy of the Brain, Containing a Paper Read before the Royal Society on the 14th of May, 1829, and Some Remarks on Mr. Charles Bell's Animadversions on Phrenology* (1830). On Bell (1774–1842) M.R.C.S. 1799, F.R.S.E. 1811, F.R.S. 1826, see: *DNB, DSB*.

Kidd, *On the Adaptation of External Nature to the Physical Condition of Man, Principally with Reference to the Supply of His Wants, and the Exercise of Intellectual Faculties* (1833; 3rd ed., 1834), pp. 59–73; this was attacked by John Elliotson in *Lancet*, 22 Feb. 1834, p. 835.

44. Jeffrey, "Phrenology" (review of Combe's *System of Phrenology*, *Edin. Rev.*, 44 (1826), 253–318; idem, "Note to the Article on Phrenology," *Edin. Rev.*, 45 (1826), 248–53. Replied to in *Letter from George Combe to Francis Jeffrey, Esq. in Answer to His Criticism on Phrenology* [from *Phren. J.*, 4 (1826/7), 1–82] (Edin., 1826; 2nd ed., 1826); and Combe, "Second Letter to Francis Jeffrey ...," *Phren. J.*, 4 (1826/7), 242–51. See also: *Facts in Favour of Phrenology: two letters to a friend in Oxford in reply to the strictures of the Edinburgh Review* (Macclesfield, 1826). On Jeffrey (1773–1850), who spent much of his leisure time studying science and was a member with Brown and Bell in the Academy of Physics in Edinburgh, see: *DNB*.

45. Hamilton's papers to the Edin. Roy. Soc. on 19 Dec. 1825 and 6 Feb. 1826 "On the Practical Conclusions from Gall's Theory Regarding the Functions of the Brain" were never published, nor were the papers given on 2 Apr. 1827 and 18 Feb. 1829, but his observations appeared later in various publications: "Account of Experiments on the Weight and Relative Proportions of the Brain, Cerebellum, and Tuber Annulare, in Man and Animals, under Various Circumstances of Age, Sex, Country, etc." which was the preface to Alexander Monro, *The Anatomy of the Brain* (Edin., 1831); "Remarks on Dr. [Samuel] Morton's Tables on the Size of the Brain,"*Edin. New Phil. J.*, 48 (1850), 330–3; and "Researches on the Frontal Sinuses, with Observations on Their Bearing on the Dogmas of Phrenology," *Med.Times*, 12 (1845), 159, 177, 371. Parts of these papers are given in Hamilton, "Phrenology," app. II of *Lectures on Metaphysics and Logic*, ed. Rev. H. L. Mansell and John Veitch (Edin., 1859), I, 404–44, where it is noted that he had intended in 1829 to collect his arguments under the title *The Fictions of Phrenology and the Facts of Nature* (p. 424n).
    The Major phrenological reply was given by Hewett C. Watson, review of "Sir William Hamilton's Prefix to Alexander Monro's *The Anatomy of the Brain* (1831)," *Phren. J.*, 7 (1831/2), 434–44; and see also: "Cruelty to Animals: Sir William Hamilton's experiments," ibid., 7 (1831/2), 427–33. Hamilton's views had earlier been made public in the anonymous *Sir William Hamilton and Phrenology: an exposition of phrenology; shewing the complete inefficacy of the objections lately advanced in the Royal Society, and the real grounds on which the system ought to be assailed* (Edin., 1826) which was discussed and refuted by Andrew Combe in a letter to the editors of the high Tory *Edinburgh and Leith Advertiser, Phren. J.*, 4 (1826/7), 100–3; and further in *Correspondence Relative to Phrenology between Sir William Hamilton, Bart., Dr. Spurzheim, and Mr. George Combe, in January, February, and March, 1828* (Edin., 1838), part of which had been published in the *Caledonian Mercury* – originally published in *Phren. J.*, 4 (1826/7), 377–407, and "Renewed Correspondence," ibid., 5 (1828/9), 1–69, 153–8.

46. Stone, [(?1793–1854), M.D. Edin. 1813, student pres. Edin. Roy. Med. Soc.,] *Evidences against the System of Phrenology, Being the Substance of a Paper Read at an Extraordinary Meeting of the Royal Society of Edinburgh* (Edin., 1828); idem, *Observations on the Phrenological Development of Burke, Hare, and Other Atrocious Murderers ... : presenting an extensive series of facts subversive of phrenology, read before the Royal Medical Society of Edinburgh* (Edin., 1829); the latter had been prompted by [G.Combe], "Phrenological Observations on the Cerebral Development of William Burk [*sic*] executed for Murder at Edinburgh ... and on the Development of William Hare, His Accomplice, Read to the Phrenological Society, 5th February, 1829," *Phren. J.*, 5 (1828/9), 549–72; and was followed by G. Combe, "Evidences against Phrenology, by Thomas Stone," *Phren. J.*, 5 (1828/9), 264–73; idem, "Answer to 'Observations ... by Thomas Stone' " *Phren. J.*, 6 (1829/30), 1–14 (also published as a pamphlet, 1829) and resulted in Stone, *A Rejoinder to the Answer of George Combe, Esq. to "Observations ... Murderers"* (Edin., 1829). See also [James Kennedy], "Remarks on the 'Evidence against the System of Phrenology. By Thomas Stone,' " *Lon. Med. & Surg. J.*, 1 (1828), 153–65, 249–65, 349–62, 435–50, and 2 (1829), 46–59, 130–46, 507–30 (a scathing attack on Stone); and William Rathbone Greg, *Observations on a Late Pamphlet by Mr.Stone* (Edin., 1829).

47. Magendie [1783–1855] (on craniology with notes by Milligan in) *An Elementary Compendium of Physiology; ... translated from the French, with copious notes and illustrations by E. Milligan* (Edin., 1823). "On the whole," said Milligan, "facts seems to go against the phrenologist: [Gall's] doctrine has now been submitted to the expense of the world for nearly thirty years, yet in all that period ... no one scientific person of *eminence* has appeared in its defence' (pp. 437–9). Replied to in "Dr. Milligan vs. Phrenology," *Phren. J.*, 1 (1823/4), 490–2; and John Elliotson, "The Arguments of Dr. Magendie and Dr. Bostock against Prenology, Read to the London Phrenological Society, 3 Dec. 1827," *Phren. J.*, 5 (1828/9), 92–102; and see: Milligan, "Theory of the Frontal Sinuses," *Trans. Prov. Med.*

& *Surg. Ass.*, 1 (1833), 59–67; Neville Wood, "Some Remarks on a Review of a Paper on Phrenology, by Dr. Milligan," *Analyst*, 2 (1835), 314–17; and, reviewing Edward Barlow's paper on phrenology (see: below, note 68) and Milligan's antiphrenological reply in *Trans. prov. Med. & Surg. Ass.*, "Provincial Medical Association," *Lancet*, 6 July 1833, pp. 461–4. Milligan (1784–1833), thought to have been educated in Ireland, was lecturer on physiology and therapeutics in Edinburgh in 1823.

Flourens [1794–1867], *Examen de la phrénologie* (Paris, 1842; Eng. trans. Charles de Lucene Meigs, Phil., 1846). Flourens was the favored pupil of Cuvier and probably the most successful physiologist of the first half of the C19. Though he paid Gall the compliment of having understood better than anyone before him that the brain was the organ of mind, he opposed phrenology as fatalistic, materialistic, anti-Christian, antisocial, and a science of nothingness. Committed to rehabilitating the mind–body dualism, he dedicated his book to Descartes.

Rudolphi [1771–1832], *Grundriss der Physiologie* (Berlin, 1821–8). Replied to in [Andrew Combe], "Professor Rudolphi and Phrenology," *Phren. J.*, 1 (1823/4), 592–9. See also: "Cranioscopie" in *Encyclopädisches Wörterbuch der medicinischen Wissenschaften* (Berlin, 1832), 590–611, which is drawn from the writings of Busch, Gräfe, Hufeland, Link, and Rudolphi and contains three pages of bibliography on early French and German works.

Sewall [1787–1845], *An Examination of Phrenology; in two lectures, delivered to the students of the Columbian College, District of Columbia, February 1837* (Washington, D.C., 1837; London, 1838; rev. 2nd ed., Boston, 1839). Replied to by Charles Caldwell, *Phrenology Vindicated, and Antiphrenology Unmasked* (N.Y., 1838) which was reviewed in *Phren. J.*, 11 (1838), 427–9. See also the review of "Sewall's Examination" in *Medico-Chirurgical Rev.*, 27 (1837), 159–60.

Bostock, "Of Craniology and Physiognomy," in his *An Elementary System of Physiology* (1827), III, 264–90, was a candid and seemingly fair explanation of the science's shortcomings with an excellent discussion on materialism (for criticism see Elliotson, above); Bostock had been more hostile twenty years earlier in his review of Crabb Robinson's "Some Account of Dr. Gall's New Theory of Physiognomy," *Monthly Rev.*, 55 (1808), 36–9. On Bostock, see: below, Chapter 2, note 27.

Copland, "The Doctrines of Gall" in appendix to A. Richerand, *Elements of Physiology*, trans. G. J. M. De Lys (2nd ed., 1829), pp. 686–9. See also: "Of Phrenology" in his *Dictionary of Practical Medicine* (1858), vol. 2, 501–5. On Copland, see: below, Chapter 2, note 26.

Prichard, *Diseases of the Nervous System* (1822), chap. 1; idem, "Temperament" in John Forbes, Alexander Tweedie, and John Conolly, eds., *Cyclopedia of Practical Medicine* (1833–5), vol. 4, pp. 165–74; and idem, "Supplementary Note on Peculiar Configurations of the Skull Connected with Mental Derangement, with Observations on the Evidence of Phrenology, and on Opinions Respecting the Functions of the Brain," in his *A Treatise on Insanity* (1835), 461–83; of the latter the reviewer in *Br. & For. Med. Rev.* noted: "Admitting the justness of Dr. Pritchard's remarks, we do not think them subversive of the phrenological doctrines": 7 (1839), 46. See also: [Andrew Combe], "Dr. Prichard and Phrenology," *Phren. J.*, 2 (1824/5), 47–55; idem, "Cyclopedia of Practical Medicine: Dr. Prichard and phrenology," *Phren. J.*, 8 (1832/4), 649–57; idem, "Remarks on Dr. Prichard's Third Attack on Phrenology, in his 'Treatise on Insantiy,' " *Phren. J.*, 11 (1838), 345–58; and Edmond Sheppard Symes, abstract of address to the LPS containing strictures upon Prichard's article (as published in *Prov. Med. & Surg. J.* and copied into *Phren. J.*, 1 May 1844), *Zoist*, 2 (1845), 448–49. For discussion on Prichard and phrenology see: William F. Bynum, "Time's Noblest Offspring: the problem of man in the British natural historical sciences, 1800–1863," Ph.D. thesis, Cambridge, 1975, pp. 215–22.

Brande, "Phrenology," in his *Dictionary of Science, Literature, and Art* (1842), 925–6. On Brande (1788–1866), see: *DNB*, *DSB*, and Morris Berman, *Social*

Change and Scientific Organization: the Royal Institution, 1799–1844 (Ithaca, N.Y., 1978).

48. "The Champions of Phrenology," *Atlas*, 19 July 1829, in *Complete Works of William Hazlitt*, ed. P. P. Howe (1934), vol. 20, 254–5.

49. *Phren. J.*, 11 (1838), 263. See also: "Phrenology and the Medical Profession," ibid., 13 (1840), 128–42. In the LPS in 1825 there were 28 physicians and surgeons in a total membership of 72, and three years later 50 in a total membership of 134; in the Sheffield society, one-half the members were medical men in the 1820s; the Dublin society in 1836 was said to be almost wholly composed of medical men; in the EPS one-third were medical men in 1826; and in the newly formed Leamington and Warwick Phrenological Society in 1835 there were 10 medical men among 26 members. *Lancet*, 21 April 1827, p. 80; Hewett Cottrell Watson, *Statistics\of Phrenology: being a sketch of the progress and present state of that science in the British Islands* (1836), pp. 124, 166–7; *Phren. J.*, 3 (1825/6), pp. 259–61; I. Inkster, "A Phase in Middle Class Culture: phrenology in Sheffield, 1824–1850," *Trans. Hunter Arch. Soc.*, 19 (1978), 273–9 at p. 276.

50. Abernethy was no phrenologist; indeed, he foresaw "nothing but mischief" if the system became widely known. Yet his confession that he could offer no rational objection to Gall and Spurzheim's physiology gave the doctrine one of its greatest boosts: *Reflections on Gall and Spurzheim's System of Physiognomy and Phrenology, Addressed to the Court of Assistants of the Royal College of Surgeons in London, in June 1821* (1821). Cooper's published works and biography express no debts to phrenology, but it was reported in *Lancet*, 13 Jan. 1827, p. 480 that he had pronounced Spurzheim's new works on phrenology "calculated to fix immortality" on Spurzheim. Lawrence, although never lecturing exclusively on phrenology, incorporated and to a great extent popularized the ideas of Gall and Spurzheim through his *Lectures on Comparative Anatomy, Physiology, Zoology, and Natural History of Man* (1819), where he observed that no one could refuse Gall's theory "patient enquiry, careful observation, and unprejudiced reflection" and praised it as opening up wonderful new terrain (pp. 237–8). On Cooper, Abernethy, and Lawrence's relative support for phrenology in 1816, see: Spurzheim to Thomas Forster, 5 Nov. 1816 in Forster Papers: Bodleian Library, Oxford: MS Eng. Letters, c.200, f.181.

51. "Dr. Gall's Lectures on the Physiology of the Brain," *Weekly Medico-Chirurgical & Phil. Mag.*, 1, 2 (May/Apr. 1823), serially.

52. For major phrenology articles in *Medico-Chirurgical Rev.*, see: 4 (1817), 53–63, 117–34; n.s. 3 (Mar./May 1823), serially and published separately as *Review of "Observations on Phrenology"* (1823); 4 (1824), 847–82; 5 (1826), 437–69 (the quotation is from p. 437); 11 (1829), 193–6; 14 (1831), 321–2; 15 (1831), 172–4; 22 (1835), 121–3; 26 (1837), 225–32; 28 (1838), 225–52; n.s. 4 (1846), 447–63. Established by Johnson in 1816, the *Review*'s circulation was estimated at twenty-five hundred before its amalgamation with the *Br. & For. Med. Rev.* in 1848. For Johnson's public endorsement of phrenology, see his testimonial to Combe in *Testimonials on Behalf of George Combe as a Candidate for the Chair of Logic in the University of Edinburgh* (Edin., 1836), p. 67. For phrenology articles in the *Br. & For. Med. Rev.*, see: 10 (1840), 474–85; 13 (1842), 527–8; 16 (1843), 81–110; 22 (1846), 230–1; and the major articles by A. Combe (1846) and D. Noble (1842) cited below. For samples of the *Lancet* on phrenology, see: 1 & 15 Feb. 1824, 162–5, 224–7; 14 Aug. 1824, 203–10; 4 Sept. 1824, 298–302; 13 & 20 May 1826, 200–11, 234–44; 4 & 11 July 1829, 435–8, 468–75; 19 Jan. 1832, 532–5; 27 Dec. 1834, 500–3; and below, note 56. *London J.* estimated *Lancet*'s weekly circulation at eighty-five hundred: 1 (1845), p. 431. For evidence of Wakley's LPS membership, see *Lancet*, 4 Sept. 1824, p. 298. The *DNB* has entries on Johnson (1777–1845) M.D. St. Andrews 1821; Forbes (1787–1861) M.D. Edin. 1817; and Wakley (1795–1862).

53. Henry William Dewhurst, *A Letter to the Right Hon. Robert Peel . . . on Some of the Impediments, Defects, and Abuses, Existing in the Present System of Medical Education: with suggestions for their removal and correction* (1828), pp. 21–2.

54. See: Elliotson, "St. Thomas Hospital Lecture: a case of monomania and phrenology," *Lancet*, 30 Apr. 1831, 135–44; see also: "Account of the Schools of Medicine in London, Session 1833–34," *Lancet*, 28 Sept. 1833, p. 7, and "List of Lectures at the London Medical Schools, Session 1831–32," *Lancet*, 1 Oct. 1831, pp. 13–16; J. W. Crane, "State of Phrenology in Great Britain" [answers to questions of the French minister of commerce respecting the progress of phrenology in Britain with notes by the *Lancet*, reporter], *Lancet*, 22 June 1833, pp. 407–8; and J. F. Clarke, *Autobiographical Recollections of the Medical Profession* (1874), pp. 125–6. Elliotson refers to phrenology in his translation of Blumenbach, *The Institutions of Physiology* (3rd ed., 1820), pp. 32–4, in his *The Principles and Practice of Medicine* (1839), 606–43, and in his *Human Physiology* (5th ed., 1835), II, 1147–62. On Elliotson, see: Chapter 2, note 34; on Grainger (1801–65) M.R.C.S. 1822, see: *DNB*.

55. On Sleigh (1797–1863) M.R.C.S. 1816, see: below, Chapter 2, note 43; on Wilson (1809–84) M.R.C.S 1831, see: *DNB*; on South (1797–1882) M.R.C.S. 1819, see: *DNB*. It is not clear whether Green (1791–1863), whose niece South married, was himself a proponent of phrenology in the 1820s. He does not appear among those present at the meetings of the LPS; but in illustrating Gall and Spurzheim's method of brain dissection he can be seen as strengthening the claim made in the *Globe* in March 1825 (q. in *Phren. J.*, 2 [1824/5], p. 488): "Whatever difference of opinion there may be as to Phrenology, there can be no doubt, we think, as to the superiority of the mode of dissection which Drs. Gall and Spurzheim have recourse to over that which has been hitherto practiced in the anatomical schools." Yet, as indicated by *Phren. J.*'s reprinting of this statement (and ones similar to it), through recognized technical expertise, authority was gained for phrenology as a whole, and general awareness of Gall and Spurzheim and their doctrine enhanced.

56. *Lancet*, 16 Apr.–24 Sept. 1825; 25 June–17 Sept. 1836; Spurzheim's lectures were delivered in the Crown and Anchor Tavern (capacity twenty-five hundred persons) after negotiations conducted by the phrenologist James Deville.‡ Broussais's lectures were delivered in the University of Paris.

57. On Billing (1791–1881) M.D. Trinity 1818, F.R.C.P. 1819, F.R.S. 1844, and on Winslow (1810–74) M.R.C.S. 1835, see: *DNB*. Wright (1791–1859) M.D. Edin. 1813, who joined the LPS Apr. 1826 and was sometime pres., was appointed resident apothecary superintendent of Bethlem Asylum 1819 but was dismissed for drunkenness in 1830. Streeter (1802–73) LSA 1823, M.R.C.S. 1824, F.R.C.S. 1852, the son of a physician, member of the Russell Inst., and author of medical works, became a devoted phrenologist after attending Spurzheim's lectures in 1825 (J. F.Clarke, *Med. Times & Gaz.*, 2 [1873], 51–2); in a prefatory letter to the 2nd ed. of Samuel Solly's *Human Brain* (1847) Streeter describes the early British reception of Gall and Spurzheim's ideas. J. Moore (d. 1855) M.D. Glas. 1814, Edin. 1815, Paris 1818, physician to the Freemasons' Royal Female Asylum and consulting physician to the Queen Charlotte Lying-in Hospital, joined and was sec. to the LPS in 1824 (later pres.); he was also a member of the PA. E. Moore (1794–1858) M.D. Edin. 1827, M.R.C.S. 1815, sen. surg. Plymouth Dispensary for Diseases of the Eyes, medical author, naturalist, and geologist, joined the LPS May 1824. On Hayes (1769–1830) M.R.C.S. prior to 1822, who joined the LPS Apr. 1825 and who turned from medicine to commerce, see: obituary, *Phren. J.*, 6 (1829/30), 500–3.

58. Greenhow (1791–1881) M.R.C.S. 1814, F.R.C.S. 1843, sen. surg. Newcastle Infirmary, was chairman of the Newcastle Phren. Soc. 1836; Thompson (1793–1876) M.D.Edin. 1820, was hon. phys. Sheffield Gen. Infirmary 1831–66 and a leading figure in the Sheffield Phren. Soc.; Mackintosh (d. 1837) F.R.C.S.E. and medical author was one of the presidents of the Edinburgh Ethical Soc. for the Practical Application of Phrenology; Macdonald (1804–74) M.D.Edin. 1832 gave ten lectures on phrenology at the Portland St. School of Medicine, Glasgow 1841.

59. On Butter (1791–1877) M.R.C.S. 1811, M.D. Edin. 1822, F.R.S. 1820, who

joined the EPS Feb. 1822 and the LPS Mar. 1825, see: *DNB*; information is wanting on both Jones and Henry; Barlow (1779–1844) M.D. Edin. 1803, who was also one of the founders of the Bath Lit & Phil, was converted to phrenology after Spurzheim's lectures in Bath in 1814; he became a member of the LPS Nov. 1826 and of the PA; his *An Apology for the Study of Phrenology* (Bath, 1825) was dedicated to G. Combe.

60. On Conolly (1794–1866) M.D. Edin. 1821, F.R.C.S. 1844, med supt. of Hanwell 1839–44, see: *DNB*; Ellis (1790–1839) M.R.C.S. 1800, M.D. St. Andrews 1818, med. supt. Wakefield Asylum 1818–20, Hanwell 1831–8, established a Phrenological society while at Wakefield and phrenologically delineated his patients. John Robertson Sibbald (1799–1868) L.R.C.S.E. 1818, F.R.C.S.E. 1829, who joined the EPS Apr. 1821 and was elected a corresp. member of the LPS Jan. 1827, was surgeon to the Royal Magdalane Asylum. For other phrenological alienists, see: my "Phrenology and British Alienists," esp. pp. 4–7.

61. For Clark (1788–1870) M.R.C.S.E. 1809, M.D. 1817, F.R.S. 1832, and his close friend A. Combe (1797–1847) M.D. Edin. 1825, F.R.C.P.E. 1833, the brother of G. Combe, see: *DNB*. See also: *DNB* on Knighton (1776–1836) M.D. Aberdeen, F.R.C.S. c. 1810, an early enthusiast of phrenology who introduced Lord Byron to Spurzheim in 1814 for Byron's phrenological delineation. Stewart, surgeon R.N., was physician extraordinary to the duke of Sussex in 1836 when he supplied Sir George MacKenzie with a testimonial on the value of phrenology: *Documents Laid Before the Rt. Hon. Lord Glenelg . . . Relative to the Convicts Sent to New South Wales* [46 testimonials] (Edin., 1836).

62. Winslow, *The Principles of Phrenology as Applied to the Elucidation and Cure of Insanity: an essay read at the Westminster Medical Society, January 4th 1832* (1832), p. 11. See also: Spurzheim, *Observations on the Deranged Manifestations of the Mind or Insanity* (1817), and A. Combe, *Observations on Mental Derangement* (Edin., 1831).

63. James G. Davey, *On the Nature, and Proximate Cause of Insanity* (1853), p. 26n. Davey (1813–95) I.S.A. 1833, M.R.C.S. 1836, was house surgeon at Hanwell under Conolly and subsequently medical superintendent of the female side of Europe's largest asylum, Colney Hatch, Middlesex.

64. *Brain and Its Physiology* pp. 123–4 (This is one of the most useful sources for the scientific–medical debates over phrenology.)

65. "Phrenology," *Lancet*, 19 Mar. 1825, p. 348.

66. Review of "Spurzheim on Education," *New Edin.Rev.*, 1 (1821), 311–334 at p. 327. This journal was edited by Richard Poole (1783–1871) M.D. St.Andrews 1805, successor in 1839 to W. A. F. Browne at the Montrose Asylum, a member of the EPS, editor of the first four numbers of *Phren. J.*, and author of the article "Phrenology" in *Ency. Edinesis* (Edin., 1816–27).

67. Disney Alexander,[‡] *A Lecture on Phrenology, as Illustrative of the Moral and Intellectual Capacities of Man* (1826), p. 2.

68. Uwins, *Treatise on Disorders of the Brain*, pp. 95–6. idem, "Phrenology," pt. 33, vol. 17, *London Ency.* (1829), 259–74; idem, "Phrenology," *New Monthly Mag.*, 34 (1832), 445–55 (this journal was then under the editorship of Edward Bulwer-Lytton and the member of the LPS, Samuel Carter Hall). On Uwins (1780–1837) M.D. Edin. 1803, physician to various London dispensaries, who was appointed in 1828 to the Peckham Lunatic Asylum, see: *DNB* and J. F.Clarke, *Recollections*, p. 234. For Barlow's confession of faith in phrenology see: Barlow, "An Address Delivered at the First Anniversary Meeting of the Provincial Medical and Surgical Association, July 19th, 1833," *Trans. Prov. Med & Surg. Ass.*, 2 (1834), 1–31 at pp. 27–8.

69. *Homoeopathy and Allopathy or Large, Small, and Atomic Doses?* [1836], p. 4n.

70. Michael Ryan, "Physiology, Phrenology, Materialsim, Immaterialism of the Mind, By the Editor," *Lon. Med. & Surg. J.*, 3 (1829), 44–51 at p. 49. See also: Dr. Michael Ryan versus Phrenology" [in his *Manual of Medical Jurisprudence* (1831), pp. 6–18], *Phren. J.*, 7 (1831/2), 366–8; and *Lancet*, 25 Oct. 1831. On Ryan (1800–41), see: *DNB*. John Kidd in public and Duglad Stewart in private

both maintained that phrenology had a mischievous, dangerous tendency: Kidd, *Course in Comparative Anatomy*, p. 72; Stewart, in the letter from Spurzheim to Forster cited above (note 50).

71. On Paracelsus in this connection, see: ref. in W. F. Bynum, "Health, Disease, and Medical Care," in Rousseau and Porter, *Ferment of Knowledge*, 211–53 at p. 253; for Marcuse, see: Herbert Marcuse "Industrialization and Capitalism in the Work of Max Weber" in his *Negations* (Boston, 1968), 201–26 and the introductory remarks to its republication in J. L. Dolgin, et al., eds. *Symbolic Anthropology* (N.Y., 1977), p. 364; for similar from Sir James Fraser, see: Mary Douglas, *Purity and Danger; an analysis of concepts of pollution and taboo* (1978), p. 24. See also: Hans Vaihinger, *The Philosophy of "As If,"* trans. C. K. Ogden (1968), pp.84, 108; Lucien Goldmann, *The Hidden God*, trans. P.Thody (1964), p. 48; and Nigel Harris, *Beliefs in Society: the problem of ideology* (Harmondsworth, 1968), p. 15.

CHAPTER 2: *The social sense of brain*

1. *Philosophisch-medizinische Untersuchungen über Natur und Kunst im Kranken und gesunden Zustande des Menuschen* (Vienna, 1791). Like Freud, Gall wished to put an end to the high-handed generalizations of the philosophers: J. C. Marshall, "Freud's Psychology of Language," p. 354.

2. See: "Some Particulars Respecting Gall," *Zoist*, 2 (1845), 455–65; J. Fossati, "Discourse Pronounced over the Tomb of Dr. Gall, 27 Aug. 1828," *Phren. J.*, 5 (1828/9), 580–4; *Times* (London), 27 Aug. 1828, p. 2; *Lon. Med. Gaz.*, 2 (1828), 477–8; R. M. Young's entry on "Gall," in *DSB*; and Marquis F. de Moscati, "On the Character and Phrenological Organization of Dr Gall," *Lancet*, 22 June 1833, 399–403.

3. The epigraph of the phrenological journal *Zoist*, (1843–56) edited by W. C. Engledue and John Elliotson.

4. Anon., *Sir William Hamilton and Phrenology* (Edin., 1826), p. 11; and *Zoist*, 1 (1843), 22.

5. Erna Lesky, "Organology of Franz Joseph Gall" in her *The Vienna Medical School* pp. 4–8; and J. Y. Hall, "Gall's Phrenology: a romantic psychology," *Stud. Romanticism*, 16 (1977), 305–17 at p. 306. For a useful introduction to the metaphysics of the romantics, see: H. W. Piper, *The Active Universe* (1962).

6. Erna Lesky, "Gall and Herder," *Clio Medica*, 2 (1967), 85–96; G. Morin, "Gall et Goethe," *Paris médical, partie paramedicale*, 72 (1929), 425–32; and George Henry Lewes, *The Life and Works of Goethe* (1855), II, p. 325.

7. On Flaxman and phrenology see: Henry Crabb Robinson, *Diary, Reminiscences, and Correspondence*, ed.Thomas Sadler (1869), II, p. 310; on Swedenborgians and phrenology see: Peter J. Lineham, "The English Swedenborgians, 1770–1840: a study in the social dimensions of religious sectarianism," Ph.D. thesis, Sussex, 1978, pp. 445–7; on Coleridge see: Trevor Levere, "Coleridge and the Human Sciences: anthropology, phrenology, and mesmerism," in M. Hanen et al., eds., *Science, Pseudoscience and Society* (Waterloo, Ont. 1980), 171–92. Coleridge's literary executor was the student of German idealism and friend of phrenologists J. H. Green (see: above, Chapter 1, note 55). Charles Augustus Tulk (1786–1849), a friend of Flaxman, Coleridge, and William Blake and a leading London Swendenborgian, frequently held the office of president of the LPS in the 1820s and 1830s. He was also M.P. for Sudbury 1820–6 and for Poole 1841; a magistrate for Middlesex 1836–47; and chairman of the Committee of Management of the Hanwell Lunatic Asylum 1839–47. His phrenological views may be seen in a ms in the Swedenborg Society of London (A/83), "Aphorisms on the Laws of Creation as Displayed in the Correspondences that Subsist between Mind and Matter," c. 1843. Other Swedenborgian phrenologists were J. P. Greaves (below, Chapter 8), J. I. Hawkins,‡ and D. G. Goyder.‡

8. For the supporters of phrenology most of the biographical information derives from their publications, especially from the *Phren. J.*, the list of *Testimonials to*

Combe, and the 46 testimonials to the utility of phrenology supplied to Sir G. S. Mackenzie in his *Documents Laid before Lord Glenelg* (1836). Additional information comes principally from *Lancet*; *Br. Med. J.*; *London and Provincial Medical Directory* (from 1845); *Index-Catalogue of the Library of the Surgeon-General's Office, United States Army* (from 1880); *List of Graduates in Medicine in the University of Edinburgh from 1705 to 1866* (Edin., 1867); *A List of the Members of the Royal College of Surgeons in London* (from 1805); *A List of Persons Who Have Obtained Certificates of Their Fitness and Qualification to Practice as Apothecaries from August 1, 1815 to July 31, 1840* (1840); Frederic Boase, *Modern English Biography*; Richard Hunter and I. MacAlpine, *Three Hundred Years of Psychiatry* (1963); and J. F. Clarke, *Autobiographical Recollections* (1874). Invaluable for Sheffield and Edinburgh, respectively, are I. Inkster, "Phrenology in Sheffield," and S. Shapin, "Phrenological Knowledge." More especially for the opponents of phrenology, information is drawn from (in addition to the already cited *DNB* and *DSB* entries) *The Record of the Royal Society of London* (4th ed., 1940); *Proceedings of the Royal Society of London*; *Proceedings of the Royal Society of Edinburgh*; *Memoirs of the Wernerian Natural History Society* (1808–38); *Lives of the Fellows of the Royal College of Physicians of London, 1826–1925* ed. G. H Brown (1955); Plarr's *Lives of the Fellows of the Royal College of Surgeons of England* (1930); W. Innes Addison, *The Matriculation Albums of the University of Glasgow, 1728–1858* (Glasgow, 1913); George Burchnell and T. U. Sadleir, *Alumni Dublinieness* (Dublin, 1935); J. A. Venn, *Alumni Cantabrigienses*, pt. II, 1752–1900 (Cambridge, 1952); Joseph Foster, *Alumni Oxonienses, 1715–1886* (1888); Jack Morrell and Arnold Thackray, *Gentlemen of Science: early years of the British Association for the Advancement of Science* (Oxford, 1981). For the members of phrenological societies, see: "List of Members of the Phrenological Society," *Phren. J.*, 3 (1826), 476–81; "Names of Members and Visitors, Inspecting the Casts etc. Belonging to the Phrenological Society, 1822–1846" (MS, Gen. 608: Edin. Univ. Lib.); "London Phrenological Society," *Panoramic Miscellany*, [I] (31 Jan.–30 June 1826); for the LPS, *Lancet* (1824–37) and *Phren. J.*, 5 (1828/9), 70–82; *Fourth Annual Report of the Sheffield Phrenological Society* (Sheffield, 1846), p. 12; for sources on PA members see: below, Chapter 3, note 85.

9. William Weir, letter to editor, *Phren. J.*, 11 (1837), 90. On the age of the supporters of Darwin and of reductionist biology in Berlin, see, respectively: J. W. Burrow, *Evolution and Society* (Cambridge, 1966), p. 42 (who observes that Charles Lyell's endorsement of Darwin's idea was apparently considered "heroic" in view of his age and standing in society); Everett Mendelsohn, "Revolution and Reduction: the sociology of methodological and philosophical concerns in nineteenth century biology," in Y. Elkana, *Interaction between Science and Philosophy*, pp. 407–27.

10. See: Christopher Hill, *The World Turned Upside Down* (Harmondsworth, 1975), p. 366 et passim; Timothy Lenoir, "Generational Factors in the Origin of Romantische Naturphilosophie," *J. Hist. Biol.*, 11 (1978), 57–100. Cf. Herbert Moller, "Youth as a Force in the Modern World," *Comp. Stud. Soc. & Hist.*, 10 (1968), 237–60 at p. 255 (who observes that in England in 1840 the age group 15 to 30 numbered 77 for every 100 outside it); and Lewis S. Feuer, "The Generational Basis for Ideological Waves," in his *Ideology and the Ideologists* (Oxford, 1975), 69–95.

11. Lenoir, "Generational Factors," p. 59.

12. Cf. Terry Parssinen's observation that of the 110 British members of the EPS in 1826, 29% are found in either the *DNB* or Boase's *Modern English Biography*, while in the LPS at the same time, when there were 72 members, the comparable figure was 26%: "Phrenology Movement," *J.Soc. Hist.*, 7 (1974), 15n.

13. Among all other phrenologists the following are known to have been educated at either Oxford or Cambridge: Arthur and Sir Walter Trevelyan, both EPS members; Robert Everest, EPS member in 1821; Richard Whately (see: below, note 16), and Charles Tulk, John Harris (1804–48) M.B. Camb. 1830 was a corresp. member of the LPS while a student at Trinity College.

14. Another R.N. surgeon who was a corresp. member of the LPS was John P. Porter (1771–1855), who rose to be med. supt. of the convict hulks in Portsmouth and was a cofounder of the Portsmouth and Portsea Lit & Phil.

15. Charles Gibbon, *The Life of George Combe* (1878), I, p. 318; and A. C. Grant, "George Combe and the 1836 Election for the Edinburgh University Chair of Logic," *The Book of the Old Edinburgh Club*, 32 (1966), 174–84. See also *Testimonials to Combe* and *Testimonials in Support of Sir William Hamilton's Application for the Chair of Logic and Metaphysics* (Edin., 1836). Combe wrote to his brother Andrew that he was offering himself for the chair "not in expectation of success, but to bring forward phrenology": 9 April 1836, Combe Papers, NLS 7386 ff 531.

16. On Wheatstone (1802–75), who joined the LPS in 1825 and was active in it in the 1830s, see: *DNB* and *DSB*. Among all other active British phrenologists, it has been determined that the following held academic posts at other times: John P. Nichol (1804–59), professor of astronomy at Glasgow; the Rev. David Welsh (1793–1845), professor of church history at Edinburgh in 1831, by which time he had broken with the EPS, although he retained his interest in phrenology; James L. Drummond (1783–1863), professor of anatomy and botany in Belfast Royal Inst. and president of the Belfast Natural History (and Phrenological) Society; Richard Whately (1787–1863), Drummond Professor of Political Economy at Oxford 1829–31 and archbishop of Dublin 1831–53. Whately had a phrenological cast of his head made while at Oxford but did not become an enthusiast until after reading Combe's *Constitution of Man* in 1832. (See Gibbon, *Life of Combe*, I, pp. 259–60 and below, Chapter 3, note 45.).

17. Samuel Solly (1805–71) was the only other medical lecturer to be a fellow of the Royal Society of London while advocating phrenology fron inside the medical establishment. The son of a merchant, he studied under Benjamin Travers at St. Thomas's and became surgeon and lecturer there in 1853 and president of the Royal Medical and Chirurgical Society in 1867. He had been inspired by Spurzheim's's dissection of a brain at St. Thomas's in 1823, but (and for this reason is not included in our sample) was not completely converted to phrenology until some time after 1836 (the year he became an F.R.S.), when he witnessed convincing craniological demonstrations. He joined the PA and, in 1843, he served on its committee; he publicly avowed himself a phrenologist in his lecture on the brain to the Royal Institution, 16 Feb. 1844. See his *The Human Brain* (2nd ed., 1847), pp. x–xiii.

    Other supporters of phrenology who were fellows of the Royal Societies of London or Edinburgh were Bryan Donkin (1786–1855) F.R.S. 1838, engineer and inventor; William Elford Leach (1790–1836) F.R.S. 1817, assistant keeper of the natural history department of the British Museum and the donor of a large collection of crania to the EPS in 1837; Charles Tulk F.R.S. 1824; Richard Beamish‡ F.R.S., civil engineer and lecturer; Patrick Neill, F.R.S.E. 1814, Edinburgh printer, and secretary of the Wernerian Soc. 1820; John Shank More, F.R.S.E. 1820, advocate; Robert Hamilton,F.R.S.E. and F.R.C.S.E. 1821; William Bonar,F.R.S.E. 1823, banker; Capt.Thomas Brown, F.R.S. and member of the Wernerian Soc.; Capt.Daniel Ross,R.N., F.R.S. 1822, a member of the LPS.

18. Browne, for example, sought to omit reference to phrenology in his *What Asylums Were, Are, and Ought to Be* (Edin., 1837) for which he was chastised by Andrew Combe; see: G. Combe, *The Life and Correspondence of Andrew Combe, M.D.* (Edin., 1850), pp. 280–1. On Lawrence, see: Owsei Temkin, "Basic Science, Medicine, and the Romantic Era," in his *The Double Face of Janus and Other Essays* (Baltimore and London, 1977), 345–72 at p. 357; on Cooper, see: B. B. Cooper, *The Life of Sir Astley Cooper* (1843), II, pp. 296–7.

19. Cited in G. N. Cantor, "Edinburgh Phrenology Debate," p. 204. See also: B. Spector, "Sir Charles Bell and the Bridgewater Treatises," *Bull. Hist. Med.*, 12 (1942), 314–22.

20. On the Lawrence–Abernethy dispute see: Temkin, "Basic Science," esp. at pp.

347–9, 357–9; "Abernethy, Lawrence, etc. on the Theories of Life," *Quart. Rev.*, 22 (1819), 1–34. For the phrenologists' views on the dispute, see: *Phren. J.*, 1 (1823/4), pp. 120–46; and Robert Macnish, *An Introduction to Phrenology* (2nd ed., 1837), p. 9. The strongly antimaterialist Rev. Thomas Rennell, the Christian advocate at Cambridge who spoke out against Lawrence in *Remarks on Scepticism* (2nd ed., 1819), was held by Thomas Forster ("Cranioscopophilus") to have been a craniologist before discovering that Gall's doctrine was philosophically materialist: "Phrenology: the Wernerian Society of Edinburgh, and the Phrenological Societies of Edinburgh and London," *Lancet*, 13 Jan. 1827, 479–80 at p. 480.

21. On this problem, see: Robert K.Webb, *Harriet Martineau, a Radical Victorian* (1960), p. 363, and in relation to individuals and institutions involved with early C19 science, see: Cannon, *Science in Culture*, p. 229.

22. Anon., *Sir William Hamilton and Phrenology*, p. 29, cited in Shapin, "Phrenological Knowledge" p. 239; and idem., "The Politics of Observation," in Wallis, *Margins of Science*, p. 170. On the history of the early C19 decline in metaphysics, see: Hugh Miller, "The Idealistic School," in *Essays Historical and Biographical, Political and Social, Literary and Scientific* (4th ed., Edin., 1870), 431–41; and see: Chapter 3, note 18.

23. Karl Mannheim, "Conservative Thought," in *Essays on Sociology and Social Psychology*, ed. P. Kecskemeti (1953), 74–164 at p. 76.

24. Arnold Momigliano, *J. Roman Stud.*, 30 (1940), 77 cited in L. Pyenson, " 'Who the Guys Were,' " p. 155; cf. Shapin and Thackray, "Prosopography as a Research Tool."

25. Charles Rosenberg, "Sexuality, Class, and Role in Nineteenth-Century America," *Amer. Q.*, 25 (1973), 132. See also: the concluding remarks of Paul Forman in his classic social study of "Weimar Culture, Causality, and Quantum Theory, 1918–1927," *Hist. Stud. Phys. Sci.*, 3 (1971), 1–115; and D. Layder, "Problems in Accounting for the Individual in Marxist–Rationalist Theoretical Discourse," *Br. J. Sociol.*, 30 (1979), 149–63. On the indivisibility of the social and psychology, see: J. F. C. Harrison, *The Second Coming: popular millenarianism, 1780–1850* (1979), p. 220.

26. Copland, M.D. Edin. 1815, F.R.S. 1833, F.R.C.P. 1837, attempted but failed to secure a medical position in London; after a stay in Africa he came back to London and, after serving as a hack medical writer, eventually secured a post as lecturer at the Little Dean Street Medical School and then at Middlesex Hospital. See *DNB*. Much of his antagonism to phrenology appears to have stemmed from an unsatisfactory phrenological delineation he received (see: his *Dictionary of Practical Medicine* [1832], vol. 2, p. 503n); It was under his editorship of the *London Medical Repository* between 1822 and 1827 that phrenology came under attack.

27. On Bostock, see: *DNB* and *DSB*; on Roget, see: Emblem, *Roget*.

28. On Hamilton (who accused Thomas Brown, postumously, of being a republican and borrowing from Condillac and De Tracy) see: *DNB* and *DSB*; on Jeffrey, see: *DNB*. Elliotson and Conolly were on the Council of the SDUK; Clark, Billing, and Conolly were on the Senate of London University. It is also worth noting that friendly relations often existed between phrenologists and antiphrenologists in private: hence Spurzheim was among Charles Bell's guests in 1816, George Combe dined with Dugald Stewart in 1826, and it was Jeffrey who introduced the visiting Audubon to the phrenologist James Simpson in 1826. See: Gordon Taylor and E. W. Walls, *Sir Charles Bell* (Edin., 1958), p. 69; and *Audubon and His Journals*, ed. M. R. Audubon (N.Y., 1960), I, pp. 161, 191.

29. For Kidd's social and intellectual circle, see: Pietro Corsi, "Natural Theology, the Methodology of Science, and the Question of Species in the Works of the Reverend Baden Powell," D.Phil thesis, Oxford, 1980. Further problems surround the inclusion of John Barclay among the antiphrenologist since his views (esp. in *Inquiry Concerning Life and Organization*) tended to the side of Lawrence and phrenological materialism; indeed, according to Forster, Barclay defended

the system upon hearing Forster lecture on it in Edinburgh in 1816: "Phrenology: the Wernerian Society," p. 479.

30. In addition to the studies on Sheffield and Edinburgh by Inkster and Shapin, see: my "The Politics of Brain: phrenology in Birmingham," *Bull. Soc. Social Hist. Med.*, no. 32 (1983), 34–6.

31. See, respectively: Sir George Lefevre, "Drs Gall and Spurzheim: phrenology," in his *The Life of a Travelling Physician* (1843), I, p. 150 (Lefevre also thought him "kind and benevolent," contrasting him to Gall, whom he thought "betrayed a disbelief in every thing, and even in his own system. . . . In conversing with several of the French professors upon this subject, I found them unanimously of this opinion. *"S[purzheim] croit au moins a tout ce qu'il dit, comme un bon enfant. Gall n'y croit pas un mot."* Such was the opinion in Paris."); Spurzheim to William Rathbone, 12 June 1831 (Bodleian Lib., MS Autog. f.181–2), and the several letters from Spurzheim to Forster between 2 Feb. 1815 and 13 Feb. 1817 (Forster papers, Bodleian Lib., MS Eng. lett c.200 f.173–89); John Elliotson, *Human Physiology* (5th ed., 1835), pp. 1159–60n.; idem, "Announcement of the Death of Dr Spurzheim, to London Phrenological Society," *Lancet*, 29 Dec. 1832, pp. 427–32; "Death of Spurzheim," *Phren. J.*, 8 (1832/4), 126–43; Marquis F. de Moscati, "Biographical Paper on the Character and Phrenological Organization of Dr Spurzheim, to the London Phrenological Society," *Lancet*, 12 Jan. 1833, pp. 493–8; G. Combe, *Life of Andrew Combe*, pp. 203–4; Spurzheim, *Education: Its elementary principles founded on the nature of man* (Manch., n.d.), p. 52; Robert Owen, *A Dialogue on Three Parts* (Manch., 1838), p. 11. The only biography of Spurzheim is the slim volume by the phrenologist Andrew Carmichael, *A Memoir of the Life and Philosophy of Spurzheim* (Dublin, 1833). For the American sources on Spurzheim see: the *DSB* entry by A. A. Walsh and idem, "Johann Christoph Spurzheim and the Rise and Fall of Scientific Phrenology in Boston, 1832–1842," Ph.D. thesis, New Hampshire, 1974; idem, "The American Tour of Dr Spurzheim," *J. Hist. Med & Allied Sci.*, 27 (1972), 187–205; and idem, "Phrenology and the Boston Medical Community in the 1830s," *Bull. Hist. Med.*, 50 (1976), 261–73.

32. *Notebooks*, 3, p. 4355, and *Table Talk*, 2 (July 1830), q. in Levere, "Coleridge and the Human Sciences," pp. 182–5. Coleridge was attracted to Gall and Spurzheim's doctrine from his aversion to sensationalist psychology, his Platonist anti-Cartesian interest in the unity of man, mind, and nature, and his rejection of empiricist philosophy. His hostility to the doctrine by 1833 (at the same time that he became hostile to fragmentation in the physical sciences) is testimony to how these features of the doctrine and philosophy could be seen to have by then become truncated as phrenology popularly manifested itself as merely a form of materialist psychological reductionism.

33. In the preface to his *The Anatomy of the Brain*, Spurzheim offers the most explicit comments on his estrangement from Gall; but see also: Spurzheim, *Physiognomical System*, p. vii; his notes to *Phrenology Article of the Foreign Quarterly Review* by Richard Chenevix (1830), pp. 11, 62; and de Moscati, "Spurzheim."

34. For an excellent recent study of Elliotson which offers psychological insights, see: J. Miller, "A Gower Street Scandal," *J. Roy. Coll. Phys.*, 17 (1983), 181–91. Miller's article largely supercedes the sources I have relied upon: *DNB*; *Reece's Monthly Gaz. Health*, 14 (Dec. 1829), 753–4; *Court Mag.*, 6 (April 1835), 175; *Lancet*, 8 June 1833, 341–4; *J. Mental Health*, 14 (1868), 428–30; G. Rosen, "John Elliotson, Physician and Hypnotist," *Bull. Hist. Med.*, 4 (1936), 500–3; Harley Williams, "John Elliotson," in *Doctors Differ* (1946); and Fred Kaplan, Introduction to *John Elliotson on Mesmerism* (N.Y., 1982). I am grateful to Irving Loudon for calling my attention to Elliotson's height. For Elliotson's attitude to Spurzheim, see: *Human Physiology*, pp. 1159–60n. He first met Gall in London 1824 at James Deville's phrenology shop and later, in the company of Sir Astley Cooper, at St. Thomas's Hospital; he subsequently visited him in Paris in 1826 and 1827 (ibid., p. 1147).

35. *A Treatise on Naval Discipline; with an explanation of the important advantages which*

naval and military discipline might derive from the science of phrenology. To which are added phrenological deductions from the cerebral development of J[oseph] H[ume], Esq. (1825). It is possible that Ross joined the EPS at the invitation of Sir George Mackenzie (on whom see: below), for in 1821 Mackenzie published in Danish a translation of the account in High German by C. W. Harnisch of [*Travels near Iceland the Bay of Baffin in Search of Discovering a Northwest Passage by Greenland in the Year 1818 by John Ross*]. This at least would have provided an occasion for coming into contact.

36. *DNB*. I am grateful to Clive A. Holland, Archivist, Scott Polar Research Institute, Cambridge, and to Admiral M. J. Ross for supplying me with information on Ross. I am also grateful to Constance Martin for her helpful suggestions. (Capt. Daniel Ross, R.N. of the LPS was unrelated to John Ross.)

37. Susan Cannon, "The Cambridge Network," in *Science in Culture*; she refers to Ross on p. 44.

38. Although Ross's antipathy of Hume bore directly on Hume's opposition to the establishment of an astronomical observatory at the Cape of Good Hope, it is unlikely that Ross would have made the remarks he did had he been in sympathy with Hume's populous politics. Indeed, Ross refers to Hume as a "notorious" man "better equipted for private than public life." *Treatise on Naval Discipline*, pp. 35–9. On phrenologists and prison discipline, see: below, Chapter 4, notes 68, 70.

39. Ibid., p. 23.

40. Ibid., p. 33. Ross is referring to certain prominent members of the Evangelical party of the Scottish Church who defended phrenology against the charge of materialsm and fatalism in order to deploy it as a rationalization of their reactionary views on human depravity and the regenerating power of Gospel in relation to reigning views and tendencies within the Established Church. Some of these persons were later to be involved in the Disruption of the Scottish Church in 1843, but by that time they had dissociated themselves from phrenology and had denounced Combe's phrenological philosophy as a revival of the materialsim of French infidels. See: below, Chapter 4, note 89.

41. See: Sabine, *Remarks on the Account of the late Voyage* (1819); and Ross, *Explanation of Capt. Sabine's Remarks* (1819).

42. Twenty-two of Ross's later phrenological delineations are housed in the Scott Polar Research Institute, Cambridge.

43. Hence the involvement with phrenology, especially in the early 1820s, of all sorts of cantakerous, bitter individuals whose politics were anything but liberal. E.g.: William Willcocks Sleigh, an exceedingly vain, reactionary, and viciously paranoid figure who was John Epps's first phrenological contact in London in 1821–2 (*Diary of Epps*, pp. 70, 109–11; Sleigh's personally and politically revealing *Letter to the Independent Governors of St George's Hospital* [1827]); and Dr. Frederick Leo, an apparantly "vain and egotistical" old-generation evangelical of German extraction – see: *The Letters of Thomas Babington Macaulay*, ed. Thomas Pinney, vol. 4 (Cambridge, 1977), pp. 234–5.

44. Cf. the reactions to head readings by Forster (below), R. Cobden (Chapter 4, note 99), H. Martineau (Chapter 4, note 57), J. Copland (above, note 26), S. Solly (above, note 17), and R. Carlile (Chapter 7, note 22). On MacKenzie's turning to phrenology see: *DNB*; Gibbon, *Life of Combe*, I, pp. 109 ff.; MacKenzie, *An Essay ... on taste*, pp. v, 2, 287–301.

45. See: MacKenzie, *Three Lectures ... for the use of Mechanics' Institutions* (Edin., 1839); idem, *General Observations on the Principles of Education: for the use of mechanics' institutions* (Edin., 1836); "Correspondence between Sir George S. MacKenzie and Duglad Stewart, 1821," *Phren. J.*, 7 (1831/2), 303–9.

46. "Essay Read by Sir Geo. S. MacKenzie, Bart., to the Royal Society of Edinburgh, Jan. 1830," *Phren. J.*, 6 (1829/30), 332–43, 355–65 (the presentation was between 8 Dec. 1829 and 1 Feb. 1830: Shapin, "Phrenological Knowledge," p.231 n.); and *Scotsman*, q. in *Phren. J.*, 6 (1829/30), 363–4. For phrenological rhetoric on the elitism in Royal Societies, see: G. Combe, "Letter on the Prejudices of the Great in Science and Philosophy against Phrenology; addressed to the editor of

the *Edinburgh Weekly Journal,*" *Phren. J.*, 6 (1829/30), 14–38; 10 (1837/8), 623–9; and 11 (1838), 13–22.

47. Berman, *Royal Institution,* pp. 38, xxi.

48. See: entry in *DNB*; Chenevix receives brief and inadequate entry in the *DSB.* Much of his early career can be traced through his correspondence with Sir Joseph Banks and Sir Charles Blagden: usefully abstracted in *The Banks Letters,* ed. Warren R. Dawson (1958). There are twenty-eight papers by him listed in the *Roy. Soc. Cat. Sci. Papers*; the *Wellesley Index to Victorian Periodicals* lists six *Edin. Rev.* articles by him and two in *Quart. Rev.* on subjects ranging from poetry and shipwrecks to industry and cookery.

49. *Phren. J.*, 6 (1828/9), 158–60; Chenevix, "Phrenology," *Foreign Q. Rev.*, at p. 15 of the pamphlet edition with notes by Spurzheim (see note 51).

50. See: M. C. Usselman, "The Wollaston/Chenevix Controversy over the Elemental Nature of Palladium: a curious episode in the history of chemistry," *Ann. Sci.*, 35 (1978), 551–79; Chenevix, "On Mesmerism Improperly Denominated Animal Magnetism," *Lon. Med. & Phys. J.*, n.s. 6 (Mar.–Sept. 1829) serially.

51. David Uwins was among those who confessed that Chenevix's article was the source of his conversion to phrenology: [Uwins], "Phrenology," *London Ency.* (1829), p. 272. Spurzheim obtained Chenevix's permission to have the article printed as a pamphlet (*Phrenology Article of the Foreign Quarterly Review* by Richard Chenevix [1830]) with twelve pages of his own notes; this was then republished in America in 1833 and was translated into German in 1838 by the geologist Carl Bernhard Cotta (1808–79). Further reference is to the 1830 edition, hereafter *Phrenology Article.*

52. *Phren. J.*, 6 (1829/30), 604; *Zoist,* 1 (1843), 58–64, 88–9.

53. See: Erwin Ackerknecht, "German Jews, English Dissenters, French Protestants: nineteenth-century pioneers of modern medicine and science," in Charles Rosenberg, ed., *Healing and History* (N.Y. and London, 1979), 86–96. For Chenevix's hatred of Germans, see: *Banks Letters,* p. 96; idem, "On Mesmerism," p. 220; Chenevix, *Remarks upon Chemical Nomenclature, According to the French Neologists* (1802). On the reactionary political significance of German chemistry, see: Lenoir, "Generational Factors," pp. 78–9. Chenevix himself drew the analogy between phrenology and the earlier revolution in chemistry in which he had been involved: *Phrenology Article,* pp. 57–8.

54. See: J.W. Crane, "State of Phrenology in Great Britain," p. 408.

55. In addition to his own *DNB* entry and that on Benjamen Furly, see: *DNB* entries on his father Thomas Furly Forster (1761–1825), his grandfather Edward Forster (1730–1812), his great uncle Benjamen Forster (1736–1805), and his uncles Benjamen Meggot Forster (1764–1829) and Edward Forster (1765–1849).

56. *Phil. Mag.*, 45 (Jan. 1815), 63. Forster received his Cambridge University M.B. in 1818.

57. Forster, *Recueil de ma vie, mes ouvrages, et mes pensées opuscule philosophique* (3rd ed., Bruxelles, 1837), pp. 16–18; the first edition, entitled *Recueil des oeuvrages et pensées d'un physician et metaphysicien,* was published in Frankfurt in 1836; idem, *Facts and Enquiries Respecting the Source of Epidemia . . . to Which Are Added Observations on Quarantine and Sanitory Rules* (3rd ed., 1832), p. 15; idem, *A Collection of Letters on Early Education, and Its influence in the Prevention of Crime* (2nd ed., 1844), p. v; *Phren. J.*, 7 (1831/2), 192 (the first ten volumes of *Phren. J.*, in Cambridge University Library are from Whewell's library). Forster's paper to the Wernerians greatly upset the society, though, according to him (*Recueil de ma vie,* p. 18), some of them later became "the greatest phrenologists in Edinburgh." True to Royal Society standards, the official proceedings of the Wernerian Soc. record, for the first time: "At this meeting, no public business": *Memoirs of the Wernerian Natural History Society for the Years 1811–1816* (Edin., 1818). p. 659. See also: [Forster], "Phrenology: the Wernerian Society," pp. 479–80. On Spurzheim's theatrics, see: "Edinburgh Dissection of the Brain," *Phil. Mag.*, 48 (1816), 153; Carmichael, *Memoir of Spurzheim,* pp. 18–23; Gibbon, *Life of Combe,* I, pp. 94–5; Combe, *Essays on Phrenology* (Edin., 1819), pp. ix–xiv.

According to a report on the LPS in *Lancet*, Forster became a "corresponding member" of the society. It seems more likely, however, that he did not choose membership but rather was, as he claimed in his autobiography, elected an "honourary member." I have found no evidence that he actually attended the meetings of the society, although the reports in *Lancet* are not complete. It is unlikely that he did attend, for after 1818 he resided in Hartwell Sussex and, for reasons of his wife's health and his daughter's education, spent much of his time on the Continent.

58. Preface to the first volume. Forster coined the word *phrenology* (i.e., *phren*, "head"; *logos*, "discourse") in his 'Observations on a New System of Phrenology; or, the anatomy and physiology of the brain of Drs Gall and Spurzheim," *Phil. Mag.*, 45 (Jan. 1815), 44–50; a month later the article appeared in *Pamphleteer*, vol. 5, 219–44 and, with additions, was published separately in 1815 with "phrenology" replaced in the title by "zoonomy." On the word, see: Eric T. Carlson and Patricia S. Noel, "Origins of the Word 'Phrenology,' " *Amer. J. Psychiatry*, 127 (1970), 694–7.

59. See: I. Inkster, "Science and Society in the Metropolis: a preliminary examination of the social and institutional context of the Askesian Society of London, 1796–1807," *Ann. Sci.*, 34 (1977), 1–32. *Phil. Mag.*, established in 1798, absorbed William Nicholson's *Journal of Natural Philosophy, Chemistry, and the Arts* in 1802; on Tilloch, who retained editorial control until 1821, see: *DNB*; *Mechanics' Oracle* [of which he also was editor] 1 (1825), 220; *Phil. Mag.*, 65 (1825), 134–5; *Gents. Mag.*, 95 (1825), 276–81; *Imperial Mag.*, 7 (1825), 208–22; *Annual Biography and Obituary*, 10 (1826), 320–34.

60. *Phil. Mag.*, 39 (1812), 142–50, q. in Inkster, "Askesian Soc.," p. 9. Tilloch appears to have gravitated to more radical bourgeois groupings after he was forced to withdraw from election to an F.R.S. because of Bank's suspicion of his political views; see: Paul Weindling, "Science and Sedition: how effective were the acts licensing lectures and meetings, 1795–1819?" *Br. J. Hist. Sci.*, 13 (1980), 139–53 at p. 149.

61. On the Philosophical Society's lectures on phrenology between 1811 and 1815, see: Inkster, "Askesian Soc.," p. 12. The *Phil. Mag.* was among the first journals in Britain to report on Gall and Spurzheim's doctrine; see: "A Short View of the Craniognomic System of Dr Gall, of Vienna. By L. Bojanus, M.D." [extracted from the *Magazin Encyclopedique*, no.4], *Phil. Mag.*, 14 (1802), 77–84, 131–8. In 1809 *Phil. Mag.*, 35, pp. 303–5 printed the French Institute's report on Gall and Spurzheim's *Memoir* and added that all had agreed that in many respects their doctrine was "clearer and more intelligible" than all the systems that had preceded it. A further report on the progress of the doctrine appeared in "Craniology," *Phil. Mag.*, 36 (1810), 77–8. A forty-page serialization of "Messrs Gall and Spurzheim's System of Craniology" began in July 1814 and ran to Feb. 1815. See also: vol. 46 (July & Nov. 1815), 9–11, 398; 49 (June 1817), 457; 52 (Oct. 1818), 300; 54 (Sept.–Nov. 1819), 226–7, 252–64, 324–35; 57 (Mar. & June 1821), 222–6, 449–53. The support for phrenology came to an end in 1822 when Richard Taylor and Richard Phillips took over as editors.

62. "Of the Physiology of Certain Disorders of Health Founded on a Knowledge of the Proportionate Development and Functions of the Special Organs of the Mind," *Phil. Mag.*, 45 (1815), 132.

63. See Richard Carlile to Forster, 16 Sept. 1826, Forster Papers, Bodleian Library, Oxford, MS Eng Lett, c.200 f.173–89. In *Recueil de ma vie*, p. 13, Forster regretted that his confidences with Abernethy, which began in 1811, ended in 1823 with the publication of *Somatopsychonoologia* (see: below, note 73). Abernethy accepted Forster as a student at St. Bartholomew's in 1815 and shared his opposition to spirituous liquors and meat eating.

64. Cited in *Recueil de ma vie*, p. 16. Cf. the accusation that Forster was the "obsequious disciple" of Spurzheim merely "puffing" his ideas: review of "*Sketch of the New Anatomy ...* by Thomas Forster," *Monthly Rev.*, 77 (1815), 165–7. Forster's *Observations on the Casual and Periodical Influence of Particular States of the Atmosphere on Human Health and Disease, Particularly Insanity* (1817) was dedicated

to Spurzheim, but within the decade (to Elliotson's delight) Forster had come
to regard Spurzheim as an egotist and intellectual thief: Elliotson, *Human Physiology*, pp. 1159–60n.

65. *DNB*; *Recueil de ma vie*, p. 17 – *which* rules were objected to is never specified.

66. *Facts and Enquiries*, p. 76; *Recueil de ma vie*, p. xi.

67. "J'ai été écolier, academicien, musicien, physicien, métaphysicien, enthusiaste,
voyaguer, aéronaute, phrénologiste, poète et philosophe!" *Recueil de ma vie*, p.
31. See also: Forster to Charles Daubeny, 9 May 1832, q. in Morrell and Thackray, *Gentlemen of Science*, p. 277.

68. Cannon, *Science in Culture*, p. 59. From an early date Forster advocated the
Pythagorean doctrine of Sati, or universal immortality. "That phrenology necessarily leads to Materialism," wrote Frederick Lange, "is obviously false. Phrenology, if it were scientifically justified, might not only be excellently supported
on Kant's system, but it may, in fact, be harmonised with those obsolete ideas
according to which the brain is related to the 'soul,' much as a more or less
perfect instrument is the person playing it. It is always noteworthy, however,
that our Materialists ... have expressed themselves surprisingly in favour of
phrenology." *History of Materialism* (1881), III,p. 118.

69. *Recueil de ma vie*, pp. xx, xviii. Knowingly, perhaps, he may have been echoing
his ancestor Benjamen Furly, who had involved himself with the ideas of van
Helmont, the Hermetic philosopher and alchemist; see: Margaret Jacob, *The
Radical Enlightenment: pantheists, freemasons, and republicans* (1981), p. 212. In 1830
Forster edited the family inheritance from Furly: *Original Letters of Locke, Algernon
Sidney, and Anthony Lord Shaftesbury*.

70. *A Biographical Memoir of George Canning Prime Minister of Great Britain* (Brussels,
1827); *England's Liberty and Prosperity under the Administration of the Duke of Wellington, based on independence of election* (2nd ed., Colchester, 1830).

71. *Recueil de ma vie*, p. 116. Shortly after, Forster moved to Bruges which, with
its English College, was a haven for English Catholics. Forster is not referred
to in John Bossy, *The English Catholic Community, 1570–1850* (1975), but it is
worth noting in passing Bossy's observations on the doctrinal similarities between Quakerism and Catholicism, pp. 392 ff. Joseph Gillow, *Bibliographical
Dictionary of English Catholics* (1886), II, pp. 318–24, has a useful entry on Forster.

72. *Recueil de ma vie*, p. 20, pp. xiv–xv. Forster was thus restating the objection, of
Schelling and other (esp. German) romantics in the 1810s, that Gall's system put
too many constraints on the soul's freedom: see J. Hall, "Gall's Phrenology,"
p. 310.

73. *Somatophychonoologia; showing that the proofs of body, life, and mind, considered as
distinct essences, cannot be deduced from physiology, but depend on a distinct sort of
evidence; being an examination of the controversy concerning life carried on by Laurence
[sic], Abernethy, Rennell, and others. By Philostratus* (1823). See also Temkin, "Basic
Science," p. 356.

74. *Recueil de ma vie*, p. 116. "The truth is," he wrote, "the Protestant Reformation
in England was a revolution which getting suddenly warped by interested people
and also by fanatics operated in favour of riches and hypocrisy, and one which
shut the poor man out of every innocent enjoyment of life, with which the old
Catholic Church had amply provided him" (p. 110).

75. On this Lukácsian point see Peter Hamilton, *Knowledge and Social Structure* (1974),
p. 69.

76. Such has been said of Rousseau in Colin Wilson's article "Man is born free, and
he is everywhere in chains," in Ronald Duncan and M. Weston-Smith, eds.,
Lying Truths: a critical scrutiny of current beliefs and conventions (Oxford, 1979), p.
5.

CHAPTER 3: *The rites of passage*

1. *Phrenology Article* (1830), p. 7.

2. "Craniology," *Portsmouth, Portsea, and Gosport Literary Register*, I (1823), 71–83,
at p. 71.

3. Carmichael, *Memoir of Spurzheim*, p. 27; J. N. Hays, "Science in the City: the London Institution, 1819–1840," *Br. J. Hist. Sci.*, 7 (1974), 146–62 at p. 150. Spurzheim first lectured at the London Institution in May 1826; his second course of twelve lectures were delivered in Apr. 1827.

4. J. W. Crane was largely correct in informing the French minister of commerce that phrenology was "very largely discussed" in all but a few philosophical societies: "State of Phrenology in Britain," pp. 407–8. Although the Liverpool Royal Institution turned down G. D. Cameron's offer of phrenology lectures in 1825 on the grounds that "phrenology is not yet sufficiently established as a science," two years later it granted rooms for the Liverpool Phrenological Society: G. W. Roderick and M. D. Stephens, "Nineteenth Century Ventures in Liverpool's Scientific Education," *Ann. Sci.*, 28 (1972), 61–86 at p. 65; H. C. Watson, *Statistics of Phrenology*, pp. 146–7.

5. *Philomathic J. & Lit. Rev.*, 3 (July 1825), 98–144. The Philomathic Institution was established in Burton Street in 1807 with the object of promoting science and literature, "general improvement of intellectual powers," and to "extend knowledge and improve ability"; it met weekly and excluded discussion of religion and party politics; membership was two guineas per annum: James Jennings, *A Lecture on the History and Utility of Literary Institutions* (1823), p. 51n. Like other institutions of its kind, the Philomathic Institution had its phrenological enthusiasts, especially in Robert Maugham, a solicitor and member of the LPS who wrote *The Outlines of Character* (1823). In the four volumes of the *Philomathic J.* (1824–6) there were seven major articles on phrenology, all favorable to it.

6. For Gramsci's use of "organic crisis," see: *Selections from Prison Notebooks*, ed. and trans. Q. Hoare and G. N. Smith (1971), p. 210 ff.; and R. Q. Gray, "Bourgeois Hegemony in Victorian Britain," in Jon Bloomfield, ed., *Papers on Class, Hegemony, and Party* (1977), p. 76; see also: Karl Mannheim, "The History of the Concept of the State as an Organism: a sociological analysis," in his *Essays* (1953), pp. 165–82.

7. "The Peculiarities of the English," p. 60; on "class" as a happening, see ibid., p. 85, and idem, "Eighteenth-century English Society: class struggle without class?" *Social Hist.*, 3 (1978), 133–65 at pp. 146–50.

8. For one of the first major statements on science as a social resource in the Lit & Phils, see: A. Thackray, "Natural Knowledge in Cultural Context: the Manchester Model," *Amer. Hist. Rev.*, 79 (1974), 672–709; for subsequent literature and sources, see: Ian Inkster and Jack Morrell, eds., *Metropolis and Province: science in British Culture, 1780–1850* (1983).

9. Hays, "London Institution"; see also: J. R. McCulloch, *A Discourse Delivered at the Opening of the City of London Literary and Scientific Institution, 30 May 1825* (1825), esp. at p.12; "City of London Institution," *Panoramic Misc.*, 1 (28 Feb. 1826), 208–14; and Shapin and Thackray, "Prosopography as a Research Tool," p. 7. On the history of the notions of "pure" and "applied" science, see: E. Mendelsohn, "Social Construction," p. 22.

10. For the respective sociological and anthropological literature, see: I. Inkster, "Marginal Men: aspects of the social role of the medical community in Sheffield, 1790–1850," in John Woodward and David Richards, eds., *Health Care and Popular Medicine in Nineteenth Century England* (1977), 128–63; Douglas, *Purity and Danger* (1970), esp. pp. 115–17; and Victor Turner, *The Ritual Process* (Harmondsworth, 1974), esp. pp. 80 ff.

11. I. Inkster, "Introduction: aspects of the history of science and science culture in Britain, 1780–1850 and beyond," in Inkster and Morrell, *Metropolis and Province*, pp. 40–41. See also: R. S. Neale on the "uneasy class" in "Class and Class-Consciousness in Early Nineteenth Century England: three classes or five?" *Vict. Stud.*, 12 (1968), 4–32, esp. at pp. 14 ff.

12. Cited in J. V. Pickstone, "The Professionalization of Medicine in England and Europe: the state, the market, and industrial society," *J. Japan. Soc. Med. Hist.*, 25 (1979), 1–31, at p. 13; see also: K. Figlio, "Chlorosis and Chronic Disease in

Nineteenth Century Britain: the social construction of somatic illness in a capitalist society," *Social Hist.*, 3 (1978), 167–97 at p. 176. For the medical profession
generally in our period, see: M. Jeanne Peterson, *The Medical Profession in Mid-
Victorian London* (Berkeley, 1978).

13. See: Philip Elliott, *The Sociology of the Professions* (1972); and Brian Heeny, *A
Different Kind of Gentleman: parish clergy as professional men in early and mid-Victorian
England* (Springfield, Ohio, 1976), esp. pp. 4–5. On the growth of the profes-
sionals in absolute numbers, see: Richard Altick, *The English Common Reader*
(Chicago, 1963), p. 83.

14. See, for example: the middle-class confidence seeking of Sir Anthony Carlisle
(pres. College of Surgeons) in *Practical Observations on the Preservation of Health
and the Prevention of Disease* (1838), p. ix. The Anatomy Act and the cholera
outbreak of 1832 further cut into public confidence in medicine; see: F. K.
Donnelly, "The Destruction of the Sheffield School of Anatomy in 1835: a
popular response to class legislation," *Trans. Hunter Arch. Soc.*, 10 (1975), 167–
72; M. J. Durey, "Bodysnatchers and Benthamites: the implications of the dead
body bill for the London schools of anatomy, 1820–42," *London J.*, 2 (1976),
200–25; idem, *The Return of the Plague: British society and the cholera, 1831–2*
(Dublin, 1979).

15. On the preponderant role of medical men in the Lit & Phils, see: Inkster, "Mar-
ginal Men," pp. 137 ff.; Thackray, "Manchester Model," pp. 684–5; and S.
Shapin, "The Pottery Philosophical Society, 1819–1835: an examination of the
cultural uses of provincial science," *Sci. Stud.*, 2 (1972), 311–36 at pp. 324–5.
Among the medical supporters of phrenology involved in founding or directing
Lit & Phils were E. Barlow in Bath, J. Fife in Newcastle, G. C. Holland in
Sheffield, G. Miller in Emsworth, Hants, John Porter in Portsmouth.

16. Obituary, *Br. Med. J.*, 19 Dec. 1868, p. 650.

17. In its "Introductory Statement" of November 1823, *Phren. J.*, asserted: "The
respect now paid to [phrenology] is the result of a REVIVAL, – a revival by
men of philosophical habits": p. v.

18. De Moscati, "Character of Gall," *Lancet*, 22 June 1833, p. 399. Harriet Martineau
depicted the familiar early C19 disdain for metaphysics, when she compared
Dugald Stewart to Gall in her *A History of the Thirty Years Peace* (1846/8; 1877
ed.), II, p. 363. For classic expressions of this disdain in phrenological writing,
see: W. C. Engledue, *Zoist*, 1 (April 1843), p. 6; John Slade, *Colloquies: Imaginary
conversations between a phrenologist and the shade of Dugald Stewart* (1838); "Correspondence between Academicus and Consiliarius [i.e., W. P. Alison and P.
Neill] on the comparative merits of phrenology and the mental philosophy of
Reid and Stewart," *Phren. J.*, 10 (1836/7), 301–37; G. Combe, "Dialogue between
a Philosopher of the Old School and a Phrenologist," ibid., 1 (1823/4), 65–72,
200–17; idem, "Address to Students of Logic and Moral Philosophy," *Phren. J.*,
6 (1829/30), 191–200 (these articles by Combe were all selected for reprinting in
Robert Cox, ed., *Selections from the Phrenological Journal* [Edin., 1836]). On the
methodological differences between phrenologists and antiphrenologists, see P.
M. Roget, "Phrenology," *Ency. Brit.*, p. 469; and Shapin, "Phrenological
Knowledge," pp. 236–7.

19. *Testimonials to Combe* (Edin., 1836), p. 55.

20. For an example of phrenologist likening metaphysics to alchemy, see: review,
"*Illustrations of Phrenology* . . . by Sir G. S. Mackenzie," *Edin. Monthly Rev.*, 5
(1821), p. 94.

21. The rule itself could be discredited by quoting Bacon, as in the following from
a Birmingham phrenologist attacking the Oxford academic elite: "To use the
words of Lord Bacon, 'the exercise' which these Oxonians fulfil, 'fitteth not the
practice or the image of life, 'but 'doth pervert the motions and faculties of the
mind, and not prepare them.' " He also accused the Oxonians of being priest-
ridden. [Joshua Toulmin Smith], "On the Progressive Diffusion of Phrenology,"
Phren. J., 10 (1836/7), 346–52 at p. 405. On naïve empiricism validating egalitarian resistence in Jacksonian America, see: J. Higham, "The Matrix of Spe-

cialization," in A. Oleson and J. Voss, eds., *The Organization of Knowledge in Modern America, 1860–1920* (Baltimore, 1979), 3–18 esp. at p. 8.

22. Cf. the interest in phrenology by some Owenite socialites (Chapter 8). The educationalist and supporter of Robert Owen, James Jennings,‡ though favorable to phrenology in some respects, criticized phrenologists for not paying sufficient attention "to our ordinary and simple SENSATIONS; and I think that our first steps in such inquiries ought always to be directed to these: for all that we know must be derived through the medium of what are usually called the SENSES – namely, *Seeing, Hearing, Smelling, Tasting, Feeling.*" *An Inquiry Concerning the Nature and Operations of the Human Mind in Which the Science of Phrenology, the Doctrine of Necessity, Punishment, and Education are Particularly Considered: a lecture delivered at the Mechanics' Institution, London* [with additional notes by J. Deville‡] (1828), p. 23.

23. *Educ. Mag. & J. Christian Philanthr. & Publ. Utility* (May 1835), p. 307.

24. E.g.: Richard Church, *Presumptive Evidence of the Truth and Reasonableness of Phrenology: a lecture delivered before the members of the Chichester Literary and Philosophical Society, January 11th, 1833* (Chichester, 1833), p. 111; James D. Green, *An Address Delivered at the Anniversary Celebration of the Birth of Spurzheim, and the Organization of the Boston Phrenological Society, December 30, 1836* (Boston, 1836), p. 14; and Robert Chambers in his testimonial to Combe, printed in *Testimonials to Combe*, p. 55.

25. Contempt for the dead languages was peppered throughout phrenological literature; see esp.: Charles Caldwell, *Thoughts on Physical Education, and the True Mode of Improving the Condition of Man; and on the study of the Greek and Latin languages*, with notes by Robert Cox and a recommendatory preface by George Combe (Boston, 1834; Edin., 1836, 1844); [William B. Hodgson], *"Classical" Instruction: its uses and abuses, reprinted from the Westminster Review for October 1853*; see also: Henry Cockburn on the anti-Latin crusaders in his *Journals* (Edin., 1874), I, entry for 5 Oct. 1834, p. 70, and Douglas's comments on this manifestation of antiritualism as a form of order seeking in *Natural Symbols: explorations in cosmology* (Harmondsworth, 1973), pp. 19 ff.

26. Cited in R. Yeo, "Scientific Method and the Image of Science, 1831–1891," in Roy MacLeod and P. Collins, eds., *The Parliament of Science: the British Association for the Advancement of Science, 1831–1981* (1981), 65–88 at p. 65. See also: Daniel Noble, "Sketch of the Accordance between the Inductive Philosophy of Bacon and the Aptitude of the Human Intellect, as demonstrated by Phrenology," *Phren. J.*, 10 (1836/7), 190–201. On Bacon's antischolasticism, see: Robert Mandrou, *From Humanism to Science, 1480–1700*, trans. B. Pearce (Hassocks, Sussex, 1978), pp. 202 ff.; see also: Merton, *Science in Seventeenth Century England*, esp. p. 97; and William Leiss, *The Domination of Nature* (N.Y. 1972), pp. 73 ff. On "Baconianism" or Bacon as a prophet of an *image* of secular scientific and social progress, see: Roszak, *Where the Wasteland Ends*, pp. 148–9; Morrell and Thackray, *Gentlemen of Science*, pp. 268–92; Cannon, *Science in Culture*, pp. 59, 73, 228 ff.

27. In the general this was a part of Max Horkheimer's critique of positivism; see: Martin Jay, *The Dialectical Imagination* (1973), p. 62.

28. Bronislow Malinowski, *Magic, Science, and Religion and Other Essays* (1948; 1974); Talcott Parsons, *The Social System* (1951); cf. J. Powles, "On the Limitations of Modern Medicine," *Science, Medicine, and Man*, 1 (1973), 1–30 at p. 20.

29. G. Combe, "Objections to Phrenology," in his *Elements of Phrenology* (9th ed., Edin., 1862), p. 211.

30. "Observations on the Recent Improvements and Discoveries in the Anatomy and Physiology of the Brain. By a medical correspondent," *Gents. Mag.*, 89 (suppl., 1819), 608–9; see also: the supporting articles: review of "Maugham's *Outlines of Character*," 93 (Feb. 1823), 149–51; and "On the Advantages of Phrenology," 94 (April 1824), 301–3.

31. Daniel Ellis, *Life of Gordon*, p. 42.

32. Gordon, "Doctrines of Gall and Spurzheim," p. 251.

33. Roland Barthes, "The Brain of Einstein," in his *Mythologies*, trans. A. Lavers (St. Albans, Herts. 1976), 68–70.
34. "Dr.Spurzheim's Lectures," *Monthly Mag.*, 59 (June 1825), p. 401n. Chenevix may have been referring to this when he claimed that "some persons accuse Dr Spurzheim of having abandoned the Baconian severity of his predecessor, and of indulging himself in a priori hypotheses": *Phrenology Article*, p. 22.
35. For a list of Gall's original German terms, see, ibid., p. 24. For a comparison between George Combe's essentially Spurzheimian labels for the mental organs and those of Gall (as represented by Bojanus and Villers in 1802) see: "Combe's Phrenology," *Nat. Mag. & Monthly Critic*, 2 (1838), 103–19 at p. 107; see also: Robert Cox, "Objections to Dr. Spurzheim's Classification and Nomenclature of the Mental Faculties," *Phren. J.*, 10 (1836/7), 154–64.
36. "Introductory Statement," *Phren. J.*, 1 (1823/4), iv.
37. The only occasion during its twenty-four years of publication in which it was run without a loss was in 1831–2. Hewett Watson, shortly before taking over the editorship and moving it to Thames Ditton, complained, "It has never been very popular, even among phrenologists, and has been much complained of as representing the feelings and ideas of its conductors [i.e., Combe and intimates in Edinburgh] rather than those of the phrenological public": *Statistics of Phrenology*, p. 14; and see: Sidney Smith, "Correspondence with the Editor of the Phrenological Journal," *Phren. J.*, 10 (1836/7), 658–64. But Watson's attempts to reach a broader readership were hardly more successful, and his editorship, in turn, was criticized by other phrenologists, e.g., T. S. Prideaux, *Strictures on the Conduct of Hewett Watson, FLS in His Capacity of Editor of the Phrenological Journal* (Ryde, 1840). In 1843 the copyright was repurchased by the Combes and Robert Cox assumed editorship: Gibbon, *Life of Combe* (1876), I, pp. 161–2, 247.
38. See, for example: "Phrenological Quacks," *Phren. J.*, 9 (1834/6), 517–19; "On the Requisites for the Advance of Phrenological Science: – Manipulators," ibid., 13 (1840), 97–119; "Phrenological Manipulators," ibid., 12 (1839), 346–50; ibid., 18 (1845), 238; and ibid., 19 (1846), 197; *Phren. Almanac*, 1 (1842), p. 12n.; "Phrenological Quackery," *Phren. Almanac & Phren. Ann.*, 4 (1845), 17–22; "Phrenology: phrenological quacks," *Medico–Chirurgical Rev.*, 24 (Jan. 1836), 207–8; *Aldine Mag.*, 19 Jan. 1839, p. 120. In order to safeguard the livelihoods of "respectable" popularizers of phrenology, it was proposed by W. A. F. Browne in 1835 that special diplomas be issued to bona fide lecturers: *Minute Book of the Edinburgh Phrenological Society*, 3 Dec. 1835 (MS, Edin. Univ. Lib: Gen. 608/2). A decade later a similar proposal was made and seriously entertained by the phrenologists of Sheffield: *Third Annual Report of the Sheffield Phrenological Society . . . during Session 1844–5* (Sheffield, 1845), p. 6, *Phren. J.*, 18 (1845), 285; and *People's Phren. J.*, 1 (1843), 178. The same problem of protecting trade led to the formation of the International Psychoanalytic Association in the mental C20: H. A. Murray, "Sigmund Freud, 1856–1939," *Amer. J. Psychol.*, 53 (1940), 134–8 at p. 135; and Ernest Jones, *Life of Sigmund Freud* (1953), p. 257.
39. Steven Marcus, *The Other Victorians* (1966), p. 283. An example of the effect is provided in the *Elgin Courier*, which commented upon the phrenology lecturer, J. Boyd, "It is grievous to find such attempts to destroy and render ridiculous an important science": 24 July 1846, q. in *Phren. J.*, 19 (1846), p. 383; see also: *Physician*, 10 Nov. 1832, p. 10; *Analyst*, (Nov. 1839), p. 337.
40. While Elliotson was "always to be seen in prisons and madhouses examining prisoners' heads" (*The London Journal of Flora Tristan, 1842*, trans. J. Hawkes [1982] p. 120), and Combe carried out masterful delineations on prisoners in Newcastle and Dublin and wrote on phrenological delineations for hiring persons of trust in insurance companies and for selecting servants (*Phren. J.*, 9 [1834/6], 519–26, 14 [1841], 297–310, 6 [1829/30], 211–22; but cf. Combe, "On the Best Means of Making Converts to Phrenology," ibid., 2 [1824/5], 130–1), Sir George Mackenzie collected an impressive list of forty-six testimonials on the value of phrenology for delineating the heads of criminals so they could more efficiently

be shipped to Australia (*Documents laid before Lord Glenelg*). The examples among lesser phrenologists may be multiplied. A similar difficulty faced some persons writing for the Society for the Diffusion of Useful Knowledge: On the one hand they wanted to keep their science lessons simple in order to convey certain values to the working class, while on the other they did not want to lose respect among scientific peer groups who might label their efforts declamatory and unscientific; such a problem obviously confronted the botanist John Lindley. See: J. N. Hays, "Science and Brougham's Society," *Ann. Sci*, 20 (1964), 227–41 at p. 239.

41. *Cheltenham Looker-on*, 27 Mar. 1841, n.p.: see also: *Analyst*, 9 (Nov. 1839), 337.

42. Page xiii; cf. the attempt of C17 astrologers to overcome the imputation of their godless fatalism or mechanical necessarianism: Bernard Capp, *English Almanacs, 1500–1800: astrology and the popular press* (Ithaca, N.Y., 1979), chap.5.

43. "Introductory Statement," p.xiii; for a nearly identical statement, see Barlow, *Apology for Phrenology*, pp. 17–24.

44. As q. in *Analyst*, 1 (Aug. 1834), 56. For other examples, see: William Robinson Lowe, "Lecture VI: phrenology in relation to religion," 18 Dec. 1839, in his *Lectures on Popular and Scientific Subjects Delivered at Various Literary Institutions* (Wolverhampton, 1857), pp. 186–213; [John Epps], *Internal Evidences of Christianity Deduced from Phrenology. By Medicus* (Edin., 1827). See also: John C. Tomilson, "The Science of Phrenology Consistent with the Doctrine of Christianity; a letter addressed to Dr Spurzheim," *Pamphleteer*, 26 (1826), 415–25; [George Lyon], "On the Harmony of Phrenology with the Scriptual Doctrine of Conversion," *Edin. Christian Instructor*, 22 (Dec. 1823), 803–18; [John Hamilton], "On the Accordance with Subsists between Phrenology and the Scriptural Doctrine of Regeneration," *Phren. J.*, 1 (1823/4), 555–70; Charles Cowan, *Phrenology Consistent with Science and Revelation* (Reading, [1841]); John Maclean, *The Testimony of Phrenology to the Truth of Revelation* (Leith, 1858); and Lot Mason, *Harmony of Phrenology and the Bible* (Leeds, [c. 1858]). Among the rational religionists phrenologists were also the Unitarians Joshura Toulmin[‡] and W. Hawkes Smith,[‡] the dissenters H. G. Wright, Mrs. Pugh, Samuel Eadon,[‡] John White,[‡] and John Wilson,[‡] the Anglican Rev. Henry Clarke,[‡] and the Boston Baptist Joseph Warne, whose *On the Harmony between the Scriptures and Phrenology* (Edin., 1836) first appeared as an appendix to the American school's edition of the *Constitution of Man*.

45. Whately claimed that the "religious and moral objections against the phrenological theory are utterly futile": q. in Gibbon, *Life of Combe*, I, p. 275; *Protestant Mag.* attacked one of its fellows for attacking phrenology, saying, "Men, equally pious and learned, equally judicious, and certainly as unprejudiced have arrived at an opposite conclusion": 4 Aug. 1842, p. 272; the American Congregationalist Henry Ward Beecher confessed that phrenology underlay his whole ministry: q. in *Zoist*, 13 (Oct. 1855), 282–4; the *Nonconformist* in 1843 went so far as to give the phrenological characteristics of strikers' delegates in the manufacturing districts: 14 June 1843, q. in W. B. Hodgson, "Progress of Phrenology," *Phren. J.*, 16 (1843), 408. The bishops of Durham and Norwich attended phrenology lectures in London in 1839 (David deGiustino, *Conquest of Mind* [1975], p. 122), and the High Church *Christian Remembrancer* confessed its support: 6 (Dec. 1843), 661–76. It was common for clergymen to stand up in support of phrenology at the conclusion to lectures. Nor was it only among the defenders of orthodoxy that this harmony was declared; the militant Yorkshire radical and former weaver Joseph Barker pointed out that phrenology militated against "existing systems of theology ... but not with religions" and tended to "make people infidels in the false systems of men, in the interventions and traditions of our unenlightened elders; but it no way interferes with the doctrine of God or his Providence, of human duty or human destiny": "Phrenology," *The People*, 1 (1848), 122.

46. But see, for example: *London Pioneer*, 1 (28 May 1846), 76.

47. Page xiii; and see: "Abuses of Phrenology," *Christian Remembrancer*, 22 (Nov. 1840), 682.

48. See, for example: "Phrenological Controversies," *Phren. J.*, 10 (1836/7), 150–3;

and "Recent Attacks on Phrenology," ibid., 11 (1838), 260–6. On intellectual insurgents' understanding of their opponents' subjectivism, see: Lucien Goldmann, *The Hidden God* (1977), p. 163; and David Ingleby, "Understanding 'Mental Illness,' " in D. Ingleby, ed., *Critical Psychiatry: the politics of mental health* (Harmondsworth, 1981), 23–71 at p. 26. Closer to home, within the current debate between intellectualist and social historians of science, as Charles Rosenberg has appreciated, "To deny the transcendence of scientific knowledge is ... a political act. The contextual approach to science is a social tool as well as an epistemology, taking knowledge which had seemed eternal, disinterested, inevitable and arguing that it was provisional, interested, a result not of the iron logic of eternal ideas, but of particular mundane interests." "Nature Decoded," *Isis*, 8 (1980), 291–5 at p. 294.

49. See: "The Pope versus Phrenology," *Phren. J.*, 10 (1836/7), 600–2.
50. *Phrenology Article*, p. 20.
51. See: G. Combe, "Letter on the Prejudices of the Great in Science and Philosophy against Phrenology," *Phren. J.*, 4 (1829/30), 14–38, 18–7; Spurzheim to vice-chancellor of Oxford, 17 Nov. 1830: Bodleian MS Top. Oxf. b.23, f.301(d); and "March of Intellect, and Suppression of Phrenology, at the King's College," *Lancet*, 7 Jan. 1832, pp. 519–20.
52. See: "Cruelty to Animals: Sir William Hamilton's experiments," *Phren. J.*, 7 (1831/2), 427–33; on the practicality of phrenology as a part of its rhetoric of appeal to the middle classes, see, for example: "Practical Phrenology," *Phren. J.*, 3 (1825/6), 410–19, 514–22; Spurzheim, "Usefulness of Phrenology," in his *Outlines of Phrenology* (1829), pp. 77–101; and Barlow, *Apology for Phrenology*, pp. 24–32 (cf. the literature on the practical applications of phrenology directed at popular audiences, cited below, Chapter 6, note 25).
53. *Phrenology Article*, p. 55.
54. R. F. Jones, *Ancients and Moderns* (2nd ed., 1965); and C. C. Gillispie, "The *Encyclopédie* and the Jacobin Philosophy of Science: a study in ideas and consequences," in Marshall Clagett, ed., *Critical Problems in the History of Science* (Madison, Wisc., 1959), 255–89. Cf. R. Mcaulay, "Velikovsky and the Infrastructure of Science: the metaphysics of a close encounter," *Theory and Society*, 6 (1978), 313–42; W. F. Cannon, "The Uniformitarian–Catastrophist Debate," *Isis*, 51 (1960), 38–55; D. MacKenzie and B. Barnes, "Scientific Judgement: the biometry–Mendelism controversy," in Barnes and Shapin, *Natural Order*, 191–210.
55. Cf. Tom Paine on the nature of "crises," cited in E. Mendelsohn, "Revolution and Reduction," p. 414.
56. In particular, G. Cantor, who explains the Edinburgh phrenology debates in terms of "incommensurable" theological, philosophical, anatomical, physiological, and methodological positions. "So many and so deeply held forms of incommensurability," he concludes, "ensured that there was minimal interaction between the two parties" with neither side significantly altering the others' views. "Edinburgh Phrenology Debate," p. 217.
57. This dialectical approach to the history of ideas may border on and even lead into what has been depicted in the history of science (by Rosenberg, "Nature Decoded," p. 294) as the substitute dilemma for the internalist's world of cognitive events – "an interpretive wilderness in which everything is potentially relevant to everything else." This is hardly a reason for not pursuing a dialectical understanding, however, especially since it is clear that to "see only cause here, effect there" is, as Engels remarked, "an empty abstraction.... metaphysical polar opposites exist in the real world only during crises ...; the whole vast process goes on in the form of interaction – though of very unequal forces, the economic movement being by far the strongest, the primary and most decisive ...; in this context everything is relative and nothing is absolute"; Letter to Conrad Schmidt, 27 Oct. 1890, in Marx and Engels, *Selected Correspondence* (3rd ed., Moscow, 1975), p. 402.
58. Mannheim, "Conservative Thought," in *Essays* 74–164, esp. pp. 74–9. For an

illuminating deployment of the concept of "styles of thought" to a similar problem, see: J. Harwood, "The Race–Intelligence Controversy: a sociological approach," *Social Stud. Sci.*, 6 (1976), 369–94 and 7 (1977), 1–20.

59. George Lyon, "Essay on the Phrenological Causes of Different Degrees of Liberty Enjoyed by Different Nations," *Phren. J.*, 2 (1824/5), 598–619 at p. 599.

60. *Examiner*, 30 Oct. 1831, n.p.

61. "The Phrenological System," *London Mag.*, 6 (Sept. 1822), 197–204 at p. 198. See also: *Edin. Monthly Rev.*, 3 (Feb. 1820), 123–45 and 5 (Jan. 1821), 90–108; "Phrenology," *Metropolitan Q. Mag.*, 2 (1826), 56–71; and Walt Whitman as q. in Madeleine B. Stern, *Heads and Headlines: the phrenological Fowlers* (Norman, Okla., 1971), p. 100.

62. *Monthly Rev.*, 94 (Apr. 1821), 396; see also: *Quart. Rev.*, 13 (Apr. 1815), 159; "Craniology," *Oxford Ency.* (Oxford, 1828), vol. 2, 708–10; *Medico-Chirurgical Rev.*, 3 (Mar. 1823), 897–8; *Christian Remembrancer*, 6 (Dec. 1843), 661.

63. "Combe's Constitution of Man, 4th ed.," *Br. & For. Rev. or European Q. J.*, 12 (1841), 142–80 at p. 142.

64. *Hampshire Telegraph*, 28 Mar. 1842, q. in *Phren. J.*, 15 (1842), 279.

65. *Southern Lit. Messenger*, 2 (March 1836), 286, q. in T. Stoehr, "Physiognomy and Phrenology in Hawthorne," *Huntington Lib. Q.*, 37 (1974), 355–400 at p. 360.

66. "Phrenology and Its Applications," *Union*, 1 (June 1842), 75–7 at p. 75.

67. *Christian Teacher*, 2 (1836), 603–4.

68. See: W. C. Engledue, "Messrs. Forbes, Wakley, and Co., the Antimesmeric Crusaders," *Zoist*, 4 (Jan. 1847), 584–601; and R. M. Glover, "Lectures on the Philosophy of Medicine, Delivered in the Lecture Room of the Literary and Philosophical Society, Newcastle, Lecture VI: quackery ... pseudo science: phrenology, mesmerism, hydropathy, tee-totalism, vegetarianism, homoeopathy," *Lancet*, 11 Jan. 1841, pp. 34–38. In this way former medical supporters of phrenology united with others in the profession who had previously been seeking professional respectability through the attack on quackery – see, in particular: James L. Bardsley, *Observations on Homoeopathy and Animal Magnetism ... a lecture introductory to a course on the practice of medicine* (Manch., 1838). Among distinguished physicians involved with phrenology who came out against homoeopathy in the 1840s and 1850s were James Inglis[‡] and Charles Cowan. John Epps expressed the feelings of other phrenologists with different social interests, however, when he wrote that Wakley "is like the City Corporation in their upholding the Smithfield nuisance: he has a vested interest in the abuse [of homoeopathy]": letter to J. Gardiner, May 1851, in *Diary of Epps* [1870], p. 488.

69. The EPS formally excluded theological discussion from their meetings on 15 Apr. 1830 (after much religious discussion had disrupted their meetings): "*Minute Book of the Phrenological Society.*" Subsequently, however, it was decided that "phrenology, by unfolding the elements of the human mind, brings all the general principles and applications of morals and politics within the range of the science," and therefore only good could come from such discussions, if "kept to general conclusions." *Phren. J.*, 8 (1832/4), 192. Cf. the Philomathic Institution's similar realization of the need to admitt discussion on religion and politics: cited in P. Weindling, "Science and Sedition," p. 10.

70. Richard Winter Hamilton, *An Essay on Craniology: being the substance of a paper submitted to the Philosophical and Literary Society, Leeds, December 2, 1825* (1826), p. 23. On the EPS see: Gibbon, *Life of Combe*, I, pp. 129, 134; *Phren. J.*, 3 (1825/6), 476–81. Elitist pretentions are manifest in "Sketch of Laws for a Phrenological Society," ibid., 2 (1824/5), 241–5. Roughly one-third of the phrenological societies were in Scotland and one-third in the north of England; twenty were in the south of England, and three were in Ireland: Watson, *Statistics of Phrenology*, pp. 218–19. As the Birmingham phrenologist Joshua T. Smith[‡] pointed out, however, "It is not by ascertaining the number of existing Phrenological Societies, that any just estimate of our number can be formed. Vast numbers of

phrenologists have a strong objection to this mode of propagating their science": "On the Progressive Diffusion of Phrenology," p. 406.

71. Circular for the institution, c. 1840, bound with MS papers relating to the Liverpool Mechanics' Institution, 1777–1850: Br. Lib. 8364. b.24.

72. "On the Moral Application of Phrenology," *Christian Observer*, 29 (May 1829), 294–5 at p. 294.

73. J. Stevenson Bushnan, "Nature of Thought: phrenology," in his *The Philosophy of Instinct and Reason* (Edin., 1837), 240–65 at pp. 261–2.

74. Quoted in Watson, *Statistics of Phrenology*, p. 124; on the quiet proceedings of the Glasgow Phrenological Society, see: D. G. Goyder, *My Battle for Life: the autobiography of a phrenologist* (1857), p.286.

75. Watson, *Statistics of Phrenology*, pp. 11–12; *Phren. J.*, 13 (1840), 109.

76. On the Geological Society, see: Cannon, *Science in Culture*, p. 161; on the institutionalization of science as a factor undermining scientistic vigour, see: Joseph Ben David, *The Scientist's Role in Society*, p. 78; and see: I. Inkster, "The Social Context of an Educational Movement: a revisionist approach to the English Mechanics' Institutes, 1820–1850," *Oxford Rev. Educ.*, 2 (1976), 277–307 at p. 284.

77. See: "Warwickshire Natural History and Archaeological Society," *Analyst*, 5 (1836), 305 (John Conolly played a leading role in this and the previous phrenological society); Neville Wood, "Phrenological Society of Warrington," *Naturalist*, 3 (Feb., Apr. 1838), 108–9, 205–6; 4 (Dec. 1838), 152–53; 5 (July 1839), 38; "Blackburn Phrenological and Geological Society," *Naturalist*, 5 (Apr. 1839), 376; *Phren. J.*, 14 (1841), 19; and on Belfast, Watson, *Statistics of Phrenology*, pp. 115–17; and see: *Phren. J.*, 12 (1839), 100. In 1842 *Phren. Almanac* could locate only eight surviving phrenological societies: Aberdeen, Ayr, Dumfries, Edinburgh, Glasgow, Heybridge, London, and Warrington (pp. 60–1). In fact, there were many more than this, as *People's Phren. J.* pointed out (4 Feb. 1843, p. 12), but most were in mechanics' institutes and the like, were differently organized, and had different objectives and social functions; see: Chapter 5.

78. "Phrenological Societies," *Phren. J.*, 13 (1840), 388–9 at p. 388.

79. See: Morrell and Thackray, *Gentlemen of Science*, esp. the section "Phrenology and the Unwelcome Sciences," pp. 276–81; MacLeod and Collins, *Parliament of Science*; and Cannon, *Science in Culture*, chaps. 6, 7.

80. I. Todhunter, *William Whewell* (1876), II, p. 293, cited in the discussion on the BAAS in W. H. G. Armytage, *The Rise of the Technocrats: a social history* (1965) p. 95. See also: M. Berman, " 'Hegemony' and the Amateur Tradition in the British Science," *J. Soc. Hist.*, 8 (1975), 30–50 at pp. 37 ff.; and Gillispie, *Genesis and Geology*, pp. 188 ff. Among BAAS ideologues was David Brewster (1781–1868) who, as coeditor of *Phil. Mag.* after 1832, insured that there would be no further articles on phrenology. He attacked phrenology in his review of *Vestiges* in *North Br. Rev.* in 1845, though it was not until 1863 that he wrote specifically against phrenology: "On the Characteristics of the Age," *Good Words*, [1] (1863), 7–13; and see: [Hector McLean], *A Reply to Sir David Brewster's Strictures on Physiognomy and Phrenology by E.M'G.* (Glasgow, 1863); and Cornelius Donovan, *The Ethnological Society and Phrenology: a paper entitled "Physiognomy Popular and Scientific" with report of the Discussion* (1864).

81. For the denunciation of the BAAS, see: "The Phrenological Association," *Phren. J.*, 12 (1839), 29–41: according to which there were no fewer than sixteen phrenologists or supporters of phrenology among the sectional office holders at the BAAS meeting of 1838. Among phrenologists who were BAAS members were G. Combe, Sir James Clark, W. H. Crook,[‡] Richard Evanson, Thomas Forster,[‡] W.R. Lowe,[‡] Mackenzie,[‡] T. S. Prideaux,[‡] and H. C. Watson.[‡] J. Q. Rumball[‡] was the author of a pamphlet *On the Claims Which Phrenology Has to Be Considered a Science: addressed to the British Association assembled at Plymouth, 1841* (Plymouth, 1841).

82. Discussion of phrenology went on mainly in the sections devoted to statistics, medicine, natural history, and (later in the century) anthropology; see: *Phren.*

J., 9 (1834/6), 120–6; 11 (1838), 92–4, and 20 (1847), 187; *Standard*, 25 Aug. 1828, p. 1; *Athenaeum*, 1837, p. 752–3; and Dr J. Thurnam, "On the Scientific Cranioscopy of Professor Carus," *Report of the 14th Meeting of the British Association Held at York, September 1844*, p. 86.

83. Quoted in *Edin. New Phil.J.*, 7 (1834), 372.

84. Mackenzie's proposal appeared in the *Phren. J.*, in Mar. 1835; in August that year the Dublin Phrenological Society made a similar proposal: Gibbon, *Life of Combe*, II, p. 101. For the private meeting and rebuff, see: Morrell and Thackray, *Gentlemen of Science*, p. 279. Cf. the association proposed by J. P. Greaves, cited below: Chapter 8, note 85.

85. The three hundred names have been gathered from *Phrenological Association: report of the Committee of the 4th session, held in London, in June 1841. Proceedings ... laws, and list of members* (1841); in conjunction with "The Phrenological Association," *Phren. J.*, 12 (1839), 29–41; "Report of the Proceedings of the Phrenological Association, at its Third Annual Session at Glasgow, in September 1840," ibid., 14 (1841), 1–63; and "Phrenological Association," *Lancet*, 5, 12 June and 17 July 1841. Cf. the occupational breakdown of the EPS in 1826 compared with the Edin. Roy. Soc., in Shapin, "Phrenological Knowledge," p. 229.

86. Morrell and Thackray, *Gentlemen of Science*, p. 280; and "Proceedings of the Phrenological Society [*sic*] at Glasgow in September Last," *Medico-Chirurgical Rev.*, 34 (Jan. 1841), 289–92.

87. See: "Dr Elliotson vs. Spurzheim and the Phrenologists of Britain," *Phren. J.*, 11 (1838), 225–47. Among the dissenters from Elliotson's group in London were Sir James Clark and Henry Holm who, along with others, formed their own private phrenological society in 1832: *Phren. J.*, 19 (1846), 288.

88. "Yes!" asserted Engledue. "The wedge has been introduced and it must be driven home. Opinions have been promulgated, and they must be countenanced and enforced." *Cerebral Physiology and Materialism: with the results of the application of animal magnetism to the cerebral organs ... with a letter from Dr Elliotson, on mesmeric phrenology and materialism* (1842), p.26 (the address originally appeared in *Med. Times*, 6 [2 July 1842], 209–14, which was quoted with comments in *Phren. J.*, 15 [1842], 291–318).

89. "The Declaration of Expediency," *Zoist*, 1 (July 1843), 148–60; "Materialism and the Phrenological Association," *Phren. J.*, 16 (1843), 40–59; Sir George MacKenzie, "The Split in the Phrenological Association," ibid., 15 (1842), 343–6; and "Phrenology and Mesmerism," *Lancet*, 25 June 1842, p. 459. Among the signatories were Charles Bray, James Silk Buckingham, William Gregory, Sir Walter Trevelyan, Arthur Trevelyan, and Richard Beamish. Another phrenological association was proposed by John Alexander Ellis in *Med.Times*, 6 (27 Aug. 1842), 342–3; see also: "New Phrenological Society," *Lancet*, 13 Aug. 1842, p. 702. For the sixth meeting of the PA, see: *Phren. J.*, 17 (1844), 414; and *Zoist*, 1 (Oct. 1843), 227–46.

90. "True and False Phrenology," *Br. & Foreign Med. Rev.*, 14 (July 1842), 65–85 at p. 70.

91. See, for example: Noble, "An Essay on the Application of Phrenology to the Investigation of the Phenomena of Insanity," *Phren. J.*, 9 (1834/6), 447–59; idem, "An Essay on Temperaments Read before the Manchester Phrenological Society, April 30, 1834," ibid., 9 (1834/6), 109–18; idem, *An Essay on the Means, Physical and Moral of Estimating Human Character* (Manch. 1835); idem, *An Inquiry into the Claims of Phrenology, to Rank among the Sciences: a paper read before the Literary and Philosophical Society of Manchester Nov. 17th, 1837* (Manch. 1837); idem, "On the Quality of Brain, as Influencing Functional Manifestation. Read before the Manchester Phrenological Society, Oct. 8th, 1838," *Phren. J.*, 12 (1839), 121–34; and ibid., 10 (1836/7), 190–201, 11 (1838), 312–14, 12 (1839), 206–12.

92. *Phren. J.*, 13 (1840), 387, Cf. "Mr L. Burke's Lectures, London Mechanics' Institution," *People's Phren.J.*, 1 (1843), 201; and Henry Clarke, "Professional Phrenologists and Party Phrenologists," *Phren. J.*, 18 (1845), 237–40 at p. 240.

93. See: *Strictures on Anti-Phrenology* . . . Roget (1838); and "Hamilton's Prefix to Monroe's *Anatomy*," *Phren. J.*, 7 (1831/2), 434–4.

94. See: *Testimonials in Favour of Hewett Cottrell Watson as a Candidate for a Chair of Botany in Ireland* [1846].

95. See: "Phrenological Collections," *J. Health & Dis.*, 4 (1848), 49–54 at p. 52.

96. True confessions are given in Noble, *Elements of Psychological Medicine* (1853), pp. x–xi, 36–8. For Carpenter's views, see: "Mr Noble on the Brain and Its Physiology," *Br. & For. Med. Rev.*, 22 (Oct. 1846), 488–544 (a review of Noble's *The Brain and Its Physiology* [1846], which Combe had inspired Noble to write as a refutation of Carpenter's views). See also: "Noble and Walkott on Phrenology," *Dublin Q. J. Med. Sci.*, 3 (Feb. 1847), 148–54; T. S. Prideaux and W. C. Engledue, *A New Year's Gift for the Medical Profession. Dr. Carpenter and the Antiphrenological Physiologists; Messrs. Forbes, Wakley and Co., the antimesmeric crusaders* (1847); and Bruce Haley, *The Healthy Body and Victorian Culture* (Cambridge, Mass., 1978), pp. 36–7.

97. Charles Cowan's rejection of phrenology in 1845 upon taking in M. P. J. Flourens's criticisms parallels Noble's rejection and was referred to by him: paper read to the Reading Pathological Society, *Prov. Med. & Surg. J.* (16 Apr. 1845), cited in Noble, *Brain and Its Physiology*, p. 359. For the withdrawal from active participation in science by "demarginalizing" groups, see: Inkster, "Askesian Society," p. 27 ff; idem, "Marginal Men," pp. 149 ff.; idem, "Phrenology in Sheffield," p. 278; Thackray, "Manchester Model," pp. 696 ff.; Lenoir, "Generational Factors," p.465; Mandrou, *Humanism to Science*, p. 138.

98. See: Andrew Combe, *Phrenology: its nature and uses: An address to the students of Anderson's University at the opening of Dr Weir's first course of lectures on phrenology in that institution, January 7th 1846* (Edin., 1846); *Lancet*, 10 Jan. 1847, pp. 61–4; *Br. & Foreign Med. Rev.*, 22 (July 1846), pp. 230–1; *J. Health & Dis.*, 1 (1846), 232; Gibbon, *Life of Combe*, II, pp. 210–11.

99. Travers, *The Physiology of Inflammation* (1844), p. 44, q. in *Medico-Chirurgical Rev.*, n.s. 1 (1845), 369.

100. Brodie, "Phrenology," in *Psychological Inquiries* (1854) 220–32 and at pp. 33–104, 262–4 (and see: Cornelius Donovan, *Reply to Sir B. Brodie's Attack on Phrenology, in His "Psychological Inquiries"; being a lecture delivered at the Marlebone Institution* [1857], Lefevre, "Phrenology," in *An Apology for the Nerves* (1844), 58–74; and "Drs Gall and Spurzheim: phrenology," in his *The Life of a Travelling Physician* (1843), I, 144–51 (criticized in *Zoist*, 2 [Jan. 1845], 462–4); Skae, "Phrenology" [review of James Straton, *Contributions to the Mathematics of Phrenology* and of Noble's *The Brain and its Physiology*], *Br. Q. Rev.*, 4 (Nov. 1846), 397–419 (replied to by Straton in *Phren. J.*, 20 [1847], 36–48 and by Combe in *Lancet*, reprinted in *Phren. J.*, 20 [1847], 63–80; see also: Skae's reply, *Lancet*, 31 July 1847, 123–6, and Combe to Skae, *Lancet*, 21 Aug. 1847, 194–6). For Brande and Flourens's critiques, see: Chap. 1, note 47; on Skae, see: F. Fish, "David Skae, MD, FRCS, Founder of the Edinburgh School of Psychiatry," *Med. Hist.*, 9 (1965), 36–53.

101. For Weber on the intrinsic value freedom and ethical neutrality of science, see: Herbert Marcuse, "Industrialization and Capitalism in the Work of Max Weber," in *Negations* (Boston, 1968), 201–26.

102. On the contrary, because of phrenology's methodological conformity to the image of science, little reference could be made to it by contemporaries writing on the difference between "genuine science" and "pseudoscience": e.g., G. Cornewall Lewis, *An Essay on the Influence of Authority in Matters of Opinion* (1849; 2nd ed., 1875), p. 53; [Elizabeth Eastlake], "Physiognomy," *Quart. Rev.* 90 (1851), 62–91 at p. 62; and Henry Dircks, *Scientific Studies, II, Chimeras of Science: astrology, alchemy, squaring the circle, perpetuum mobile, etc.* (1869), esp. pp. 41, 80.

103. J. W. Hudson, *History of Adult Education* (1851), p. 167; and "Decay of Literary and Scientific Institutions," *London Pioneer*, 2 (9 Dec. 1847), 536.

104. Indeed, it became possible for a person such as John Forbes to renew his acquaintance with phrenology and to lean heavily on the Combean expression of it to advocate social harmony among the working class: Forbes, *Of Happiness*

in Its Relation to Work and Knowledge: an introductory lecture delivered before the members of the Chichester Literary Society and Mechanics' Institute, October 25th, 1850 (2nd ed., 1867), esp. pp. 13–15. See also: "Combe on the Constitution of Man," *Medico-Chirurgical Rev.*, 23 (1835), 361–70 (where it is implied that no intelligent doctor could possibly not read it); "Combe on Moral Philosophy," ibid., 35 (1841), 68–80, 353–76; Andrew Combe, "Phrenology," *Br. & For. Med. Rev.*, 9 (1840), 190–215; and J. G. Davey, "G. Combe and His Writings: a lecture delivered at Bristol," *J. Mental Sci.*, 10 (1864), 168–94.

CHAPTER 4: *George Combe and the remolding of man's constitution*

1. "George Combe," in *Biographical Sketches, 1852–1875* (new ed., 1877), 265–77 at p. 265.
2. William Ellis to Combe, 30 Oct. 1853, Combe Papers, NLS 7333/87.
3. Charles Gibbon, *The Life of Combe* (1878) I, pp. 55 ff. (the first 68 pages, to 1804, are from the autobiography that Combe never lived to complete).
4. Ibid., I., pp. 51, 17, 53; Combe, *The Life and Correspondence of Andrew Combe, M.D.* (1850), pp. 8, 22.
5. Abram's more outgoing manner might be taken as confirming the repression in the family home: According to George Combe, it was only after Abram left home for London for the first time that he discovered "that life could be enjoyed without infringement of morality." [G. Combe], *The Life and Dying Testimony of Abram Combe in favour of Robt. Owen's Views of Man and Society*, ed. Alexander Campbell (1844), p. 6.
6. Silvan S. Tomkins, *Affect, Imagery, Consciousness* (N.Y., 1963), pp. 132–56, cited in Thomas J. Scheff, "Labelling, Emotion, and Individual Change," in Scheff, ed., *Labelling Madness* (Englewood Cliffs, N.J., 1975), p. 83. See also Jenny Cook-Gumperz, *Social Control and Socialization: a study of class differences in the language of maternal control* (1973). Cf. R. P. Neuman, "Masturbation, Madness, and the Modern Concepts of Childhood and Adolescence," *J. Soc. Hist.*, 8 (1975), 1–27; and Lloyd de Mause, ed., *The History of Childhood* (N.Y., 1974).
7. Combe, *Life of Andrew*, pp. 8, 21.
8. Ibid., p. 4; Charles Mackay, "George Combe," in his *Forty Years' Recollections of Life* (1877), II, 241–70 at p. 245; Elizabeth Eastlake to Miss Laura Browne, Edinburgh, 5 Nov. 1842, in *Journals and Correspondences of Lady Eastlake*, ed. Charles E. Smith, (1895), I, p. 31; Robert Cooper, "Autobiographical Sketch," *National Reformer*, 11 (1868), 373.
9. Gibbon, *Life of Combe*, I, pp. 281–8; de Guistino, *Conquest of Mind*, p. 5. For an example of Combe's alleged lack of Amativeness deployed to give sting to an attack on his social views, see: A. J. Hamilton to Combe, 16 May 1824, Combe papers, NLS 7213/46–7; and Elliotson, *Human Physiology* (5th ed. 1835), p. 1156n.
10. Combe, *Life of Andrew*, pp. 9–10; Gibbon, *Life of Combe*, I, pp. 9, 12–13, 37–42.
11. The idea of cosmologies as lived and therefore changing with us is a theme prevalent in the work of Douglas; see, for example; "Couvade and Menstruation," in her *Implicit Meanings* (1975), 60–72 at pp. 60–1; Walzer, "Puritanism as a Revolutionary Ideology," *History and Theory*, 3 (1963), 58–90. See also: Raymond Firth, "Religious Belief and Personal Adjustment," in his *Essays on Social Organization and Values* (1964), 257–93.
12. Gibbon, *Life of Combe*, I, p. 16.
13. Martineau, *Autobiography* (1877), 3 vols; and R. K. Webb, *Martineau* (1960); Bray, *Phases of Opinion and Experience during a Long Life: autobiography* [1888]; Giles St. Aubyn, *A Victorian Eminence: the life and works of Henry Thomas Buckle* (1958); J. D. Y. Peel, *Herbert Spencer: the evolution of a sociologist* (1971); *Diary of John Epps* [1870]; F. N. Egerton, "Hewett Cottrell Watson," *DSB*; and *Life and Letters of William Ballantyne Hodgson*, ed. J. M. D. Meiklejohn (Edin., 1883).

14. Gibbon, *Life of Combe*, I, p. 16, my emphasis; see also p. 51, and his letter to Robert Chambers q. on pp. 296–7.

15. Ibid., p. 11. The illness, at about age ten, brought Combe back home from the various aunts and uncles with whom he had been boarded. He remained at home until he passed his examinations to be admitted as a Writer to the Signet in January 1812, aged twenty-four. It may be significant that during his illness one of his mother's servants was led to remark: "O, laddie, you should never marry," which in turn may have had something to do with Combe's confiding in Dr. Spurzheim before marriage and, of course, to the lack of offspring. Ibid., p. 284.

16. Ibid., I, pp. 60–5, 82; Combe, *Life of Abram*, p. 22. But cf. his apparent kindnesses to his sister Anne's family (Robert, [Sir] James, and [Dr.] Abram Cox) after Robert Cox senior had died in 1815, noted in Benjamin Wm. Crombie, "George Combe," in *Modern Athenians* (Edin., 1882), 161–5.

17. Bruce Mazlish, *James and John Stuart Mill: father and son in the nineteenth century* (1975), p. 57.

18. See: Martin Jay, *The Dialectical Imagination* (1973), p. 126. John Stuart Mill commented on "that rarity in England, a really warm hearted mother" and on the difference it would have made to his own life in *The Early Draft of John Stuart Mill's Autobiography*, ed. Jack Stillinger (Urbana, Ill., 1961), p. 184. For an only slightly overdrawn fictional depiction of the Calvinist mother and her relations with her children, see Charles Kingsley, *Alton Locke, Tailor and Poet: an autobiography* (1849), chap. 1.

19. Mazlish, *James and John Stuart Mill*, pp. 7–8 emphasizes that generational conflict was "pivotal" and "as important as class conflict"; see also: the review of Mazlish by J. Hamburger in *History and Theory*, 15 (1976), 328–41, esp. p. 335.

20. Gibbon, *Life of Combe*, I, pp. 94–5, and Combe, *A System of Phrenology* (Edin., 1825), preface. The latter was the retitled 2nd edition of the *Essays on Phrenology* (Edin., 1819), which became a two-volume work in its 4th edition of 1836 and had reached a 10th edition by 1863.

21. Gibbon, *Life of Combe*, I, pp. 73–83, 171, and II, p. 5. On his pride and concern with his early essays, see: ibid., I, p. 99.

22. Ibid., I, p. 75. On Lyell, see: Cannon, *Science in Culture*, p. 151; and R. Porter, "Charles Lyell: the public and private faces of science" (typescript, 1980). On Robert Chambers's confession that "it was my design from the first to be the essayist of the middle class," see: William Chambers, *Memoir of William and Robert Chambers* (Edin., 1884), p. 240.

23. Somewhat precociously in "On the Philosophy of Dugald Stewart, Esq., and Comparison betwixt It and the System of Gall and Spurzheim," *Lit. & Stats. Mag. Scot.*, 3 (Feb. 1819), 34–51.

24. "Materialism and Scepticism," *Phren.*, I (1823/4), p. 140.

25. Gibbon, *Life of Combe*, I, pp. 72–3. Combe was a member of a Cobbett Club in Edinburgh, and in 1809 he assisted in the formation of a Cobbett Club near Stirling. Henry Holland, studying medicine in Edinburgh around this time, recollected "the eagerness with which Cobbett's 'Register' was looked and read on every day of its publication." *Recollections of Past Life* (1872), p. 21 n.

26. Combe, *On the Relation between Science and Religion* (Edin., 1847; 4th ed. 1857), pp. xii, ix.

27. Carlyle, "Sign of the Times," *Edin. Rev.*, 49 (1829), 439–59 at p. 442; and see: Raymond Williams, *Culture and Society, 1780–1950* (1963), pp. 85–90.

28. The idea that symbols act to conceal as well as to reveal was apparently put forward by Carlyle in *Sartor Resartus* (see: Raymond Firth, *Symbols Public and Private* [1973], p. 15); with specific reference to maps and pictorial sets of symbols, see: Barry Barnes, *Interests and the Growth of Knowledge* (1977), pp. 4–7 et passim. Also useful in this connection is Ian G. Barbour, *Myths, Models, and Paradigms: the nature of scientific and religious language* (1974), esp. pp. 27–8, 69–70.

29. See: C. Hill, "William Harvey and the Idea of Monarchy," *Past & Present*, no.

27 (1964), 54–72, repr. in Charles Webster, ed., *The Intellectual Revolution of the Seventeenth Century* (1974), 160–81; and Critchley, *Banquet of the Brain.*

30. For a tribal example of the head's celebration (during a crucial period in the history of the Fipa peoples of East Africa), see: Roy Willis, *Man and Beast* (1974); for industrializing Britain, see: S. Shapin and B. Barnes, "Head and Hand: rhetorical resources in British pedagogical writing, 1770–1850," *Oxford Rev. Educ.*, 2 (1976), 231–54; see also: Alfred Sohn-Rethel, *Intellectual and Manual Labour* (1978).

31. See: M. Neve and R. Porter, "Alexander Catcott: glory and geology," *Br. J. Hist. Sci.*, 10 (1977), 37–60, esp. pp. 47–8. See also: R. Porter, "The Terraqueous Globe," in Rousseau and Porter, *Ferment of Knowledge*, 285–324 at p. 300; and on the use of geological strata imagery among the Victorian educated: John Fowles, *The French Lieutenant's Woman* (1969), chap. 8, esp. p. 54.

32. James Wilkinson, *The Human Body and Its Connexion with Man* (1851), p. 1, who in the same passage refers to wisdom being the "machinery answering to faculty." But only rarely in phrenological literature was the assumptive metaphor spelled out literally; normally the faculties were portrayed as muscles, although the whole was frequently spoken of as an "organized system": e.g., Spurzheim, *Elementary Principles of Education* (2nd ed., 1828), pp. 56–7. For stimulating and perceptive insights on the body metaphor, see: J. Miller, "The Dog beneath the Skin," *Listener*, 88 (20 July 1972), 74–6; and Mary Douglas, *Purity and Danger* and *Natural Symbols.*

33. See: Piper, *Active Universe*, pp. 7–8; also Donald A. Schon, *Displacement of Concepts* (1963), esp. p. 144; and J. C. Marshall, "Minds, Machines, and Metaphors," *Soc. Stud. Sci.*, 7 (1977), 475–88. On organicism in relation to mechanism, see: H. Scott Gordon, "Alfred Marshall and the Development of Economics as a Science," in R. N. Giere and R. S. Westfall, eds., *Foundations of Scientific Method: the nineteenth century* (Indiana U.P., 1973), 234–58, esp. at p. 244; and K. Deutsch, "Mechanism, Organism, and Society: some models in natural and social science," *Phil. of Sci.*, 18 (1951), 230–52.

34. For an excellent illustration of the body as machine, see: frontispiece to the *London Med. & Surg. J.*, 4 (1835). For what was omitted from this conception of organism, see: Mannheim, "Concept of State as an Organism," in *Essays* (1953), esp. at pp. 177–8.

35. On the latter, see: Désirée Hirst, *Hidden Riches: traditional symbolism from the Renaissance to Blake* (1964), chap. 10 and p. 12.

36. See: George Canguilhem, *Le Normal et le pathologique* (2nd ed., Paris, 1972); Frank E. Manuel, "From Equality to Organicism," *J. Hist. Ideas*, 17 (1956), 54–69, repr. in his *Freedom from History and Other Untimely Essays* (1972); K. Figlio, "The Metaphor of Organization: an historiographical perspective on the biomedical sciences of the early nineteenth century," *Hist. Sci.*, 14 (1976), 17–53; Cynthia Russett, *The Concept of Equilibrium in American Social Thought* (New Haven, 1966); R. Cooter, "The Power of the Body: the early nineteenth century," in Barnes and Shapin, *Natural Order*, pp. 73–92. Cf. Bentham on the "false and extravagant" ideas arising from the biological metaphor: Halévy, *Philosophical Radicalism*, p. 500.

37. R. M. Young, "The Development of Herbert Spencer's Concept of Evolution," *Actes du XIᵉ Congres International D'Histoire des Sciences* (Warsaw, 1967), II, 273–8 at p. 274. Spencer submitted papers on the function of various phrenological faculties to *Phren. J.* but had them turned down; they were subsequently published in *Zoist*, I (1844), 369–85, 2 (1844), 186–9, 316–25. The design for his "cephalograph" is appended in his *Autobiography* (1904), II, pp. 540–3; on his introduction to phrenology, see: vol. I, pp. 200–3, 225–8, 540. See also: his *Principles of Psychology* (1855), p. 607; Peel, *Spencer*, pp. 10–11; and Bernard Hollander, "Herbert Spencer as a Phrenologist," *Westminster Rev.*, 139 (1893), 142–54. On Saint-Simon's debt to Gall, see: B. Haines, "The Inter-Relations between Social, Biological, and Medical Thought, 1750–1850: Saint-Simon and Comte," *Br. J. Hist. Sci.*, 11 (1978), 19–35, esp. p. 20; and on Saint-Simon, see

also: Frank Manuel, *The New World of Henri Saint-Simon* (Cambridge, Mass., 1956); idem, "Henri Saint-Simon on the Role of the Scientist," in *Freedom from History*, pp. 205–18. On Comte and phrenology, see: E. Littre, "Du tableau cerebral, ou modification apportee par M. Comte au system phrenologique de Gall," in *Auguste Comte et la philosophie positive* (Paris, 1863), 538–52; Bernard Hollander, "Comte's Analysis of the Human Faculties," repr. in *Proceedings of the Aristotelian Society*, Nov. 1891, n.p.; John Ingram, *Human Nature and Morals According to Auguste Comte with Notes Illustrative of the Principles of Positivism* (1901), which was largely taken up with a discussion of Gall's faculty divisions and Comte's reliance on them; J. Greene, "Biology and Social Theory in the Nineteenth Century: Auguste Comte and Herbert Spencer," in Clagett, *Critical Problems*, pp. 419–46, esp. pp. 425, 444, 453 (Green details the relevant passages on Gall from Comte's *Cours de philosophie positive*). On the clash over phrenology between Comte and J. S. Mill, see: Iris W. Mueller, *John Stuart Mill and French Thought* (Urbana, Ill., 1956), pp. 107–12; and Mazlish, *James and John Stuart Mill*, pp. 260–1.

38. See: N. J. Demerath and R. A. Peterson, eds., *System, Change, and Conflict: a reader on contemporary sociological theory and the debate over functionalism* (1967); H. E. Barnes, "Representative Biological Theories of Society," *Sociol. Rev.*, 17 (1925), 120–30, 182–94, 294–300; R. Harrison, "Functionalism and Its Historical Significance," *Genetic Psychol. Monographs*, 68 (1963), 387–423; D. Martindale, ed., *Functionalism in the Social Sciences: the strength and limits of functionalism in anthropology, economics, political science, and sociology*, Monograph 5, American Academy of Political and Social Science (Phil., 1965); Emile Durkheim, *The Division of Labour in Society* (1893), trans. G. Simpson (1933, repr. 1964); A. R. Radcliffe-Brown, "The Concept of Function in Social Science," in his *Structure and Function in Primitive Society* (1952); Herbert Spencer, "The Social Organism," *Westminster Rev.*, (1860), repr. in his *Essays: scientific, political, and speculative* (1901), I, 265–307; R. M. Young, "Functionalism" (typescript, 1971).

39. "Phrenology," in his *Biographical History of Philosophy* (2nd, rev. ed., 1857), 629–45 at pp. 632, 640; and (this chapter, supposedly written at George Eliot's insistence, was extensively rewritten as "Psychology Finally Recognised as a Branch of Biology: the Phrenological hypothesis") in the 3rd ed. (retitled *The History of Philosophy from Thales to Comte*, vol. I [1867], vol. II [1871]), II, 394–435 at p. 410. See also: Lewes, "Psychology: a new cerebral theory," in his *Comte's Philosophy of the Sciences* (1853), 213–32.

40. "Phrenological Fallacies," *Atlas*, 5 July 1829, repr. in *Works*, vol. 20, pp. 248–53.

41. This strikingly unanthropological and historically doubtful assertion (cf. behavior during periods of very rapid change in Russia, Cuba, and China) is made by Robin Horton, "African Traditional Thought and Western Science," *Africa*, 37 (1967), repr. in M. D. F. Young, ed., *Knowledge and Control* (1971), 206–88, at p. 224.

42. "Fourier's Theory," *Democratic Review*, I (Mar 1850), p. 383. Although Fourier believed that everything he wrote came out of his own head (see: David Zeldin, *The Educational Ideas of Charles Fourier* [1772–1837] [1969], pp. 13–14), there is no doubt that his use of "faculties" was phrenologically derived. Given our interpretation of the mediations of phrenology, the case for arguing that Fourier was a precursor of "Taylorism" is strengthened precisely *because* his ideas originated "within the worker's psyche": cf. J. Beecher and R. Bienvenu, *The Utopian Vision of Charles Fourier* (1972), p. 46.

43. This was the motto of the neo-Owenite journal *Spirit of the Age* (1848–9), edited by G. J. Holyoake.

44. Pope, *Essay on Man*, IV, II, 49 ff., q. in Arthur O. Lovejoy, *The Great Chain of Being: a study of the history of an idea* (1936; Cambridge, Mass., 1957), p. 206. Uncritical of Lovejoy's concept but useful for the British context is W. F. Bynum, "The Great Chain of Being after Forty Years: an appraisal," *Hist. Sci.*, 13 (1975), 1–28.

45. On the division of labor as a cohesive mechanism, see: Durkheim, *Division of Labour*, pp. 54–63. For Durkheim the extending division of labor was the moving power of progress, since after ruptures in the social mass it functioned to establish equilibrium (ibid., p. 270).
46. See: Combe, "Letter on the Functions of Concentrativeness," *Phren. J.*, 2 (1824/5), 246–50. On phrenological nomenclature, see: above, Chapter 3, note 35; phreno-mesmerism was to be the source for innumerable additions: The American La Roy Sunderland, for example, in his *New Theory of Mind: Pathetism* (Boston and London, 1851), added, among many others, the organs of Contentment, Modesty, and Piety. (Sunderland is usually accredited the first person to proclaim the link between phrenology and mesmerism, around 1841.)
47. Shapin, "Phrenological Knowledge," pp. 239–40; and idem, "Politics of Observation," pp. 149 ff. In addition to the sources on the debate over the frontal sinuses given above (Chapter 1, notes, 45, 47), see: Thomas Stone, "On the Frontal Sinus," *Edin. New Phil. J.*, 14 (1833), 82–9; and, with a rather different view on the matter, George Murray Humphry, *A Treatise on the Human Skeleton* (Cambridge, 1858). Phrenologists allowed that the mental organs were not confined to the surface of the brain (see Spurzheim, *Physiognical System*, p. 239), but claimed that it was there that they were manifested for observation.
48. R. Macnish, *Introduction to Phrenology*, p. 17.
49. See: Robert J. Lifton, *Boundaries: psychological man in revolution* (N.Y., 1970), pp. 54–5, 85; R. Firth, *Essays*, p. 234; C. Geertz, "Ideology as a Cultural System," p. 61; Douglas, *Natural Symbols*, p. 98; and Malinowski, *Magic, Science, and Religion*, p. 101.
50. The title was subsequently modified to *The Constitution of Man Considered in Relation to External Objects*; an American schools edition (first published in Albany in 1836) altered the latter part of the title to ... *in Relation to the Natural Laws*, and it was with that title that Cassell republished the book in New York in 1893. Unless otherwise stated, all reference is to the 6th edition, 1836.
51. "The Excursion," *Poetical Works*, ed. T. Hutchinson, rev. ed. edited by E. de Selincourt (Oxford, 1978), p. 590. The idea of a fit between external nature and man's internal mental nature (especially when the brain is conceived of in terms of physiological parts) is obviously a very old one and has connections with the idea of microcosm–macrocosm as regarded thus by Albertus Magnus in the C13. On the neurosis of Churchill and Newton, see, respectively: Geertz, "Ideology as a Cultural System," p. 72; and F. Manuel, *Newton*, pp. 49–51, 66, and R. S. Westfall, "Newton and Order," in Paul G. Kuntz, ed., *The Concept of Order* (1968), 77–88. On the ideologist as political metaphysician projecting his social drama isomorphically on total reality, etc. see: Lewis S. Feuer, *Ideology and the Ideologists* (Oxford, 1975), esp. p. 103.
52. Information on sales is abstracted from the advertisements to the various editions and from Gibbon, *Life of Combe*, I, pp. 262–3, 306, II, p. 274.
53. On the sales of these books see, respectively: R. M. Young, "The Impact of Darwin on Conventional Thought," p. 16; Charles Gillispie, *Genesis and Geology*, pp. 163, 172; R. K. Webb, *The British Working Class Reader, 1790–1848* (1955), p. 38; Richard Altick, *The English Common Reader*, pp. 70, 390. For reflection on the symbolic significance of an "influential book," see: Owen Chadwick, *Secularization*, pp. 171 ff. A further appropriate comparison might be made with Paley's *Evidences*, which soared through twenty-nine editions between 1794 and 1830 and then fell rapidly out of fashion, to some extent, arguably, being displaced by its Combean revisions: Hamish Swanston, *Ideas of Order* (Assen, 1974), pp. 5–6.
54. William Harral Johnson, "Death of Mr. George Combe," *Investigator, a Journal of Secularism*, 5 (1858), p. 93; also made by Martineau, "Combe," p. 265 and repeated by Morley, Charles Mackay, and many others. See also: Robert Chambers's eulogy to Combe in "George Combe," *The Book of Days* (Edin., 1864), II, 213–14.
55. "Combe's Moral Philosophy," *Spectator*, 10 Apr. 1841, p. 351.

56. "Combe," p. 276; see also: *Life and Letters of W. B. Hodgson*, p. 13. For the appropriateness of pairing Combe with Von Humboldt, see: Cannon, *Science in Culture*, chap. 3: "Humboldtian Science."

57. Morley, *Cobden* I, p. 93; Martineau, "Combe," p. 273. See also: "Mr. George Combe," *Illustrated London News*, suppl., 28 (Aug. 1858), 203–4; and William Jolly, ed., *Education: its principles and practice as developed by George Combe* (1879), p. v. Like Charles Gibbon, Jolly felt that Combe was then little known and appreciated, especially by "the class for whom he did such eminent service." Martineau's confession to Combe, "I am a thorough unbeliever in phrenology. ... Yet I read with satisfaction every word you write on your " 'science' " (letter to Combe, 24 Sept. 1841, Combe Papers, NLS 7261/58) was shared by Channing and Emerson in America (see: T. Stoehr, "Physiognomy and Phrenology in Hawthorne," p. 363), but to the vast majority of Combe's readers, the *Constitution of Man* occasioned taking phrenology seriously (e.g., Sophia Peabody Hawthorne's response cited in ibid., p. 359n.). Nor, for bourgeois ideologues, did private opinions on phrenology prevent their own public reliance on the science when convenient; Martineau, for example, exploited its authority in her *Household Education* (1849), p. 259 and relied on it extensively in her and H. G. Atkinson, *Letters on the Laws of Man's Nature and Development* (1851). At her brother James's suggestion, she had her head read in 1830 and on subsequent occasions had it read by Deville[‡] and J. D. Holm[‡]: *Autobiography*, I, pp. 393–6; Webb, *Martineau*, p. 247; and V. K. Pichanick, *Harriet Martineau* (Ann Arbor, Mich., 1980), pp. 183–97. Her faith in phrenology was cemented through her mesmeric experience in 1844; see: "Appendix" to her *Letters on Mesmerism* (2nd ed., 1845), pp. 67–70.

58. *Constitution of Man*, pp. 95, 211–12, 218–19, et passim, and 1855 ed., p. 59; letter to Welsh, 26 June 1825, q. in Gibbon, *Life of Combe*, I, p. 182.

59. *Constitution of Man* (1st ed., Edin., 1828), p. 204. Spencer explained in *The Data of Ethics* (1879), pp. iii–iv that since 1842 his aim in writing had been to make morality sacred or to give it authority in a secular world. For the background to Combe's use of nature in relation to morality, see: latter chapters of Basil Willey, *The Eighteenth Century Background* (Harmondsworth, 1972).

60. *Constitution of Man*, p. 52; see also: pp. 66–9.

61. See, in particular: chaps. 5 and 6, "To What Extent Are the Miseries of Mankind Referable to Infringement of the Laws of Nature?" and "On Punishment."

62. See, for example: William Scott, *Remarks on Mr. Combe's Essay on the Constitution of Man, and Its Relation to External Objects* (Edin., for private circulation, 1827); [Alexander Smith], "Phrenological Ethics," *Edin. Rev.*, 74 (1842), 376–414 at p. 403; "Mr. Combe's Constitution of Man Regarding the Efficacy of Prayer," *Macphail's Edin. Eccles. J.*, 14 (1853), 27–34 at p. 27; "Mr G. Combe on Education," *Free Church Mag.*, 5 (1848), 33–6 at p. 33; "The Constitution of Man, 4th edition," *Br. & For. Rev.*, 12 (1841), 142–80 at p. 172; J. L. Murphy, "Phrenology," in his *Essay Towards a Science of Consciousness* (1838), pp. 53ff. For popular examples of Combe's use of natural law, see: Edwin Lunn, *A Lecture on Prayer, Its Folly, Inutility, and Irrationality* (Manch.) [1839]), p. 5; John Scott,[‡] *Scott's Popular and Scientific Lectures* [1850]), pp. 3 ff.

63. *Vestiges of the Natural History of Creation* (2nd ed., 1844), pp. 333–4, q. in Young, "Impact of Darwin on Conventional Thought," p. 17. Chambers was converted to phrenology in 1834 after hearing Combe lecture. He provided Combe with a testimonial on the value of phrenology in 1836. See: de Giustino, *Conquest of Mind*, p. 52; *Testimonials to Combe*, p. 55. Adam Sedgwick in his review of *Vestiges* in *Edin. Rev.*, 82 (1845), 11, believed that the author thought "that Gall and Spurzheim are the only mental philosophers since the days of Plato"; others thought so too, which is why Combe was widely believed to have been the author.

64. Whewell, *Astronomy and General Physics Considered with Reference to Natural Theology* (1833; 1852), pp. 5–6; Lewes, "What Are the Laws of Nature?" in his *Problems of Life and Mind* (1874), I, 307–13, which first appeared in his *Comte's*

Philosophy of the Sciences (1853), 51–7; Carpenter, "Man the Interpreter of Nature" (presidential address to the British Association, 1872), and "Nature and Law," *Modern Rev.* (Oct. 1880), both repr. in idem, *Nature and Man* (1888); T. H. Huxley, "Scientific and Pseudo-Scientific Realism," and "Science and Pseudo-Science," both repr. in *Collected Essays*, vol. 5, *Science and Christian Tradition* (1904), esp. pp. 79, 108. For the latter, see also: O. Stanley, "T. H. Huxley's Treatment of 'Nature,' " *J. Hist. Ideas*, 18 (1957), 120–7.

65. *Nature; the Utility of Religion; and Theism* (2nd ed., 1874), p. 14. See also: E. Zilsel, "The Genesis of the Concept of Physical Law," *Phil. Rev.*, 51 (1942), 245–79. For Bentham and the philosophical radicals' thinking on natural law and its ambiguities, see: Halévy, *Philosophical Radicalism*, pp. 489 ff.

66. On the celebrated antithesis between nurture and nature, see: E. R. Dodds, *The Greeks and the Irrational* (Berkeley, Calif., 1951), pp. 182 ff., and Mary Douglas, *Cultural Bias* (1978), pp. 22 ff.; on the human compulsion for moral law as an ultimate moderator, see: Leszek Kolakowski, "The Priest and the Jester," in his *Marxism and Beyond: on historical understanding and individual responsibility*, trans. J. Zielonko Peel (1968), p. 29.

67. *Constitution of Man*, pp. 95–6.

68. Ibid., (6th ed., 1836), pp. 249, 254. Combe's reform methods were spelled out more fully in Combe and C. J. A. Mittermaier, "On the Application of Phrenology to Criminal Legislation and Prison Discipline," *Phren. J.*, 16 (1843), 1–19; Combe, *Remarks on the Principles of Criminal Legislation, and the Practice of Prison Discipline* (1854), a reworking of his "Criminal Legislation and Prison Discipline," *Westminster Rev.*, n.s., 5 (1854), 409–45; idem, "Prison Discipline," *Illus. London News*, 25 (5 Aug. 1854), 114; idem, *Thoughts on Capital Punishment* (Edin., 1847); idem, *Penal Colonies: the management of prisoners in the Australian colonies* (Edin., 1845); idem, "Instances of Successful Moral Treatment of Criminals," *Phren. J.*, 18 (1845), 205–9.

69. Whereas in the 1st edition the section "On Punishment" takes up only five pages of large type, by the 6th edition of 1836 it takes up twenty-seven pages of close print.

70. The same can be said of course of all the other phrenological interest in and writing upon criminality; see, for example: "Result of an Examination, by Mr James DeVille, of the Heads of 148 Convicts on the Convict Ship England, When About to Sail for New South Wales in the Spring of 1826," *Phren. J.*, 4 (1826/7), 467–71; G. S. MacKenzie, *Documents Laid before Lord Glenelg* ([Edin.], Apr. 1836); Marmaduke B. Sampson, *Criminal Jurisprudence Considered in Relation to Mental Organization* (1841; 3rd ed., 1851); idem, "Phrenology in Its Application to the Treatment of Criminals," *Lancet*, 5 and 12 Feb. 1842, pp. 639–43, 672–7; idem, *The Phrenological Theory of the Treatment of Criminals Defended in a Letter to John Forbes* (1843). For Lord Stanley's interest in phrenology for the classification of criminals and an example of the influence of the science upon those dealing with criminals, see: Walter Lowe Clay, *The Prison Chaplain: a memoir of the Rev. John Clay, B.D.* (Cambridge, 1861), p. 569.

71. For a summary of and introduction to Foucault, see: Edith Kurzweil, *The Age of Structuralism: Levi-Strauss to Foucault* (N.Y., 1980), esp. p. 113.

72. From his investments in the New York and Illinois railroads, Combe derived over £200 annually: de Giustino, *Conquest of Mind*, pp. 4–5. Letters on railway finance, banking, and investment abound in the Combe papers.

73. *Constitution of Man*, p. 214.

74. Ibid., pp. 215–28.

75. See: Herbert Marcuse, "The Affirmative Character of Culture," in his *Negations*, 88–133 at p. 90.

76. In this respect the *Constitution of Man* is similar to J. P. Kay[-Shuttleworth's] *The Moral and Physical Condition of the Working Classes Employed in the Cotton Manufacture in Manchester* (1832) and countless similar productions. On Kay-Shuttleworth's book, see: R. Johnson, "Educational Policy and Social Control in Early Victorian England," *Past and Present*, no. 49 (1970), repr. in Peter

Stansky, ed., *The Victorian Revolution* (N.Y., 1973), 199–226 at p. 205. For different but useful comparisons, see also: Eugene Genovese, "In the Name of Humanity and the Cause of Reform," in his *Roll Jordan Roll: the world the slaves made* (1975), 49–70; and J. Stauder, "The 'Relevance' of Anthropology to Colonialism and Imperialism," *Rad. Sci. J.*, (1974), 51–70, esp. p. 64.

77. See: G. Lichtheim, "The Concept of Ideology," *History and Theory*, 4 (1965), 164–95, esp. pp. 167–9; Leiss, *Domination of Nature*, pp. 148–51; L. R. Kass, "The New Biology: what price relieving man's estate?" *Science*, 174 (19 Nov. 1971), 781–2.

78. Combe was secretary of the Edinburgh Reform League in 1831; he spoke directly on his sociopolitical reform interests in "Parliamentary Reform Considered in Relation to the Moral and Intellectual Improvement of the People," *Phren. J.*, 7 (1831/2), 118–31, 587–97; preface and notes to E. P. Hurlbut, *Essays on Human Rights and Their Political Guaranties* (Edin., 1847); and *Our Rule in India* (Edin., 1858), among many others. In November 1830 he contemplated establishing a political journal for the "free and liberal discussion of politics, political economy, and religion" on the basis of the *Constitution of Man* but without phrenology (A. C. Grant, "George Combe and His Circle," p. 108). Before becoming the Edinburgh correspondent to the *London Courier* in 1834 Combe spelled out his political views to the editor thus: "My sentiments are Whig, and I am very much in favour of the present ministry; but in many points I go farther in favour of the people than they in their public measures can venture to proceed, but not, I hope, farther than, in their hearts, they would wish to advance. My view of human nature is that men require, 1st, knowledge, and 2d, training of their moral and intellectual faculties, before they can be trusted with power or be made the arbiters of their own destinies with advantage to themselves; but I believe that men *collectively*, when enlightened and trained, will go right and promote their own happiness; and hence that all churches and oligarchies that pretend to reign over either the minds or properties of mankind permanently ought to be overthrown, but *not till the people are* rendered rational by the means foresaid. I therefore advocate very liberal sentiments, as principles to be ultimately carried into practice, but am moderate as to the time and means": q. in Gibbon, *Life of Combe*, I, p. 302; see also I, p. 243 for his admiration of Whately's political economy; II, p. 213 for his intimacy with J. R. MacCulloch; and II, p. 244 for his friendship with William Ellis.

79. Cf. Lukács, *Class Consciousness*, esp. p. 234; Alfred Schmidt, "The Mediation of Nature through Society and Society through Nature," in his *The Concept of Nature in Marx* (1971), 63–93; Raymond Williams, "Ideas of Nature," *Times Lit. Supp.*, 4 Dec. 1970, pp. 1419–21; R. M. Young, "Evolutionary Biology and Ideology: then and now," *Science Studies*, 1 (1971), 177–206, repr. in Watson Fuller, ed., *The Biological Revolution: social good or social evil?* (N.Y., 1972), 241–82; R. M. Young, "The Human Limits of Nature," in Jonathan Benthall, ed., *The Limits of Human Nature* (1973), 235–74.

80. See: A. C. Grant, "Combe and the 1836 Election," p. 177.

81. *Constitution of Man*, p. 73. On the C19 attitude to atheism, see: J. M. Robertson, *A History of Freethought in the Nineteenth Century* (1929), pp. 70–202.

82. *[Lectures on] Moral Philosophy; or the duties of man considered in his individual, social, and domestic capacities* (Boston and Edin., 1840; 1893), p. 95. See also: *Constitution of Man*, chap. 9, "On the Relation between Science and Scripture."

83. On Chalmers's political economy, see also: his *On Political Economy in Connexion with the Moral State and the Moral Prospects of Society* (Glasgow, 1832); and idem, *The Christian and Civic Economy of Large Towns* (Glasgow, 1826). For his contribution to the debate on man's place in nature, see: R. M. Young, "Malthus and the Evolutionists: the common context of biological and social theory," *Past and Present*, no. 43 (1969), 109–45, esp. pp. 120–5. See also: [John Minter Morgan], *The Critics Criticised: with remarks on a passage in Dr. Chalmers's Bridgewater Treatise* (1834).

84. Combe, *On the Relation between Religion and Science* (Edin., 1847), pp. 37–9.

Some of Combe's naïvity is revealed in the letter he wrote to Chalmers after reading the latter's Bridgewater Treatise: q. in Gibbon, *Life of Combe*, I, p. 276.

85. See: Corsi, "Natural Theology"; and J. H. Brooke, "The Natural Theology of the Geologists: some theological strata," in L. J. Jordanova and Roy Porter, eds., *Images of the Earth* (Br. Soc. Hist. Sci. Monographs, 1979), 34–64.

86. The phrase is E. P. Thompson's: "Peculiarities of the English," pp. 60–1.

87. Cf. the situation in the C17 when, as between Puritan sects and their Anglican opponents, God and Nature together were competed for as the crucial legitimating resources: referred to in S. Shapin, "Social Uses of Science," in Rousseau and Porter, *Ferment of Knowledge*, 93–139 at pp. 115 ff.

88. Gibbon, *Life of Combe*, I, pp. 181 ff. See: William Gillespie, *An Exposure of the Unchristian and Unphilosophical Principles, Set Forth in Mr George Combe's Work Entitled "The Constitution of Man* ... *"; being an antidote to the poison of that publication* (Edin., 1836; 2nd ed., 1836); Joseph S. Hodgson, *Consideration of Phrenology in Connexion with an Intellectual, Moral, and Religious Education* (1839); C. J. Kennedy, *Nature and Revelation Harmonious: a defence of scriptural truths assailed in Mr. George Combe's work on "The Constitution of Man"* (Edin., published under the auspices of the Scottish Association for Opposing Prevalent Errors, 1846), replied to in Combe, *Answer [to] the Attack* ... (Edin., 1848; 1857); M. Ryan, "Physiology, Phrenology, Materialism, Immateriality of the Mind," 44–51; "Combe's Constitution of Man," *Presby. Rev.*, 9 (1836), 92–118; "Mr George Combe and the Philosophy of Phrenology," *Fraser's Mag.*, 22 (1840), 509–20; "Phrenology," *Christian Remembrancer*, 6 (1843), 661–76; "Combe's Reply to Kennedy's Nature ... ," *United Presby. Mag.*, 2 (1848), 64–8; William Scott, *A Few Last Words to Mr. Combe on the Subject of His Essay on the Natural Laws* (Edin., 1828); idem, *The Harmony of Phrenology with Scripture: shown in a refutation of the philosophical errors contained in Mr. Combe's "Constitution of Man"* (Edin., 1836). See also: note 62, above. These are only some of the more religiously focused attacks on the *Constitution of Man*.

89. On Chalmers's interest in phrenology, see: Gibbon, *Life of Combe*, I, p. 135. On Welsh, see: above, Chapter 1, note 31. On phrenology and the Scottish Evangelicals, see: Paul Baxter, "Combe, the Constitution of Man, and the Churches," paper delivered to Bri. Soc. Hist. Sci., July 1979, Durham; and idem, "Natural Laws and Divine Judgments: some reflections on Scottish natural theology," paper delivered to Br. Soc. Hist. Sci., Apr. 1980, Bath. Chalmers refused to lecture at the Greenoch Mechanics' Institute after Combe had lectured there, lest he be thought of as endorsing Combe's views: W. Hanna, *Memoirs of the Life and Writings of Thomas Chalmers* (Edin., 1849–52), IV, pp. 205–11.

90. Scott, *Remarks on Constitution of Man*.

91. Adam Rushton, *My Life as Farmer's Boy, Factory Lad, Teacher, and Preacher* (Manch., 1909), p. 50. A librarian of a Methodist Sunday school (c. 1837), Rushton had been censured for allowing the book on the shelves.

92. The classic examples are J. W. Draper, *History of the Conflict between Religion and Science* (1875); and A. D. White, *History of the Warfare of Science with Theology* (1896). But see also: John T. Merz, *A History of European Thought in the Nineteenth Century*, I, *Scientific Thought* (1896); John R. Beard, *Religion, Science, and Orthodoxy: their real nature and reciprocal relations* (Manch., 1861); Thomas Dick, *The Christian Philosophers; or the connection of science and philosophy with religion*, 2 vols. (Glasgow, 1869); and J. Y. Simpson, *Landmarks in the Struggle between Science and Religion* (1925). Useful secondary sources are Joseph Needham, ed , *Science, Religion, and Reality* (1925); Budd, *Varieties of Unbelief*; and Chadwick, "Science and religion," in his *Secularization*, chap. 7.

93. The phrase is from Beatrice Webb, *My Apprenticeship* (1926), p. 83, cited in Frank M. Turner, *Between Science and Religion: the reaction to scientific naturalism in late Victorian England* (New Haven and London, 1974), p. 12. For the argument that controversy over *Vestiges* can be explained in large part by its mockery of the mediating role of natural theological appeals to design, see: Brooke, "Natural Theology," p. 50. On the reaction to *Vestiges*, see: Gillispie, *Genesis and Geology*,

pp. 156–7. For a recent but interpretively dubious source on Darwinian debates, see: James R. Moore, *Post Darwinian Controversies* (1980).

94. *On the Relation between Religion and Science* (1847), p. 37. This pamphlet first appeared in *Phren. J.*, 20 (1847), 193–239 and appeared in the 9th ed. of 1857, which incorporated Combe's printed but unpublished *An Inquiry into Natural Religion, Its Foundation, Nature, and Application* (Edin., 1853) [Combe Coll., NLS] and which was dedicated to Charles Mackay, appeared with the title *The Relation between Science and Religion*. A 5th ed. of 317 pages appeared in 1872. Combe was seen by freethinkers as having done more than anyone else, save Robert Owen, for the cause of secular education and the removal of "the chimeras of special providence and efficacy of prayer": J. M. Wheeler, *Biographical Dictionary of Freethinkers* (1889), p. 85.

95. Cf. the ultrapositivist view in F. V. Konstantinov et al., "Science: its place and role in the life of society," in *Fundamentals of Marxist–Leninist Philosophy*, trans. R. Daglish (Moscow, 1974), 507–33 at p. 508; cf. also W. R. Comstock, "Consciousness, Purpose, and Mystery" [review of Harold Schilling, *Science and Religion* and *The New Consciousness in Science and Religion*], *Zygon*, 12 (1977), 390–412, esp. p. 392; and John Skorupski, *Symbol and Theory: a philosophical study of theories of religion in social anthropology* (1976), pp. 2, 18.

96. Max Weber, *The Protestant Ethic and the Spirit of Capitalism* (1904–5; trans. T. Parsons, N.Y., 1930). I have gained useful insights on Calvinism from James L. Peacock, *Consciousness and Change* (Oxford, 1975), pp. 184–95; see also: R. H. Tawney, "Calvin," in his *Religion and the Rise of Capitalism* (1926; 1975), 111–39; and David Landes, *The Unbound Prometheus* (Cambridge, 1969), pp. 21–4.

97. See: Alan Macfarlane, *The Origins of English Individualism* (Oxford, 1978).

98. *Relation between Religion and Science*, p. 12.

99. Cobden to Combe, 1 Aug. 1846, q. in Gibbon, *Life of Combe*, II, p. 218. Having abandoned phrenological satire for calico manufacture, Cobden, after reading the *Constitution of Man*, declared it a "transcript of his own familiar thoughts." He played a leading part in forming the Manchester Phrenological Society and remained a councillor of it, sending skulls back to it from Egypt and elsewhere. His faith in phrenology was cemented in 1836 after Combe delineated his head and discovered the faculty of Veneration pronounced. Ten years later he confessed to Combe, "*That* was a triumph for Phrenology, for you could have formed no such notion from anything you had seen or heard of me": q. in Gibbon, *Life of Combe*, II, p. 218. Also see: Morley, *Cobden*, I, p. 93; and de Giustino, *Conquest of Mind*, pp. 203–4.

CHAPTER 5: *The poacher turned gamekeeper: phrenologists abroad*

1. II, p. 4.
2. See, in particular: J. Harrison, *Second Coming*; and L. Barrow, "Socialism in Eternity: the ideology of plebeian spiritualists, 1853–1913," *Hist. Workshop J.*, 9 (1980), 37–69.
3. J. E. "Shepherd" Smith, "Phrenology," *Shepherd*, 1 (15 Nov. 1834), 90–2 at p. 90; "Phrenology," *Bolster's Q. Mag.*, 1 (May 1826), 179–86 at p. 179; "Lectureship of Phrenology," *J. Health & Dis.*, 1 (1846), 232; *Morning Advertiser*, 28 Nov. 1848, q. in *J. Health & Dis.*, 4 (1848), p. 78; Thomas Morgan, "Letter to H. C. Watson on the History and Statistics of Phrenology in Southampton," *Phren. J.*, 10 (1836/7), 520–25 at p. 524; ibid., 4 (1826/7), pp. 154–5; Martineau, "Combe," p. 270.
4. "Combe's Moral Philosophy," *Spectator*, 10 Apr. 1841, pp. 351–3 at p. 351.
5. [J. T. Smith], "Progressive Diffusion of Phrenology," pp. 407–8. Andrew Combe observed the same prevalence of phrenological paraphernalia in London and thought it "a sign not without meaning to reflecting minds": "Phrenology," p. 193.

6. "Phrenology and Politics," *New Monthly Mag.*, 35 (Nov. 1832), 487–8; "Phrenology: its utility and importance," *Farrier and Naturalist*, 1 (Jan. 1828), 34–5; Edward Jarman Lance, *The Golden Farmer; being an attempt to unite the facts pointed out by Nature in the sciences of geology, chemistry, and botany, with practical operations of husband men . . . increase the employment of the labourer* (1831), frontispiece; the *Non-Phrenological Essay* was by the Rev. H. H. Jones. For examples of unselfconscious use of phrenological vocabulary, see: Alexander Somerville, *Autobiography of a Working Man* (1848), p. 289; J. D. Burn, *The Autobiography of a Beggar Boy* (1855), pp. v, 20; Thomas Low Nichols, *Nichols' Health Manual; being also a memorial of the life and work of Mrs. Mary S. Grove Nichols (1810–1884)* (1887), passim.

7. By the Congregationalist Rev. J. W. Massie of Manchester, *Manchester Guardian*, 20 Dec. 1843, q. in *Phren. J.*, 17 (1844), 212. The claim was justified; among the many papers backing the science were the *Manchester Guardian, Wolverhampton Chronicle, Lincoln Mercury, West Briton and Nottingham Review, Preston Chronicle, Reading Mercury, Sheffield Independent*, and *Dumfries Courier*. The *Scotsman*, edited by Combe's friend and fellow phrenologist Charles Maclaren, was referred to by Sir William Hamilton as the "phrenologists' paper" and on one occasion was edited by Combe; Combe also contributed regularly to the *London Courier*. The *Tyne Pilot* was edited by John Connon[‡] and the *Coventry Herald and Observer* by Charles Bray.[‡] Several phrenologists wrote for the *Spectator*, and the editor of the *Chesterfield Gazette*, H. D. Inglis,[‡] wrote *A Lecture upon the Truth, Reasonableness, and Utility of the Doctrines of Phrenology* (1826).

8. 1 (4 Mar. 1843), p. 57.

9. Alexander Taylor, "Dundee Mechanics' Phrenological Society," *Phren. J.*, 3 (1825/6), 456–8 at p. 456. On other similar groups, see: below.

10. J. C. James, *Thoughts on Phrenology; being a brief dissertation on the principles and progress and tendency of that science* (1836), p. 26.

11. *Necessity of Popular Education, as a National Object* (Edin., 1834), p. 20. Leigh Hunt remarked that this was a work "indispensable to every lover of his species who can afford to purchase it"; *Analyst*, 2 (1835), 413n. Similar may be found in Henry Parr Hamilton, *The Education of the Lower Classes: a sermon* (2nd ed., 1841); or J. P. Kay[-Shuttleworth], *Condition of the Working Classes in Manchester*, the latter, by a friend and fellow educator, having doubtless inspired Simpson.

12. *Phren. J.*, 11 (1838), 222; Samuel Laing, *Atlas Prize Essay, National Distress: its causes and remedies* (1844), p. 19; Combe, q. in Gibbon, *Life of Combe*, I, p. 302 (for full text, see: Chapter 4, note 78).

13. The Stalybridge Mechanics' Institute in 1838 upon the dissolution of the Lit & Phil received all thirty-three of the latter's members into its hall along with "two human skulls and fourteen phrenological casts, [and] books on phrenology." Cited in Mabel Tylecote, *The Mechanics' Institute of Lancashire and Yorkshire before 1851* (Manch., 1957), p. 243n.

14. Page 334.

15. By the Rev. John Davies, *An Estimate of the Human Mind* (1828), I, p. 6. On the SDUK, see: F. A. Cavenagh, "Lord Brougham and the Society for the Diffusion of Useful Knowledge," *J. Adult Educ.*, 4 (1929), 3–37; Monica C. Grobel, "The SDUK, 1826–46," M.A. thesis, London, 1933; J. N. Hays, "Brougham's Society"; Elaine A. Storella, " 'O, What a World of Profit and Delight': the Society for the Diffusion of Useful Knowledge," Ph.D. thesis, Brandeis, 1969; J. G. Crowther, "Henry Brougham, 1778–1868," in his *Statesmen of Science* (1965), 7–73; Chester New, *The Life of Henry Brougham to 1830* (Oxford, 1961), chaps. 17, 18; R. K. Webb, *Working Class Reader* (1955), esp. chaps. 3, 4; and David Vincent, *Bread, Knowledge, and Freedom: a study of nineteenth-century working class autobiography* (1982).

16. See: S. Shapin and B. Barnes, "Science, Nature, and Control: interpreting mechanics' institutes," *Social Stud. Sci.*, 7 (1977), 31–74, esp. at p. 46. See also: L. Stone, "Literacy and Education in England, 1640–1900," *Past & Present*, no. 42

(1969), 69–139 at p. 91; and cf. E. P. Thompson, "Patrician Society, Plebeian Culture," *J. Soc. Hist.*, 6 (1974), 382–405 at p. 383.

17. Gibbon, *Life of Combe*, I, p. 254; *Fifth Annual Report of the Edinburgh School of Arts for 1825–6*, q. in W. H. Marwick, "Early Adult Education in Edinburgh," *J. Adult Educ.*, 5 (1932), 389–404 at p. 393; and H. C. Watson, *Statistics of Phrenology*, p. 41. It is also worth noting the complete absence of reference to phrenology in the ten volumes of the SDUK's *Q. J. Educ.* (1831–5).

18. Vol. XI, pp. 49–50.

19. Quoted in Gibbon, *Life of Combe*, I, p. 234. An EPS member, Fraser was also to become involved with Combe, Hodgson, S. Smith, Simpson, J. P. Nichol, Peter Murray, and other phrenological educators in the Edinburgh Association for Providing Instruction in Useful and Entertaining Sciences (est. 1832). See: S. Shapin, " 'Nibbling at the Teats of Science': Edinburgh and the diffusion of science in the 1830s," in Inkster and Morrell, *Metropolis and Province*, 151–78.

20. "Henderson's Bequest," *Phren. J.*, 7 (1831/2), 656: and Gibbon, *Life of Combe*, I, pp. 256–9.

21. Ibid., I, p. 263n., and advertisements in 5th and 6th editions.

22. One such hawker was James E. "Shepherd" Smith, the Calvinist-raised spiritual seeker who edited the Owenite *Crisis* and later the *Family Herald*. See: W. Anderson Smith, *"Shepherd" Smith, the Universalist: the story of a mind* (1892), p. 191.

    After the Chartist demonstration of 10 Apr. 1848 some educationalists abandoned science instruction and turned (or returned) to overt instruction in bourgeois political economy; see, for example: *The Voice of the People and the Rights of Industry* (Apr./May 1848) edited by Harriet Martineau and Charles Knight; and *Politics for the People* (May/June 1848), edited by Charles Kingsley and others. A parallel might be drawn with British imperialism, which, prior to c. 1855, followed a policy of "improvement through influence," but, when British dominance was challenged, undertook territorial aggression legitimated by racism. See: Ronald Hyam, *Britain's Imperial Century, 1815–1914* (1976).

    On "masses" as a new equivalent for the old aristocracy's fear of the "mob" and its characteristics, see: Raymond Williams, *Culture and Society*, p. 288. Charles Kingsley wrote of the years when "young [bourgeois] lads believed (and not so wrongly) that the masses were their natural enemies, and that they might have to fight, any year or any day, for the safety of their property and the honour of their sisters": q. in G. M. Young, *Early Victorian England, 1830–1865* (1934), II, p. 436; and in F. C. Mather, *Public Order in the Age of the Chartists* (Manch., 1959), p. 1.

23. E.g.: *Hoggs Weekly Instructor*, 4 (19 Dec. 1846), p. 260n.; *Mirror*, (4 Nov. 1837), p. 298.

24. "Mr. Combe's Lecture to the Mechanics of Edinburgh," *Phren. J.*, 7 (1831/2), 657–60; and Gibbon, *Life of Combe*, I, pp. 255–83. This appears to have been Combe's first venture into lecturing to working-class audiences, his first lectures (of 1822) being to small middle-class audiences. In 1835 Combe and those who came together in the Edinburgh Philosophical Association delivered penny lectures in the Cowgate Chapel, Edinburgh, under the auspices of the Society for the Diffusion of Moral and Economical Knowledge. Combe's twenty lectures on moral philosophy, which the title page of the published work claims to have been delivered to the Edinburgh Philosophical Association, were in fact delivered to the Working Mens' Association of Edinburgh in the winter of 1835–6.

25. *Journals*, I, p. 117, entry for 23 Apr. 1836. Certainly by this date the *Constitution of Man* had superceded Brougham's seminal *Practical Observations upon the Education of the People* (1825) as a source of educational inspiration and rationalization. See, for example: John Fletcher, *Discourse on the Importance of the Study of Physiology as a Branch of Popular Education* (Edin., 1836), where "bourgeois liberalism" can be seen to have fully replaced "Whig utilitarianism."

26. A. Smith, "Phrenological Ethics," p. 400; Combe, "Phrenological Analysis of Mr. Owen's New Views of Society," *Phren. J.*, 1 (1823/4), 218–37; Jeffrey,

"Phrenology," p. 253; Combe, "Education in America: State of Massachusetts," *Edin. Rev.*, 73 (1841), 486–502.

27. *Cheltenham J.*, 31 May 1841, n.p.

28. Barber's lectures were reported in the *Bristol Mercury*, 27 Nov., and 4, 11, and 18 Dec. 1841; Owen's debate with Brindley (reputedly before an audience of four thousand) had taken place in Jan. 1841 and had been chaired by the local banker, brass manufacturer, and philanthropist John Scandrett Harford. Brindley had done well in the debate with Owen, but when he debated phrenology with Barber in Bristol in Jan. 1842 his popular support fell away. I am indebted to Mike Neve for this reference.

29. *Brief Reports of Lectures Delivered to the Working Classes of Edinburgh; or, the means in their own power of improving their character and condition* [reprinted from *Edin. Weekly Chron. & Scottish Pilot*] (Edin. [1844]), p. 54. To Cockburn it seemed that in Simpson's declaration "to repress the inferior faculties, and elevate the superior – that was education" Simpson's object was to "reconcile the poor man to his condition, by explaining its necessity and uses, by showing how happiness may be extracted out of it, and how individuals may rise above it": *Journals*, II, p. 84, entry for 30 July 1844. In their obituary on Simpson, the *Spectator* breathed the liberal myth perfectly: "Wholly free from the coarseness and class-prejudice which too often characterize the advocates of popular rights, his eloquence had the refinement of high education and the impress of genuine philanthropy": 17 Sept. 1843, p. 893. See also: *National Education: report of the speeches delivered at a dinner given to James Simpson, Esq., by the friends of education in Manchester* (Manch., 1836). Along with the phrenologists Elliotson, Mackenzie, and John Clendinning and phrenologically intimate educationalists such as William Ellis, Thomas Bastard, Serjeant Adams, and Thomas Wyse, as well as G. Poulett Scrope, Charles Knight, and Thomas Coates, Simpson was a member of the Central Society for Education (the fully Victorian equivalent of the SDUK). The first publication of the CSE observed that "political economy is a subject peculiarly appropriate for the study of those who are likely to become members of Mechanics' Institutions. ... In towns where the working population forms a dense mass, – where strikes, trade unions, and combinations have been so ruinous to the merchant, the manufacturer, and the workman, – it is of the utmost importance that the principles which affect natural wealth and industry would be most thoroughly understood": Charles Baker, "Mechanics' Institutes and Libraries: from the first publication of the Central Society of Education [1837], repr. in Baker, *Contributions to the Publications of the SDUK* (1842), p. 367.

30. "Education, As It Is and as It Should Be," *Analyst*, 7 (Aug. 1837), 70. See also: H. C. Watson, "Phrenology and Political Economy," *Phren. J.*, 11 (1837/8), 201–2 and pp. 247–8; William and Robert Chambers, *Political Economy for Use in Schools and Private Instruction* (Edin., 1852). On the political economist Richard Whately and his relations with Combe, see: de Giustino, *Conquest of Mind*, p. 183, and Gibbon, *Life of Combe*, I, pp. 259–60; on the political economist William B. Hodgson, see his *Life and Letters*.

31. *Phren. J.*, 15 (1842), p. 382; Trevelyan received £41.0.2 back in 1865 when the suit in Chancery for the assets of the Queenwood Community was finished: George J. Holyoake, *The History of Co-operation* (1875), II, p. 469.

32. *Testimonials to Combe*, p. 52. See also: George Lyon, "Essay on Liberty," p. 598; and "The Press and Political Economy," *Phren. J.*, 3 (1825/6 47–51)

33. Ure, *Philosophy of Manufactures* (1835), p. 16. The book was published by the SDUK's publisher Charles Knight. It is worth noting that in 1804 Dr. Ure succeeded George Birkbeck in delivering science lectures to working men in Glasgow, out of which developed the Glasgow Mechanics' Institute in 1823. Ure, author of *A New System of Geology* (1829), a forced reconciliation of Genesis with geology, was also the principal reviewer for the Royal Institution's *Journal of Science and the Arts* and was in many respects W. T. Brande's Scottish counterpart: C. C. Gillespie, *Genesis and Geology*, p. 194; D. L. S. Cardwell, *Orga-*

nization of Science in England (rev. ed., 1972), p. 40; Berman, *Royal Institution*, p. 142.

34. Similarly, certain American policy makers on Vietnam in the 1960s thought that the only way to win the war was to change the social perception or consciousness of that stratum of Vietcong who had recently been aroused by the process of modernization and urbanization: Chomsky, "Objectivity and Liberal Scholarship," pp. 44ff. On liberalism, see: Kenneth R. Minogue, *The Liberal Mind* (N.Y., 1968). On Marx's distinction between "formal" and "real" control, see: Keith McClelland's review of Patrick Joyce's *Work, Society, and Politics* in *Hist. Workshop J.*, 11 (1981), 170–1.

35. *Constitution of Man*, p. 338. For the application of the same philosophy in the Victorian madhouse, see: Andrew Scull, *Museums of Madness* (1979), esp. pp. 71–2.

36. 1846, q. in Edmund K. Blyth, *Life of William Ellis* (1889), p. 142. Known as the founder of the Birkbeck Schools, Ellis along with J. C. Hobhouse, Charles Knight, Francis Place, Birkbeck, and Brougham was an initial subscriber to the London Mechanics' Institute.

37. Thus, wrote the Rev. Joseph Warne, a knowledge of phrenology was especially important for judges, teachers, clergymen and parents: *Phrenology in the Family; or, the utility of phrenology in early domestic education.* Reprinted from the American edition of 1830 and prefaced by "A Christian Mother" [i.e., Mrs. Johanna Graham] (Edin., 1833), p. 61. For a nearly identical statement, see: Spurzheim, *Physiognomical System*, p. 2.

38. This was self-evident to Marx and Engels when they spoke of knowledge as a dialectical function of the social relations of production, e.g., *Communist Manifesto* (1848), in *Collected Works*, vol. 6 (1976), p. 503.

39. Letter to W. B. Hodgson, 19 Aug. 1847, q. in Blyth, *Life of Ellis*, p. 58.

40. On the institutes (in addition to the secondary sources cited below in note 45), see: Cardwell, *Organization of Science*, pp. 39–44, 71–5; J. F. C. Harrison, *Learning and Living, 1790–1960* (1961), 57–89; Brian Simon, *Studies in the History of Education, 1780–1870* (1960); D. A. Hinton, "Popular Science in England". For interpretive focus, see: Thompson, *The Making of the English Working Class* (Harmondsworth, 1968), pp. 817–19; E. Royle, "Mechanics' Institutes and the Working Classes, 1840–1860," *Hist. J.*, 14 (1971), 305–21; Shapin and Barnes, "Nature and Control"; I. Inkster, "English Mechanics' Institutes"; Maxine Berg, *The Machinery Question and the Making of Political Economy, 1815–1848* (Cambridge, 1980), chap. 7.

41. *Mechanics' Mag.*, 7 (21 Apr. 1827), 246. Richard Altick puts the circulation of *Mechanics' Mag.* in 1824 at sixteen thousand: *English Common Reader*, p. 393. On Hodgskin and Robertson and the politics of mechanics' education in London, see: Iorwerth Prothero, *Artisans and Politics in Early Nineteenth Century London: John Gast and his times* (Folkestone, 1979), pp. 191–203; and Simon, *Studies in Education*, p. 216. John G. Godard in his panegyric on Birkbeck at the end of the century came out strongly against *Mechanics' Mag.* for its denial of Brougham and Birkbeck as "the fathers" of the London Mechanics' Institute. Robertson (says Godard), "annoyed by the small notice taken of his attacks . . . , descended to the most flagrant untruth, of which an illustration may be given in his allegation that the subjects to which the greatest degree of attention had been paid since the establishment of the Institution had probably been phrenology and the drama!": *George Birkbeck, the Pioneer of Popular Education* (1884), pp. 137–8.

42. "Observations on Phrenology," 3 (14 Jan. 1826), 202–4; "Outlines of Phrenology," 3 (29 Oct., 19 Nov., 10 Dec. 1825), 11–12, 49–51, 105–6. The *London Mechanics' Register* ran from Nov. 1824 to 1826, becoming then the *New London Mechanics' Register and Magazine of Science and the Useful Arts* (1827–8). Published by Cowie and Strange, it was mostly given to reprinting the lectures in the London Mechanics' Institute.

43. Brougham, *Practical Observations*, cited in Simon, *Studies in Education*, p. 216 (also pp. 215–22). However, this did not check Brougham's enthusiasm for dissem-

inating bourgeois political economy in the institutes. It was at his suggestion that William Ellis prepared lectures on political economy that were sent to every mechanics' institute (for which James Mill wanted itinerant lectures or "men of tolerable capacity trained to be good readers" to deliver them in the institutes). Alexander Bain, *James Mill: a biography* (1882), p. 389; and Berg, "Political Economy for Mechanics," in *Machinery Question*, pp. 161–6. But as Shapin and Barnes have pointed out ("Nature and Control," p. 53), "natural theological knowledge was much more frequently encountered in the Institutes than political economy, which drew analogous conclusions from 'the scientific study of natural laws,' and which might have been expected to have greater appeal to Whigs and reformers. Political economy and its 'iron laws' were indeed frequently explicitly excluded from Institutes' curricula, whereas the natural theological flavour of many courses, particularly in physiology, phrenology and, to an extent, the earth sciences is readily apparent." This may have had something to do with the effort that Brougham put into editing Paley's *Discourse on Natural Theology* (1835). See, too: "On the Study of Natural History," *Saturday Mag.*, I (7 July 1832), 3 and 7 (17 Oct. 1835), 151.

44. Subtitled *a peep at the evil intentions and the evils likely to result from the establishment of the weavers' Mechanic Institution*, as reviewed dismissively by science lecturer Charles Partington in his *Sci. Gaz.*, 16 July 1825, pp. 34–6 – a journal that a few weeks later was to print an article in praise of phrenology by F. Wood.[‡] The mechanics' institutes movement is epitomized in the efforts to establish an institute in Spitalfields, there to convert to bourgeois political economy its very worse victims. For that reason, however, the shrill rhetoric on both sides must be treated as exceptional. See: Ure, *Philosophy of Manufacturers*, pp. 453–6; for a minimally mediated attempt at ideological conversion, see: T. Hodgkin, *Lectures on the Means of Promoting and Preserving Health, Delivered at the Mechanics' Institution, Spitalfields* (1835).

45. Prothero, *Artisans and Politics*, p. 203. When the occupational statistics on the members of the London Mechanics' Institute were released in 1838 after bitter attacks by *Mechanics' Mag.*, it was revealed that of the 1,144 members, 600 could be called working-class, 289 were unaccounted for, but only one person was actually listed as a "mechanic." Skilled tradesmen, comprising about one-third of the members, fell well behind the combined figures for the working and middle classes. "Classification of the Members: London Mechanics' Institute," *Mechanics' Mag.*, 29 (11 Aug. 1838), 311–12. Similar evidence (similarly intended for rhetorical purposes) is contained in the evidence given before the following select committees: *Education in England and Wales*, 1835, VII, pp. 763–1003, esp. app. 3 with evidence from Simpson, A. J. Dorsay,[‡] Samuel Wilderspin, and Francis Place; *Arts and Manufactures*, 1835, V, pp. 375–516, esp. the evidence of Charles Toplis, vice-president of the London Mechanics' Institute; *Education of the Poorer Classes in England and Wales*, 1838, VII, pp. 157–343, esp. the evidence of Kay-Shuttleworth, p. 182, q. 73 (where it is claimed that of 1,526 members of the Manchester Mechanics' Institute only 58 were in any way connected with the mills); *Public Libraries*, 1849, XVII, pp. 1–450, esp. the evidence of Lovett, Langley, and Smiles; and *Newspaper Stamps*, 1851, XVII, esp. the evidence of Thomas Hogg, secretary of the Union of Institutes in Lancashire and Cheshire, and then W. B. Hodgson's successor at Liverpool, pp. 167–75, arguing for the repeal of the taxes on knowledge. See also: John Glyde, *The Moral, Social, and Religious Condition of Ipswich in the Middle of the Nineteenth Century* (Ipswich, 1850; repr. ed., 1971), pp. 69–70.

On the disillusionment of many artisans with the mechanics' institutes and on changes in the clientele, see: Tylecote, *Institutes of Lancashire and Yorkshire*, pp. 38–9, 87; Thomas Kelly, *George Birkbeck, Pioneer of Adult Education* (Liverpool, 1957), pp. 209 ff.; idem, *A History of Adult Education in Great Britain* (Liverpool, 1962; rev. ed., 1970), pp. 112–13, 115; Harold Silver, *The Concept of Popular Education* (1965), pp. 210–26; I. R. Cowan, "Mechanics' Institutes and Science and Art Classes in Salford in the Nineteenth Century," *Vocational Aspect*, 20

(1968), 208; A. T. Patterson, *Radical Leicester* (Leicester, 1954), pp. 235–8; J. W. Hudson, *History of Adult Education* pp. 130 ff.; Webb, *Working Class Reader*, pp. 66–74; Thomas Coates, *Report of the State of Literary, Scientific, and Mechanics' Institutions in England; with a list of such institutions and a list of lectures* (SDUK, 1841); James Hole, *An Essay on the History and Management of Literary, Scientific, and Mechanics' Institutions* (1853); and Frederick Engels, *The Condition of the Working Class in England* (1845; Eng. trans., 1892), in *Karl Marx and Frederich Engels on Britain* (2nd ed., Moscow, 1962), p. 275; cf. J. M. Ludlow and Lloyd Jones, *Progress of the Working Classes, 1832–1867* (1867), p. 169; I. Inkster, "Science and the Mechanics' Institutes, 1820–1850: the case of Sheffield," *Ann. Sci.*, 32 (1975), pp. 451–3; idem, "English Mechanics' Institutes," pp. 278–9 et passim.

46. Thomas Hogg, evidence before the *Select Committee on Newspaper Stamps* (1851), *Parliamentary Papers*, XVII, p. 175.

47. *Science and Religion*, p. 258. For the same without the phrenology, see: Richard Dawes, *An Address Delivered at the Annual Soiree of the Huddersfield Institute, December 13th, 1855* (1856), pp. 16–17; George Boole, *The Right Use of Leisure: an address, deliverd before the members of the Lincoln Early Closing Association, February 9 1847* (1847), p. 14; J. J. Garth Wilkinson, *Science for All: a lecture delivered before the Swedenborg Association* (1847), p. 7.

48. See: "Decay of Literary and Scientific Institutions," *London Pioneer*, 2 (9 Dec. 1847), 536; for an illustration of the shift in subject matter, see: G. W. Roderick and M. D. Stephens "Middle-Class Non-Vocational Lecture and Debating Subjects in 19th Century England," *Br. J. Educ. Stud.*, 21 (1973), 192–201.

    At the Manchester Mechanics' Institute, for example, lectures on physical science diminished from 235 for the period 1835–9 to 127 in 1840–4 to only 88 in 1845–9; at the Polytechnic in Birmingham, chemistry and mathematics ceased to be taught between 1845 and 1850, while photographic and phonetic societies flourished; at Aberdeen, natural philosophy and chemistry were retired for want of custom. (Hudson, *Adult Education*, pp. 130, 65, 61; see also: Altick, *English Common Reader*, pp. 202–3; and Coates, *Report on Literary Institutions*, pp. 51–62.)

49. See: "Mechanics' Institutions," *Taits Mag.*, 5 (1838), 521–6. On the reluctance of some institutes to soften their curricula, see: Dickens's fine caricature, "Dullborough Town Mechanics' Institution," in his *The Uncommercial Traveller* (1861), chap. 12.

50. E. J. Hytch[‡] noted of the London Mechanics' Institute in January 1842 that "upwards of one-third of the directors ... are avowed phrenologists; and at least one-third of the teachers profess a belief in the science." *Phren. J.*, 15 (1842), 185. In the 1830s, the chairman of the Newcastle Mechanics' Institute was the phrenologist John Fife;[‡] W. A. F. Browne[‡] was chairman of the institute in Dumfries, J. I. Hawkins[‡] of the Kentish Town Mechanics' Institute, and G. C. Holland[‡] of the Sheffield Mechanics' Institute.

51. "Phrenology," *Newcastle Chronicle*, 14 May 1836, p. 2 (emphasis added). G. J. Holyoake related the anecdote of a surgeon who, having lectured on phrenology and shown the mind's materiality, considered himself very clever in doing an about-turn with his logic to appease the enquiries of a clergyman. "His profession required a religion," Holyoake added: *Reasoner*, 5 (9 Aug. 1848), 174.

52. J. L. Dyer, "The Hitchin Mechanics' Institute," *Adult Educ.*, 23 (1950), 113–21, 212–20; John Salt, "Isaac Ironside and Education in the Sheffield Region in the First Half of the Nineteenth Century," M.A. thesis, Sheffield, 1960; Inkster, "Phrenology in Sheffield," p. 277; idem, "Science Instruction for Youth in the Industrial Revolution: the informal network in Sheffield," *Vocational Aspect*, 25 (1973), p. 94; Harrison, *Learning and Living*, p. 115. In the returns made by the literary, scientific, and mechanics' institutions in the *Census of Great Britain, 1851: education: England and Wales*, pp. 215–58, several of the mechanics' institutes were still listing phrenology lectures two and three times annually: *Parliamentary Papers* (1854), Vol. LXX.

    It should be noted as well that phrenology was not always confined to the obvious lecture category: A seemingly unconnected subject like the "Principles of Mechanics" could be a vehicle for phrenology when it contained a section on the "Brain and Nervous System – the mechanics of sensation," as did William Mackenzie's course on mechanics to the Manchester Mechanics' Institute, Apr. 1832.

53. *Q. J. Educ.*, 2 (1831), 391.

54. W. Hawkes Smith, "On the Tendency and Prospects of Mechanics' Institutions (being a portion of a lecture lately read before the Birmingham Mechanics' Institution)" *Analyst*, 2 (June 1835), 336. On Combe's lectures in Birmingham, see below, Chapter 8. Brindley was hired for 18 guineas to give a course of six antiphrenology lectures. To these Hawkes Smith replied in two further lectures, and Brindley in Jan. 1839 gave a further four lectures at the School of Arts at 3s 6d for the course or 10s 6d for a family: *Midland Counties Adver.*, 10 Jan. 1839.

55. "Phrenology: relief of the distressed operatives," a handbill dated 25 Apr. 1827, contained in *Phrenological Museum Scrap Book* [I], (MS, Edin. Univ. Libr.). Hamilton's lecture was given in a classroom in the university; Combe's lecture was attended by six hundred persons and lasted three hours: Gibbon, *Life of Combe*, I, p. 192. It was discovered by the Edinburgh Philosophical Association that of all their lectures (on chemistry, botany, geology, astronomy, physiology, etc.), those on phrenology were the best attended. See five reports of this society in NLS, Combe 4 (30–34); and Watson, *Statistics of Phrenology*, p. 131.

56. *Reasoner*, 3 (8 Sept. 1847), 82; on the Finsbury Institute, see: ibid., 4 (26 Apr. 1848), 43.

57. *Phren. J.*, 15 (1842), 86; ibid., 17 (1844), 210. One long gallery of the Manchester Mechanics' Institute was filled with busts, including a complete set displaying the individual organs and another set of the most notorious murderers – altogether, thought *Phren. J.*, the most complete and finest set of casts outside London. See also: "Mr Bally's Phrenological Gallery, Mechanics' Institution," *Manchester Guardian*, 10 Jan. 1844, p. 6; *Catalogue of the Fifth Exhibition at the Manchester Mechanics' Institution, Cooper St., Christmas, 1844–5*: "no. 6, 'Phrenological Room' "; and *Exhibition Gazette 1844–5 with a Catalogue of the Exhibition, Edited by the Manchester Mechanics' Institution* (Manch., 1845). At an earlier exhibition Bally was set up as the practical phrenologist in residence and operated a delineating booth; see: *Exhibition Gaz.*, 27 June 1840, p. 45. Tylecote refers to fifty thousand persons attending the exhibition of 1837–8: *Institutes of Lancashire and Yorkshire*, p. 180. A similar fund-raising exhibition by the Polytechnic in Newcastle in July 1840 supplied at additional cost an illustrated brochure of the exhibited casts, so that the visitor might better understand "the facts illustrative of [phrenology's] truth": prefatory remarks "To the Visitor," *Phrenology Illustrated in a Series of Profiles by J. H. Mole from the Collection of Casts Contributed to the Polytechnic Exhibition Newcastle, with Explanatory Descriptions by Alexander Falkner* (Newcastle, 1840). Similar exhibitions were held in Halifax, Huddersfield, and Bradford in 1840.

Although these exhibitions were for fund raising, they also served other functions – most obviously the celebrating of the wonders of machine technology, thereby to undermine lingering resistence to the mechanical age. See: T. Kusamitsu, "Great Exhibitions before 1851," *Hist. Workshop J.* 9 (1980), 70–89.

58. Spencer T. Hall, *The Phreno-Magnet, and Mirror of Nature: a record of facts, experiments, and discoveries in phrenology, magnetism, etc.*, 1 (1843), 66; idem, *Mesmeric Experiences* (1845), p. 21. On Wakley, see: above, Chapter 3, note 68; for Engels's opinion, see: his *The Dialectics of Nature* (1872–82; trans. & ed. C. Dutt, preface and notes by J. B. S. Haldane, 1940), pp. 299–300, where he criticizes A. R. Wallace's movement into "the world of spirits" via mesmerism. Engels had seen Hall – the "very mediocre charlatan" – in Manchester in the winter of 1843–4 and had undertaken experiments to disprove the theory, since Hall was attempting "to prove thereby the existence of God, the immortality of the soul, and the incorrectness of the materialism that was being preached at that time by the Owenites in all the big towns." (See also: Steven Marcus, *Engels, Manchester, and the Working Class* [N.Y., 1974], pp. 96–97n.) The Elliotson quotation is from

his address to the sixth annual conference of the PA, July 1847, *Zoist*, 1 (Oct. 1843), 230.

Combe hesitated and then introduced into the 5th edition of his *System of Phrenology* (1843) a chapter on "Mesmeric Phrenology." Sir George Mackenzie also came out in favor (*Phren. J.*, 16 [1843], 234–7), as did James Simpson (ibid., 16 [1843], 246–50, and 17 [1844], 261–72; T. S. Prideaux, on the other hand, remained violently opposed: "On the Fallacies of Phreno-Magnetism," *Phren. J.*, 17 (1844), 158–68, and 18 (1845), 15–31. For the opinion of Owenites, see: Chapter 8. On the popular spread of phreno-mesmerism, see also: *New Age*, 1 (10 June 1843), 44–5; *Mesmerist*, 1 (27 May 1843), 23; James Hopkinson, *Victorian Cabinet Maker: the memoirs of James Hopkinson, 1819–1894*, ed. J. B. Goodman (1968), p. 52; T. M. Parssinen, "Mesmeric Performers," *Vict. Stud.* 21 (1977), 87–104; Barrow, "Socialism in Eternity."

59. 10 Apr. 1841, p. 351.
60. Cited in Hinton, "Popular Science," p. 252.
61. Admittedly, this is a vast field in which little research has been carried out; almost alone is Ian Inkster's "A Note on Itinerant Science Lectures, 1749–1850," *Ann. Sci.*, 28 (1972), 235–6; see also: idem, "Sheffield Mechanics' Institutes," pp. 454–5. For the earlier period, see: A. E. Musson and E. Robinson, "Science and Industry in the Late Eighteenth Century," in their *Science and Technology in the Industrial Revolution* (Manch., 1969); John R. Millburn, *Benjamin Martin* (Leyden, 1976), chap. 4, "Itinerant Lecturer, 1740–55"; F. W. Gibbs, "Itinerant Lecturers in Natural Philosophy," *Ambix*, 8 (1960), 111–17; and Nicholas Hans, *New Trends in the Eighteenth Century* (1951), chap. 7, "Adult Education, Sciences, and Mathematics." For our period, see: J. N. Hays, "The London Lecturing Empire, 1800–50," in Inkster and Morrell, *Metropolis and Province*, 91–119; and for the later period, [Henry Wace], "Scientific Lectures: their use and abuse," *Quart. Rev.*, 145 (1878), 35–61. Useful for phrenology, but far from exhaustive, is the section "Phrenological Lectures" in Watson, *Statistics of Phrenology*, pp. 230–1.
62. The cabinetmaker James Hopkinson, after discovering that he had the ability to mesmerize, believed: "If I had a little more cheek, I might have come out as a public mesmerist, as I was able to produce most of the manifestations I had seen Spencer Hall do, only I was not so glib upon the tongue": *Memoirs*, p. 53. (Hopkinson, who already had "a good knowledge of Phrenology," was one of those to find the science wholly confirmed by mesmerism. He exercised his talent for three years before deciding that it weakened the intellect.) For want of a glib tongue, W. R. Henderson[‡] failed as a phrenology lecturer, and Alexander Wilson[‡] did poorly.
63. Bray to Combe, 14 Jan. 1848, Combe Papers, NLS 7391/424.
64. "The Intellectuals," in *Prison Notebooks*, p. 12.
65. Admission 2s front seats, 1s back: handbill in a collection of handbills on mesmerism and phreno-mesmerism in three boxes on "Magic & Mystery" in the Johnson Collection, Bodleian Library, Oxford. (Mr. Reynoldson was a mesmerist who lectured at the Western Institute, Leicester Sq., London and who also did "private consultations" for ills at his Portman Sq. residence: Parssinen, "Mesmeric Performers," p. 100.) Gideon Mantell, the eminently respectable popularizer of geology, attended one such lecture/demonstration in the Egyptian Hall, Picadilly, in 1852 and was shocked to find "at least 150 persons present, at 3/- 2/- and 1/- each!" "The lecturer," he added, was "a dark villainous determined looking man, with a loud monotonous voice and a continuous *utterance*." *The Journal of Gideon Mantell, Surgeon and Geologist Covering the Years 1818–1852*, ed. E. Cecil Curwen (Oxford, 1940), entry for 11 Feb. 1852, pp. 281–2.
66. In consequence of his lectures on phrenology in Glasgow, Smith relates he was "requested by a deputation of the Glasgow Total Abstinence Society, to deliver my lecture on Alimentiveness under its auspices. I did so twice to audiences of six hundred and nine hundred. By the same society in Paisley the same request was preferred, and I delivered the lecture there to about six or seven hundred":

Phren. J., 11 (1837/8), 341. Smith is later found lecturing on the corn laws in Huddersfield and elsewhere.

67. Carlyle, upon first hearing him lecture to the "rich and fair" in Kirkcaldy, thought him possessing talents, if somewhat given to "hypothesis building"; when he heard him again in 1817, he commented: "greatly past comprehension. He seemed to have taken the fly-wheel from his brain.... It appears to have knocked the bottom out of Spurzheim's doctrine in these parts." *Early Letters of Thomas Carlyle, 1814–26*, ed. Charles Eliot Norton (1886), I, pp. 135–6; see also: ibid., pp. 91–6, and II, p. 252. On Allen, see also: M. Barnet, "Matthew Allen, M.D. (Aberdeen), 1783–1845," *Med. Hist.*, 9 (1965), 16–28.

68. *Lit. Gaz.*, 5 Sept. 1829, p. 577 in reference to J. I. Hawkins[‡] and W. H. Crook.[‡]

69. *Science for All*, p. 10; Clement Wilkinson, *James John Garth Wilkinson; a memoir of his life* (1911), pp. 66–9.

70. See: Harriet Martineau's remarks on this in her *Retrospect of Western Travel* (1838), pp. 188–9, cited in Webb, *Martineau*, p. 247.

71. Combe picked up £250 for his lectures in Apr. 1836 to approximately 500 Glaswegians who each paid 10s 6d for the course; he demanded £100 for his course of sixteen 1 1/2 hour lectures in the Newcastle Lit & Phil in 1836, the highest price they had paid for a lecture up to that time. Gibbon, *Life of Combe*, I, pp. 311–12, *Forty-third Annual Report of the Newcastle Literary and Philosophical Society* (Newcastle, 1836); and Watson, *Statistics of Phrenology*, pp. 231–2. By comparison, the well-known lecturer on chemistry Peter Murray was offered by the Newcastle Mechanics' Institute for a course of six lectures only £12 12s: *Eleventh Annual Report of the Newcastle Mechanics' Institution* (Newc., 1835) p. 7. See also: the earnings of the lecturers mentioned in Inkster, "Sheffield Mechanics' Institutes," p. 463; and in Shapin, "Teats of Science," pp. 155–6. A percentage of the takings at the door could be highly profitable in some cases. If Goyder is to be believed, Crook received by these means 500 guineas for his lectures on mnemonics in the Newcastle Lit & Phil in 1832. The audience felt they had been cozened, however, and Crook refused to stay around to lecture on phrenology, "*Not now – not now,*" he said to Goyder, "*it would not take*": Goyder, *Autobiography*, pp. 250–1; Goyder himself seems never to have got above a subsistence level of income.

72. "Syllabus of a Course of Lectures on Phrenology, by Mr. Crook (Member of the Council of the London Phrenological Society, etc., etc.) to Be Delivered at the Crown and Anchor, Strand, on Mon., Tues. and Weds., the 5th, 6th and 7th of February 1827 at 7 pm": handbill in Box "Phrenology and Chirology" in J. Johnson Collection of ephemera, Bodleian Library, Oxford. Crook charged 1 guinea for a gentleman and two ladies; or alternatively 4s per lecture: *Phren. Almanac* 1 (1842), 59.

J. B. Langley in his evidence to the *Select Committee on Public Libraries* in 1849 claimed that a lecturer could earn from £500 to £1,000 per annum and that "in some places lectures have been overdone. Lecturing now having become so profitable": *Parliamentary Papers*, 1849, XVII, pp. 152–5; see also the evidence of Lovett, in ibid., p. 180. There seems little doubt that the decline in science lectures in the 1840s bore some relation to cost of lectures.

The cost of phrenology lectures to the auditor varied according to place, lecture, and seat – e.g.:

Cameron	Liverpool (Paris Rms.)	1824	1g 12 lects.
Crook	Private	1828	20g
Spurzheim	Sheffield (Tontine Rm.)	1829	2g 12 lects. or 3s each
Aitken	Dundee	1835	3d (front seats), 6d (back)
Combe	Newcastle (Lit & Phil)	1835	10s 6d per lect.
Weir	Glasgow (Andersonion Univ.)	1836	2s 6d per lect.
Brindley	Birmingham (Soc. of Arts)	1839	1s; 3s 6d for 4 lects. or 10s 6d for a whole family

Martin	Sheffield (Owenite Hall)	1840	2d per lect.
J. Wilson	Birmingham (Med. Sch.)	1842	3s per lect.
			or 15s for 6
P. Jones	London (Owenite Hall)	1840s	1d per lect.

73. Like the cost of lectures, the cost of delineations varied: John Boyd[‡] was fairly typical in charging 1s for a verbal account, 2s 6d for a written account, and 5s for a written and detailed account (written accounts were usually given in printed booklets which also gave a potted history of the science, a list of its eminent supporters, etc.). Crook[‡] in 1828 and Hawkins[‡] in 1829 both charged 2 guineas for a written delineation, 1 guinea for a verbal account; Rumball[‡] charged 5s in 1842 for a full delineation, while John Wilson[‡] could be consulted for "practical applications" for 20s, 10s, 5s, or 2s 6d; Madame Bernard in 1844 in London charged 1s, 3s, or 5s, and H. Bushea[‡] in 1846 from 2s 6d (written) to 20s (full sketch delineation and a private lecture). Alexander Verner, a practical phrenologist in Bolton at the end of the century, charged from 2s 6d for a verbal account (with advice on health) to £3 3s for a "complete and carefully written Mental and Physical analysis, recommended in extreme and dangerous cases; a minute and reliable guide for parents in training delicate or imperfectly organized children, with Self-Instructor." Like most other phrenologists at the time, Verner also did delineations from photographs for 2s 6d: *Practical Phrenology* (Bolton, 1902).

An advertisement for Donovan's London Phrenological Institute in the *People's Phren. J.* 1 (1843), 96 sums up the commercial-cum-social outlook of many itinerant phrenologists by that date: "Mr Donovan's fee from the wealthier classes is half-a-guinea at the minimum; but he is at all times glad to devote his time to the operative classes on terms suited to their means, feeling convinced that the progress of phrenology will be rather from the humbler to the higher than the contrary."

The cost of a cast of a head was usually between 1s 6d and 2s 6d; Goyder[‡] and Deville[‡] were both suppliers, as was Anthony O'Neil of Edinburgh, who sold replicas of famous heads in the Edinburgh Phrenology Museum (at 30 for £2 15s).

Craig, Crook, Goyder, Deville, Epps, and Donovan all had their "manuals" of phrenology; Combe sold 200 copies of the *Constitution of Man* at 1s 6d to the auditors of his 1831 lectures in Edinburgh (*Phren. J.*, 7 [1831/2], 657).

74. Bushea, Deville, Donovan, Falkner, Goyder, and Levison. Donovan charged 3 guineas for nine private lessons in his London Phrenological Institution (est. 1840), 5 guineas for two persons taking the lessons together, and 6 guineas for three persons. On C18 "medical institutions" and window shop museums, see: Eric Jameson [i.e., E. J. Trimmer], *The Natural History of Quackery* (1961), p. 99.

75. "The Country Phrenologists," *Inspector & Nat. Mag.*, 3 (June 1827), 151.

76. Thus did Mantell accuse the lecturer referred to above (note 65). For the contents of a conventional phrenology lecture to a mechanics' institute, see: Goyder, *Autobiography*, pp. 346–84.

77. Holyoake, *History of Co-operation*, I, p. 375; and *New Moral World* 4 (18 Nov. 1837), 28.

78. William Mattieu Williams, *Vindication of Phrenology* (1894), pp. 257–8; Eastlake, *Journals and Correspondence* (1895), I, pp. 65–6; *Crisis*, 4 (3 May 1834), pp. 32–4. Besides lecturing on "The Course of Women's Freedom," she also lectured on temperance; see: *Crisis*, 3 (1 Feb. 1834), 191; *Phren. J.*, 13 (1840), 187–8; ibid, 20 (1847), 449–50.

79. *Chapters in the Life of a Dundee Factory Boy: an autobiography* (Dundee, 1850), pp. 72–3. Another example of phrenologists inflicting their knowledge upon rural culture (symbolically, the urban–industrial present and future over the agrarian

past) is to be found in the endeavors of the Woods family of Campsall Hall, near Doncaster. In 1837 they established the Campsall Society for the Diffusion of Useful Knowledge, which endeavored to elevate the forty-odd "labourers, artisans, farmers, etc" by reading to them from the *Penny Magazine*. This soon developed into a platform for phrenology lectures by Charles Wood[‡] – lectures that were to receive glowing accounts in the *Analyst*, edited by Charles's brother Neville. See: "Campsall Society for the Acquisition of Knowledge," *Analyst*, 7 (Aug. 1837), 100; "Hints on Educational Reform in Connexion with Phrenology," *Phren. (Anthropol.) Mag. & Christian Physician*, 2 (May 1837), 256; C. T. Wood, "Society for the Acquisition of Knowledge of Campsall and Its Vicinity," ibid., 3 (Nov. 1837), 70–2; "Campsall Newspaper Club," ibid., 4 (Jan. 1839), 145–54. Nevertheless, while the urban-over-rural intentions of phrenologists are clear (Combe helped form in Edinburgh the Association for Aiding Country Lectures on Science), examples of phrenologists conscientiously taking their science into the country are not plentiful. The *Nottingham Review* stated in reference to James K. Dow's[‡] lectures on phrenology in the village of Beeston, near Nottingham, "We believe that this is the only instance in which knowledge had been thus disseminated in any village weekly": 16 Mar. 1838, p. 5.

80. E.g., James Jennings, *Inquiry Concerning Phrenology*, p. 1; or for the same, the opening line of Epps, *Manual of Phrenology* (n.d.), p. 1.

81. *Twelfth Year's Report of the Committee of the Literary, Scientific, and Mechanical Institution of Newcastle-upon-Tyne* (Newcastle, 1836), p. 6. It was regarded as consolation for not having reached the standards of Leonard Horner's Edinburgh School of Arts.

82. *Derby Reporter*, 1 Nov. 1844, q. in *Phren. J.*, 18 (1845), 91.

83. T. Morgan, "Phrenology in Southampton," pp. 520–5.

84. Cleckheaton example cited in Harrison, *Learning and Living*, p. 115; Northampton: *Mesmerist*, 1 (1 July 1843), 64. A phrenology class was established in the Manchester Mechanics' Institute in the early 1830s, in the Heybridge Institute in the early 1840s; Derby's class was established in 1832, Hitchen's in 1844, Halifax's in 1842, Leeds's about the same time, London Mechanics' Institute's in 1831, City of London Mechanics' Institute (a place for mutual instruction only, est. in 1836) in 1843 (led by W. H. Newman[‡]), Westminster Mechanics' and Literary Institute's in 1837 (led by the surgeon W. U. Whitney[‡]). The Social Institution, John Street, had a Sunday afternoon class in 1840 led by Richard Redburn (on whom see: below Chapter 8), and Lovett's National Hall, Holborn, had a class in 1843 led by Peter Jones.[‡]

85. *Phren. Almanac*, 1 (1842), p. 59.

86. The London Mechanics' Institute's class cost 6d per quarter, Southampton's 2s 6d per quarter, Social Institution's 1d per lesson or 1s 6d per quarter or 4s for 7 months, and Liverpool's 5s per annum. Members of the Dundee Mechanics' Phrenological Society paid 2s 2d per meeting until £1 had been submitted.

87. *Phren. J.*, 14 (1841), 193. The phrenologist William Mattieu Williams, later the principal of Combe's Edinburgh Secular School, was one such graduate of the class. The class is first referred to in *Phren. J.*, 7 (1831/2), 479. See also: ibid., 10 (1836/7), 742; and 20 (1847), 186.

88. The members of the class solicited Epps[‡] in 1839 and presented their requisition to the Managing Committee, signed by 430 members. The committee, however, rejected this application by a vote of 13 to 12, possibly because of Epps's radicalism or perhaps because his fee was thought too high. The members then voted unanimously to engage another phrenologist, Simon Logan,[‡] an LPS member who was then delivering highly popular lectures in various parts of the country. This proposal was carried, and Logan's three lectures were attended by upwards of 800 persons. *Phren. J.*, 12 (1839) 107, 187.

89. *Phren. J.*, 11 (1838), 218, 338; other subjects of discussion are given in the above reference. Another list of subjects discussed and the persons presenting the papers

in 1848 is given in G. Combe, R. Cox, et al., *Moral and Intellectual Science Applied to the Elevation of Society* (N.Y., 1848), p. 112. W. C. Corson's lecture "Phrenology Considered in Relation to the Soul" before the members of the Sheffield Phrenological Society in 1850 seems a familiar theme by that time in the phrenology classes: cited in Inkster, "Phrenology in Sheffield," p. 278.

90. Hytch, *Phren. J.*, 20 (1847), 186; the *British Controversialist and Impartial Inquirer* (comprised of letters primarily from members of mutual instruction societies, and aimed at that audience) virtually launched itself with the debate on "Is Phrenology True?" 1 (July/Nov. 1850), 83–228 (serially). In Hytch's opinion it was the duty of a phrenologist to act as a moral physician and not permit "the deep-seated cancer [i.e., abuse of the animal faculties] . . . to strengthen and riot in the system unmolested": "The Philosophy of Phrenology," *London Phalanx*, 1 (11 Dec. 1841), 586.

91. Shapin and Barnes, "Nature and Control," p. 57; on the "failure" of the institutes, see: Inkster, "English Mechanics' Institutes": and R. N. Price, "The Working Men's Club Movement and Victorian Social Reform Ideology," *Vict. Stud.*, 15 (1971), 117–47. Cf. Royle, "Mechanics Institutes." For Tory criticism of Brougham & Co. for passing by "the tens of thousands of coal-heavers, carmen, dustmen, bricklayers, labourers, porters, and servants and labourers of all descriptions, tailors, shoemakers, etc, etc," see: [David Robinson], "Brougham on the Education of the People," *Blackwoods*, 17 (1825), 534–51 at p. 538.

92. In the Birmingham Mechanics' Institute 240 out of a total of 485 members were under 21 years old; in the York Mechanics' Institute, 119 out of 404; in Manchester 739 members were under 21, 769 over 21; and in the Sheffield Mechanics' Institute statistics on the conversation class between June 1850 and Mar. 1851 show 308 under 21 and only 26 over 21: Coates, *Report on Literary Institutions*, pp. 19–20; and *Analyst*, 4 (Jan. 1836), 135–7. The Sowerby Bridge Mechanics' Institute (est. 1838) divided its members into three classes: first – proprietors, second – subscribers, and third – subscribers under 21; in 1840, 51 out of 153 were third-class (most trades were represented, the largest group being 16 piecers, then 10 mechanics, 8 joiners, 7 spinners, 5 fullers, 4 weavers). *Halifax Express and Huddersfield, Bradford, and Wakefield J.*, 23 May 1840, p. 2. On age, see also: Inkster, "Science Instruction for Youth," p. 94. A. R. Wallace and his brother, for example, were 13 and 18 years old when they attended the Social Institution in 1836: *My Life: a record of events and opinions* (1905), I, p. 87; Alexander Bain attended the Aberdeen Mechanics' Institute between the ages of 13 and 16: *Autobiography* (1904), p. 16. Against the argument that these youths were in the institutes more by accident than by design, we may cite the discussion in Manchester in 1839 to establish an "Institution of Practical Science" to be modeled on the Adelaide Gallery in London (est. 1830) and aimed at the "younger classes." Leading this discussion was the institute's future director, H. H. Birley, local Tory and civic worthy, infamous as leader of the charge at Peterloo two decades previously. Cited in Robert Kargon, *Science in Victorian Manchester* (Baltimore and London, 1977), p. 36.

The quotation on the superior order of worker in the institutes comes from Samuel Smiles's evidence, *Select Committee on Public Libraries, 1849*, XVII, p. 126 in reference to the 16,000 members of the Yorkshire Union of Mechanics' Institutes.

93. Hudson, *History of Adult Education*, p. vi. On the difficulty of understanding exactly which audience the managers of mechanics' institutes saw themselves as aiming at when they referred to their target as the "intelligent artisan," see: Thomas Wright, "The Working Man's Education," in his *Some Habits and Customs of the Working Classes* (1867), pp. 3–4. It should not be forgotten that the aims of middle-class educators changed between the 1820s and 1840s; see: Berg, *Machinery Question*, pp. 145–73.

94. See: Armytage, *Technocrats*, p. 105; R. Q. Gray, "Styles of Life; the 'labour aristocracy' and class relations in later nineteenth century Edinburgh," *Int. Rev.*

Soc. Hist., 18 (1973), 428–52; and cf. G. W. Roderick and M. D. Stephens, "Science, the Working Classes, and Mechanics' Institutes," *Ann. Sci.*, 29 (1972), 349–60 at p. 360.

95. Prothero, *Artisans and Politics*, p. 194; and he adds, the institutes "offered the opportunity of gratifying widely-felt needs. There was the hope of rising socially, for with industrial and commercial expansion there was an ever-growing need for educated people, not only clerks and supervisors but also manual workers. Changes in technology militated against learning in the traditional way by precept and working by the eye and necessitated the use of plans and scale drawings." For the sources of phrenology's working-class support, see: below, Chap. 6.

96. On Browne, *Phren. J.*, 12 (1839), 109; he was also highly esteemed as the chairman of the Dumfries Mechanics' Institute; see: W. H. Marwick, "Mechanics' Institutes in Scotland," *J. Adult Educ.*, 6 (1933), 292–309 at p. 296. For examples of his remarkable success as a lecturer on phrenology both before and after his appointment as superintendent of the Montrose Asylum, see: *Phren. J.*, 8 (1832/4), 571–2, 662–3; and ibid., 11 (1838), 214. On Witham: *York Herald*, 6 Aug. 1836, q. in *Phren. J.*, 10 (1836/7), 245; see also: his obituary in ibid., 18 (1845), 188.

97. *New Moral World*, 2 (18 June 1836), p. 267. The quotation and other references are from his *Necessity of Popular Education*, pp. 14, 9–11, 23. Each of his Edinburgh lectures for the Society for the Diffusion of Moral and Economical knowledge in 1835 was attended by over a thousand mainly working-class persons, and in 1844 three thousand working men solicited him to give further lectures, presenting him with lavish testimonials and a handsome purse. See: app. to his *The Philosophy of Education* (Edin., 1836), pp. 251–6, and on the SDMEK, see: above, notes 19, 24; Marwick, "Early Adult Education in Edinburgh," pp. 401–2; and Simpson, *Brief Reports*, p. 1; and see: "Proposed Testimonial to James Simpson Esq. Advocate," NLS (a sheet soliciting money to give to Simpson for all he had done for the "moral and social elevation" of the Edinburgh working class).

98. A. Tyrrell, "Class Consciousness in Early Victorian Britain: Samuel Smiles, Leeds Politics, and the Self-Help Creed," *J. Br. Stud.*, 9 (1970), 103–25 at p. 120; and see also: Harrison, *Learning and Living*, p. 53; idem, "Adult Education and Self Help," *Br. J. Educ. Stud.*, 6 (1957/8), 37–50 at p. 46. On people's colleges etc. see: "Mechanics' Institutions and People's Colleges," *People*, 2 (1850), 358; on lyceums, see: Coates, *Report on Literary Institutions*, p. 43; on Owenites' halls of science, see: A. Black, "Education before Rochdale: the Owenites and the halls of science," *Co-operative Rev.*, 29 (1955), 42–44; and Eileen Yeo, "Robert Owen and Radical Culture," in Sidney Pollard and John Salt, eds., *Robert Owen: prophet of the poor* (1971), 84–114 at pp. 90–5. On the best-known breakaway mechanics' institute (in which phrenology figured) see: "New Mechanics' Institution, Manchester," *Analyst*, 3 (Oct. 1835), 155–6; "Mechanics' Institutions," *Working Man's Friend*, 12 Jan. 1833, p. 32; and R. G. Kirby, "An Early Experiment in Workers' Self-Education: the Manchester New Mechanics' Institution, 1829–35," in D. S. L. Cardwell, ed., *Artisan to Graduate* (Manch., 1974), 87–98. For illuminating details on a mutual improvement society in the potteries in the 1840s, see: Charles Shaw, *When I Was a Child* (1903; repr. ed., 1969), chap. 23, "The Pursuit of Knowledge under Difficulties."

99. Pages 219 ff.

100. *The Life of Thomas Cooper Written by Himself* (1872), p. 169. The republican engraver James Linton advertised phrenology as one of the subjects for discussion at (and hopefully to revive) the Walthamstow Mutual Instruction Society, which he had established in 1839: F. B. Smith, *Radical Artisan: William James Linton, 1822–97* (Manch., 1973), p. 44.

101. See: J. Salt, "The Sheffield Hall of Science," *Vocational Aspect*, 12 (1960), 133–8; and Inkster, "Phrenology in Sheffield," p. 277. There were lectures in the Hall of Science (est. by I. Ironsides and Robert Owen in 1839) by Emma Martin[‡] in Dec. 1840 and G. J. Holyoake[‡] in Aug. 1841.

102. Bain, *Autobiography*, p. 26.

103. "Mutual Instruction Societies," *London Sat. J.*, 3 (29 Feb. 1840), 129–32; see also: "Useful Knowledge: with a few hints to members of mutual instruction societies," ibid., 3 (18 Apr. 1840), 232–3. On the setting up of a mutual instruction society, see: Christopher Thomson, *The Autobiography of an Artisan* (1847), pp. 335 ff.

     Goyder discovered a mutual instruction group near Scarborough where the members, having purchased some plaster casts and copies of the *Constitution of Man*, had studied the science diligently until their Methodist preacher denounced the science as infidel. Goyder assured them of the harmony between phrenology and scripture, and the group reassembled. *People's Phren. J.*, 1 (11 Feb. 1843), 60.

104. Myles, *Autobiography*, p. 73.

105. At the "Phrenological Association and Meeting," *Newcastle Courant*, 7 Sept. 1838, pt. II, p. 3. E.g.: *Selections from the Phrenological Journal*, ed. Robert Cox (Edin. and Boston, 1836) apparently sold eighteen thousand copies the first year; Robert Macnish, *Introduction to Phrenology* (1836) exhausted a first edition of two thousand in six months; Robert Hunter's anonymously published *Philosophy of Phrenology Simplified* (1836) was into a third edition and had sold four thousand by 1845; George Macnish's *Catechism of Phrenology* (1831) sold nine hundred copies during its first ten days, seventeen hundred copies by the end of three months, was into a 7th edition by 1834, and advertised the thirty-four thousandth in 1857 (noted by Robert Macnish, *The Modern Pythagorean: a series of tales, essays, and sketches, by the late Robert Macnish, LLD with the author's life by his friend D. M. Moir* [Edin., 1838], I, pp. 371 ff.). Such a successful work invited sequels: George Macnish, *Phrenology Simplified* (1836); and idem, *Science of Phrenology* (1838). In addition were the vast stock of manuals on phrenology by Epps, Spurzheim, Akin, Donovan, Deville, Bridges, Boyd, and many others. Common in journals such as the *New Moral World*, *Parthenon*, and *Reasoner* were back-page advertisements for 1d to 4d publications such as Goyder's *Epitome of Phrenology* (n.d.); idem, *Acquisitiveness* (1837); Crook's *Compendium* (1828); Edwin Saunders's *What Is Phrenology?* (1835); Engledue's *Cerebral Physiology and Materialism* (1842); Dewhurst's *Grammar of Phrenology* (1834); and John Mills's *A Catechism of Practical Phrenology* (Leeds, 1851). The demand for more serious-minded elementary texts declined after mid-century, but sales remained steady for works such as those by Bridges,[‡] A. L. Vago, J. Inwards,[‡] A. Cheetham, and above all L. N. Fowler[‡] between 1860 and 1900. At the turn of the century the "pier phrenologists" (the Ellis family at Blackpool and Morecambe, J. J. Spark at Bournemouth, and the Severns at Brighton) issued innumerable phrenological manuals, while in London Jessie Fowler[‡] (the last of the "phrenological Fowlers") and then Stackpool O'Dell of Ludgate Circus did the same.

     Mechanics' and similar institutes purchased many of the more high-minded phrenological works: The Newcastle Mechanics' Institute was fairly typical, with a copy of Combe's *System* in the library by 1827 and Combe's *Letter to Francis Jeffrey* being purchased in 1829. The eighth annual *Report* reveals the phrenologist Arthur Trevelyan the benefactor of copies of *Phren. J.* As much as 20% of the books in the Warrington Mechanics' Institute in 1847 were on phrenology; see: Hinton, "Popular Science," table V, p. 251. (Due to donations and various other factors, however, library catalogs are a poor guide to the concerns within most institutes.)

106. This decision was apparently made in 1834 just after Robert Chambers had been converted to phrenology upon hearing Combe lecture and when, as it happened, the sales of the journal had begun to slip (Altick puts the circulation in 1832 at fifty thousand [p. 393]); thereafter, to the accompaniment of a highly favorable article on phrenology (entitled "Is Ignorance Bliss?" 2 [4 Jan. 1834], 385–8), the circulation rose by ten thousand on each successive number. See: De Giustino, *Conquest of Mind*, p. 52; William Chambers, *Memoir of Robert Chambers with Autobiographical Reminiscences of William Chambers* (Edin., 1872). "I have reason to know," Robert Chambers said in his testimonial to Combe in 1836, "that

[phrenology] is making rapid progress amongst the more thinking portions of the middle and lower ranks ... tending without the sanction of the learned, to embrace the great body of the people" (*Testimonials*, pp. 55–7).

107. W. J. Linton, *James Watson: a memoir* (Manch., 1880), p. 27; *New Moral World*, 3 (4 Feb. 1837), 117. See also: the evidence of W. E. Hickson, *Select Committee on Newspaper Stamps*, p. 478, q. 3249–51, who asserted that no one earning less than 16s a week could be found taking *Chambers* or the *Penny Mag*. Robert Chambers was aware of and regretted the opinion of his journal held by radicals; he was consoled, however, by the journal's circulation and by the fact that "our labours ... are profitable beyond our hopes, beyond our wants." Letter to Leigh Hunt, q. in Chambers, *Memoir* (1884), p. 249.

108. "Phrenology," *Moral Reformer*, 1 (Mar./May 1838), 77–115 (serially); "Phrenology," *The People*, 1 (1848), 280, 297–8; "The Works of O. S. Fowler, the American Phrenologist and Physiologist," ibid., 1 (1849), 291; "All Our Faculties Should Be Cultivated," ibid., 3 (1851), 282; "The Laws of Nature and Human Nature," ibid., 1 (1848), 167; "Combe's Works," ibid., 1 (1848), 199. Barker was so enthused by Fowler's works that he published them at 2d each (on the circulation of *The People*, which was dedicated to "Phrenology, Teetotalism, Theological Reform, Dietetics ... and all that contributes to the free and full development of the whole human being and of the whole human family," see: *Life of Joseph Barker Written by Himself*, ed. John Thomas Barker [1880], p. 288, and the evidence of Abel Heywood to *Select Committee on Newspaper Stamps*, pp. 373–5); "Mr George Combe and the Philosophy of Phrenology," *Fraser's Mag.*, 22 (Nov. 1840), 509–20 at p. 509.

109. 27 Dec. 1834, q. in *Phren. J.*, 9 (1834/6), 284.

110. 27 Jan. 1838, q. in *Phren. J.*, 11 (1838), 219.

111. Cited in De Giustino, *Conquest of Mind*, p. 204.

112. Hays, "Science and Brougham's Society," pp. 231, 238; cf. A. Tyrrell, "Political Economy, Whiggism, and the Education of Working-Class Adults in Scotland, 1817–40," *Scottish Hist. Rev.*, 48 (1969), 151–65, esp. p. 155; R. Johnson, "Educational Policy and Social Control in Early Victorian England"; Simon, *Studies in Education*, p. 132 et passim; D. G. Paz, "Working Class Education and the State, 1839–1849: the sources of government policy," *J. Brit. Stud.*, 16 (1976), 129–52; Webb, *Working-Class Reader*, pp. 64–5. See also: A. P. Donajgrodski, ed., *Social Control in Nineteenth Century Britain* (1977).

113. E.g., H. F. Kearney, "Puritanism, Capitalism, and the Scientific Revolution," *Past & Present*, no. 28 (1964), 80–101, esp. p. 85. For a similar approach but without the specific anti-Marxist coloration, see: K. Fielden, "Samuel Smiles and Self-help," *Vict. Stud.*, 12 (1968/9), 155–76, who argues that because Smiles cannot be found with his hand actually in the till he was truly concerned with elevating the working class and was not engaged in defending industrial capitalism.

114. Almost all of secondary sources on adult education cited in this chapter have illustrations of such working-class "demystifications." Thompson provides many others in *The Making*, but he is also aware that "those moments in which governing institutions appear as the direct, emphatic, and unmediated organs of a 'ruling-class' are exceedingly rare, as well as transient" ... and that "attempts to short-circuit analysis end up by explaining nothing": "The Peculiarities of the English," p. 48. For an incisive comment on the non-Marxist nature of much left-wing history of the working class, see: D. Selbourne, "On the Methods of the History Workshop," *Hist. Workshop J.*, 9 (1980), 150–61.

115. *Condition of the Working Class in England*, p. 275; cf. Prothero, *Artisans and Politics*, p. 195.

116. The rhetoric of educators might lead one to suppose exceptions, however: Dr. Thomas Murray, lecturer on political economy, told Cockburn in 1838 that he had just finished twenty eight lectures to a thousand mechanics in Dunfermline who had come to his first lecture expecting to hear "the doctrines of Radicalism demonstrated; but that being interested in the principles of wages, pauperism, population, combination, machinery, free trade, emigration, etc., and not stupefied by such subjects as money, taxation, banking, etc., they not only remained

[but] ... made him double the length of the course." *Journals of Henry Cockburn*, I, pp. 177–8. On Murray's conversance with phrenology see his *Autobiographical Notes*, ed. John A. Fairley (Dumfries, 1911), pp. 51, 64, 72, 89.

117. John Foster, *Class Struggle and the Industrial Revolution: early industrial capitalism in three English towns* (1974). For references to the many outstanding reviews of Foster's book and the historical and historiographical issues raised by it, see: G. McLennan, " 'The Labour Artistocracy' and 'Incorporation': notes on some terms in the social history of the working class," *Social Hist.* 6 (1981), 71–81.

118. Indeed, we might say that in the beginning was "the word," which, once uttered, bore a value load determining the structure of future thought and the patterns and shapes of the economic structure. On "the value" as the beginning, see: R. M. Young, "The Anthropology of Science," *Sci. Stud.*, 1 (1971), 177–206. On the need to redefine "base as a human and dynamic concept," see: Raymond Williams, "Base and Superstructure in Marxist Cultural Theory," *New Left Rev.*, no. 82 (1973), 3–16; and idem, *Marxism and Literature* (Oxford, 1977), pp. 75–82; S. Hall, "Rethinking the "Base-and-Superstructure" Metaphor," in Bloomfield, *Papers on Class*, 43–72; and V. N. Volosinov, "Concerning the Relationship of the Basis and Superstructures," in his *Marxism and the Philosophy of Language*, trans. L. Matejka and I. R. Titunik (N.Y. and London, 1973), 17–24.

119. See: S. Feuchtwang, "Investigating Religion," in Maurice Bloch, ed., *Marxist Analysis and Social Anthropology* (1975), 61–81 at p. 62.

120. Luke Burke[‡] in 1864 thought that the science had become "a sort of religion" (see: C. Donovan, *The Ethnological Society and Phrenology*, p. 17); others were more certain: "Are you aware," wrote James Wordsworth to Combe in 1839, "that in your *Constitution of Man* you have given a new Religion to the world? The views of the divine government there unfolded will in time subvert all other religions, and become a religion themselves": q. in Mackay, "Combe," in his *Forty Years Recollections* (1877), II, p. 255.

121. *The Making*, esp. pp. 392–3, 437, and the section "The Chiliasm of Despair," pp. 411–40; see also: his "Time, Work Discipline, and Industrial Capitalism," *Past & Present*, no. 38 (1967), 56–97, repr. in M. W. Flinn and T. C. Smout, eds., *Essays in Social History* (Oxford, 1974), 39–77, esp. pp. 61 ff.

122. See: his 1968 postscript in *The Making*, pp. 917–23; and his review of Robert Moore, *Pit-Men, Preachers and Politics: the effects of Methodism in a Durham mining community* (Cambridge, 1974), in *Br. J. Sociol.*, 27 (1976), 387–402. See also: F. K. Donnelly, "Ideology and Early English Working-Class History: Edward Thompson and his critics," *Social Hist.*, 1 (1976), 219–38.

123. Mannheim, *Ideology and Utopia* (1936; repr. ed., 1960), p. 54: "It is only when we more or less consciously seek to discover the source of [individuals'] untruthfulness in a social factor, that we are properly making an ideological interpretation"; see also ibid., pp. 237–47.

CHAPTER 6: *Secular Methodism*

1. *Afterthoughts on Material Civilization and Capitalism* (Baltimore, 1977), p. 42.

2. See: Douglas, "Environments at Risk," in her *Implicit Meanings*, pp. 230–48; Sir Andrew Huxley, "Fact and Value Must Not Be Confused," *Times Higher Educ. Suppl.*, 7 Oct. 1977, p. 21; D. Ingleby, "Ideology and the Human Sciences: some comments on the role of reification in psychology and psychiatry," in Trevor Pateman, ed., *Counter Course: a handbook for course criticism* (Harmondsworth, 1972), 51–81 at p. 54; and Roland Barthes, "Operation Margarine," in his *Mythologies*, 41–2.

3. See: the letter from a London mechanic to Elliotson in *Zoist*, 1 (Oct. 1843), p. 273; and "Combe and the Philosophy of Phrenology," *Fraser's Mag.*, 22 (Nov. 1840), 509.

4. See: A. L. Morton "Pilgrim's Progress," *Hist. Workshop J.*, 5 (1978), 3–8. For literal evidence of artisan conflation of phrenology and Bunyan, see: Hopkinson, *Memoirs*, pp. 52–6.

5. *Reasoner*, 3 (29 Sept. 1847), 539; for other different political–religious views of

working people in specific reference to phrenology, see: W. B. (of Bradford) to Barker, *The People*, 1 (1848), 167; and *Nottingham J.*, 5 June 1840, p. 3.

6. See: E. P. Thompson, *The Making*, pp. 259, 711; and Prothero, *Artisans and Politics* pp. 5, 332–33, et passim. For a specific contextualization and discussion of the dependent artisanry, see: F. K. Donnelly and J. L. Baxter, "Sheffield and the English Revolutionary Tradition, 1791–1820," *Int. Rev. Soc. Hist.*, 20 (1975) 398–423.

7. This is not to dispute that long before the second quarter of the C19 it was possible for artisans along with some lower-middle-class and laboring elements to be alienated from the established order of society, due largely to changes in their status (as Weber suggested in his classic thesis on the origins of religious radicalism). Gwyn Williams, *Artisans and Sans-culottes: popular movements in France and Britain during the French Revolution* (1968), refers to the radicals of the 1790s as "socially displaced persons," and J. F. C. Harrison (confirming Weber) calls attention to the late C18 appeal of millenarianism among artisans, small farmers, shopkeepers, tradesmen, domestic servants, and women (*Second Coming* pp. 221–2; see also: E. J. Hobsbawm, "Religion and the Rise of Socialism," *Marxist Perspectives*, 1 (1978), 14–33 at pp. 23–4.

8. *Artisans and Politics*, p. 336.

9. See: R. Q. Gray, "Styles of Life: the 'labour aristocracy,'" pp. 436, 445; and E. J. Hobsbawm, "The Labour Aristocracy in Nineteenth-Century Britain," in his *Labouring Men* (1964), 272–315. For a detailed and sensitive treatment of the "ideological co-option" of artisans, see: Trygve Tholfsen, *Working Class Radicalism in Mid-Victorian England* (1976); see also: Geoffrey Crossick, *An Artisan Elite in Victorian Society* (1978); and R. Q. Gray, *The Labour Aristocracy in Victorian Edinburgh* (Oxford, 1976).

10. *The Works of the Late G. A. Stevens, Esq. Consisting of his Celebrated Lecture on Heads, and Songs; a new and improved edition to which is prefixed a life of the author by W. H. Badham* (1823); on Stevens, see: John Money, *Experience and Identity: Birmingham and the West Midlands, 1760–1800* (Montreal, 1977), pp. 123, 131–2. Works such as John Taylor's *Heads of All Fashions; being a plaine description or definition of diverse, and sundry sorts of heads* (1642) do not appear to have been common or to have excited much interest before the C19; cf. *Heads of the People; or, portraits of the English* (1840–1), 2 vols.

11. Over the past few years phrenology busts have appeared on the cover of the *Observer* color supplement, *Radio Times*, *New Scientist*, *Time*, *Nursing Times*, and *Newsweek*, Donald Mackay's *Brains, Machines, and Persons* (1980), and the Penguin reissue of Gilbert Ryle's *The Concept of Mind*. The use of the phrenological motif in advertising particular products is even more extensive, from the *Daily Telegraph*'s use of it for their appointments pages, to the New York Presbyterian Hospital's appeal for funds, to a water pump company's cute "Phlowology" promotion, to the American Kotex Company's use of it in the promotion of sanitary napkins.

12. Murders in particular were a focus of attention. *A Full Report on the Trial of James Blomfield Rush for the Murder of Mr Jermy and His Son, of Stanfield Hall, in the County of Norfolk*, which contained a foldout of Rush's cerebral development and a phrenological examination, was advertised as being the 50th edition (c. 1849). This is believable given Mayhew's discovery that some 2.5 million printed sheets on the Rush and Manning execution were run off, and over 1.5 million on several other executions (Webb, *Working Class Reader*, p. 31) For a typical example of the phrenological analysis of murderers, see: app. on Haggart's cerebral development written by Combe in *The Life of David Haggart Written by Himself, While under Sentence of Death* (Edin., 1821). Newspaper accounts of executed criminals frequently reported the finding of phrenologists with complete factuality and with the certainty of common understanding. A bulky scrapbook dated 1856–61 belonging to the EPS is filled with newspaper cuttings of such examinations: MS Phrenological Scrap Book (Edin. Univ. Lib.).

13. Combe advertised the dissection of a brain as a part of his course of lectures in 1823: *Prospectus of Lectures on Phrenology by Mr Combe, to be Delivered in the Clyde*

St. Hall, Commencing on Wednesday 14th May 1823. Other lecturers made do with facsimiles, often supplied by the Edinburgh firm of Anthony O'Neil & Co. (who also supplied reproductions of, among other things, "Dr. Heymor's case of a Foetus taken out of a young man at Sherborne in Dorsetshire" – advertised in *Phren. Almanac* [1842], p. 6).

14. E.g.: G. Combe and A. Combe, *On the Functions of the Cerebellum, by Drs. Gall, Vimont, and Broussais* (Edin., 1838); Orson S. Fowler, "Amativeness," in his *Works on Phrenology, Physiology, and Kindred Subjects*, ed. Joseph Barker (1851); see also: Lorenzo N. Fowler, *Marriage: its history and ceremonies with a phrenological and physiological exposition of the functions and qualifications for happy marriages* (Manch., n.d.).

15. E. T. Craig, "Palmistry and Phrenology," *Phren. Mag.*, 2 (25 Feb. 1886), 148. On the difficulties for mechanics in pursuing other science subjects, see: George Head, *A Home Tour through the Manufacturing Districts of England in the Summer of 1835* (1836), p. 202.

16. "Combe's Phrenology," *Nat. Mag. and Monthly Critic*, 2 (1838), 103–19 at p. 119; "The Immoral Tendency of Combe's 'Constitution of Man,'" *Presby. Mag.*, n.s. suppl., 4 (1836), 368–78 at p. 369; *Keene's Bath J.*, 28 Feb. 1842, n.p. See also: Phineas Deseret, *The Christian or True Constitution of Man* (1856; 2nd ed., 1858), p. 16.

17. Myles, *Autobiography*, p. 69; Bain, *Autobiography* (1904); Gutteridge, *Light and Shadows in the Life of an Artisan* (1893) repr. in *Master and Artisan in Victorian England*, ed. V. E. Chanellor (1969), 77–238 (Gutteridge never refers to phrenology, but he attended Charles Bray's Coventry Mutual Improvement Class and in the 1850s lectured on physiology). On the pursuit of scientific learning under awesome conditions, see also: William Dodd, *A Narrative of the Experience and Sufferings [of] William Dodd* (2nd ed., 1841; repr. ed., N.Y., 1968), esp. pp. 89, 307.

18. "Combe and the Philosophy of Phrenology," *Fraser's Mag.*, 22 (Nov. 1840), p. 509. Hazlitt said much the same in "Phrenological Fallacies," *Atlas*, 5 July 1829, repr. in *Works*, vol. 20, 248–53 at p. 249.

19. Editor's introduction to [James Simpson], "Phrenology," *Chambers's Information for the People*, 2 (1842), 129–60 at p. 129.

20. "On the Influence of Prejudice on the Arts," *London Mercury* [an ultraradical paper edited by John Bell], 13 Nov. 1836, n.p., adding: "All the operations of nature are characterized by simplicity and power.... The more we extend our inquiries into the laws of nature, the more do we generalize and simplify; so it is in our inquiries into the laws of mind."

21. The neoencyclopedists' language against "intellectual property" was used overtly in James Garth Wilkinson's *Science for All* (1847), pp. 3–7. Yet to be written is the late-C18–early-C19 history of the artisan involvement in scientific pursuit and invention and its closing-off (in some cases by the outright expropriation of institutions). J. L. Heilbron notes the involvement of common people in the development of electical theory in the C18 ("Experimental Natural Philosophy," in Rousseau and Porter, *Ferment of Knowledge*, 357–87 at p. 369. Robert Darnton has noted it in Mesmerism (*Mesmerism and the End of the Enlightenment in France* [N.Y., 1970]); and David Allen has observed it with respect to botany and natural history (*The Naturalist in Britain* [1976]). See also: Thompson, *The Making*, p. 322; and P. Weindling, "Science and Sedition,"p. 143.

22. In his "Essays on Phrenology, No. 1: on an organ of Sympathy, seated between Comparison and Benevolence," *Zoist*, 4 (1848), 72–85 at p. 73.

23. Sept. 1836 in *The Journals and Miscellaneous Notebooks of Ralph Waldo Emerson*, vol. 5 (1835–8), ed. Merton M. Sealts (Cambridge, Mass., 1965), p. 212; see also: similar statements made in March 1836, pp. 142, 146. A contemporary phrenologist, Sybil Leek, maintains this as a reason for turning to phrenology in the modern world: *Phrenology* (1970), p. 12. Cf. Douglas, *Purity and Danger*, p. 210, and idem, "Self-evidence," in her *Implicit Meanings*, pp. 284–5.

24. See: the passage from Jack London's autobiographical novel *Martin Eden*, q. in Budd, *Varieties of Unbelief*, p. 139.

25. On practical qua practical phrenology, see: "Uses of Phrenology," *Phren. J.*, 6

(1829/30), 320–6, 368–76, 449–50, 620–30; "Practical Utility of Phrenology," ibid., 7 (1831/2), 368–73; Joshua T. Smith, *Synopsis of Phrenology; directed chiefly to the exhibition of the utility and application of the science to the advancement of social happiness* (London and Boston, 1839); "Practical Phrenology," *J. Health*, 4 [1855], 230–1; D. G. Goyder, "Marriage Considered Phrenologically," *Phren. Ann. & Almanac*, 5 (1846), 25–31; "On the Practical Application of Phrenology in the Ordinary Affairs of Life," *Phren. J.*, 19 (1846), 223–7.

26. Colin Wilson, *The Outsider* (1956), p. 277. For the parallel with astrology, see: Capp, *English Almanacs*, and Harrison, *Second Coming*, p. 48. While Goyder's *Phren. Almanac* (1842–46) reflects its antecedents in popular literature, an attempt to conjoin phrenology with astrology was made by Lieut. Richard James Morrison (1795–1874) in his *Zadkiel's Magazine, or Record and Review of Astrology, Phrenology, Mesmerism, and Other Sciences* (Jan./Feb. 1849).

27. D. G. Goyder, *Heads of the People, 1843: measurements and manipulations of heads in 1843* (MS, Edin. Univ. Lib: Gen. 608 x [v]). Of these clients 156 were between the ages of 18 and 26; 43 females are entered, most of whom were domestics.

28. E.g.: "Friendly Computer Clarence May Hold Key to Your Future," *Calgary Herald*, 19 Mar 1979. Bushea (see Figure 7, Chapter 5) typically stressed the importance of phrenology for determining the character of wives, clerks, shop-men, and domestic servants. For an example of a small master's enthusiasm for the science as a hiring technique, see: *Phren. J.* 8 (1832/4), 425; see also: Combe, "On the Application of Phrenology to the Purposes of the 'Guarantee Society, for Providing Security for Persons in Situations of Trust, Where Sureties Are Required, on Payment of an Annual Premium,' " *Phren. J.*, 14 (1841), 297–310 (the directors of this company apparently passed a resolution adopting the aid of phrenology: *Phren. J.*, 14 [1841], 61–2); Combe, "Practical Phrenology: choosing servants by their heads: criminal legislation," *Phren.J.*, 6 (1829/30), 211–22; the section on "Choice of Servants" in *Constitution of Man*, pp. 176–9, and p. 61; H. C. Watson, "Relation between Cerebral Development and the Tendency to Particular Pursuits," *Phren. J.*, 8 (1832/4), 97–108; and E. J. Hytch, "On the Selection of Keepers in Lunatic Asylums," *Lancet*, 6 Nov. 1841, pp. 190–2. For the critique of this practice, see: below Chapter 8.

29. J. D. Holm, *Phren. J.*, 9 (1834/6), 494; Combe, *Constitution of Man*, cited in G. D. Campbell (i.e., duke of Argyll), "Phrenology: its place and relations," *North Br. Rev.*, 17 (May 1852), 41–70 at p. 59; J. N. Bailey, *Essays on Miscellaneous Subjects* (Leeds, 1842), p. 21; "Self-Knowledge," *People*, 2 (1849), 98. See also: John R. Beard, *Self Culture: a complete guide to self-instruction* (1850), esp. at p. 19.

30. Alexander Taylor, "Dundee Mechanics' Phrenological Society," pp. 456–8. Combe reprinted this letter in his *Letter to Francis Jeffrey*, pp. 7–8.

31. *The Autobiography of an Artisan* (1847), p. 116; Bray, "Phrenology and Its Applications," p. 76.

32. See, for example: J. L. Levison, *Lecture on the Hereditary Tendency of Drunkenness* (1839); De Giustino, *Conquest of Mind*, pp. 62–4; Cooter, "Phrenology and British Alienists," p. 144; and V. L. Hilts, "Obeying the Laws of Hereditary Descent: phrenological views on inheritance and eugenics," *J. Hist. Behav. Sci.*, 18 (1982), 62–77.

33. Main chapters of *Principles of Physiology* first appeared in *Phren. J.* vols. 6, 8 (1829/30, 1832–4); a 16th edition appeared in 1885, preceded by several American editions and a German trans. of 1837. Andrew Combe's *Physiology of Digestion* (1836) reached a 9th edition in 1849, while the work he regarded as his most valuable, *A Treatise on the Physiological and Moral Management of Infancy* (1840), had sold over 9,500 copies before mid-century and was to make him the Dr. Spock of the C19. The Lockean attribution comes from the fulsome tribute by John Brown, "Dr Andrew Combe," in his *Horae Subsecivae* (new ed., 1900), I, 103–32.

34. "Physical Puritanism," *Westminster Rev.*, n.s., 1 (1852), 418–19. Brown (1817–56, a cousin of John Brown and an intimate with the Combes) also observed: "The very atheism of the times, among the illuminated artisans of the times, is

all in favour of the bodily virtues now under discussion. Cleanliness and temperance are the very religion of the materialist, and should be the complement of religion for all" (ibid., p. 419). George Eliot, who had just taken up the editorship of the *Westminster*, wrote enthusiastically to Sara Hennell about Brown's contribution (see: *George Eliot Letters*, ed. G. S. Haight [1954], II, pp. 5–6). For similar appreciation, see: *London Sat. J.*, 3 (18 Apr. 1840), 259; and *Eliza Cook's J.*, 3 (7 Sept. 1850), 292.

35. Graham, *Lectures on the Science of Human Life* (People's edition, 1849), p. iii (on Graham see Stephen Nissenbaum, *Sex, Diet, and Debility in Jacksonian America: Sylvester Graham and health reform* [Westport, Conn., 1980]); review of "Smiles, *Physical Education; or, the nature and management of children, founded on the study of their nature and constitution* [Edin., 1838]," *Phren. J.*, 11 (1838), 317–20. (In connection with reviewing the publisher's copy, see: Smiles to Combe, 20 Dec. 1837, Combe papers, NLS 7244 f 10, and Combe to Smiles 22 Dec. 1837, NLS 7387 f 504.) Smiles paid handsome tribute to phrenology and Andrew Combe in "Dr Andrew Combe" in his *Brief Biographies* (Boston, 1861), 365–76. (Useful on this aspect of Smiles is T. Travers, "Samuel Smiles and the Origins of 'Self-help': reform and the new enlightenment," *Albion*, 9 [1977], 161–87.) Close companion volumes also owing much to the Combes were Amariah Brigham, *Remarks on the Influence of Mental Cultivation and Mental Excitement upon Health* (Boston, 1833); Charles Caldwell, *Physical Education* (1844) (Brigham and Caldwell were both phrenologists); T. B. Johnson, *Physiological Observations on Mental Susceptibility* (1837), G. T. Black, *The Principles of the Natural Laws of Man with the Lights Which the New Philosophy Will Shed upon the World* (1837); L. J. Beale, *The Laws of Health, in Relation to Mind and Body* (1851). Dozens of very similar works exist, most of which use Combe as their starting point. For general reflections, see: Haley, *The Healthy Body*.

36. Bain, *Autobiography*, p. 50; on the popular disdain for orthodox medicine see, for example: J. W. Lake, *Medicine Unveiled* (advertised in Holyoake's *Reasoner*, 4 [8 Mar. 1848], 30). Frederick Hollick, the student of phrenology and Owenite social missionary who turned to lecturing on physiology in America, seems to have captured the reality accurately when he said that the medical art was "relied upon blindly by a few; is distrusted by many; and by some even treated with utter contempt," in his *Neuropathy; or, principles of the art of healing the sick*, q. in *Reasoner*, 3 (20 Oct. 1847), 569. See also: *Reasoner*, 7 (1 Aug. 1849), 65.

37. Cited in James Simpson's evidence, *Select Committee on Foundation Schools and Education in Ireland, Parliamentary Papers*, XIII, pt. I (1835), p. 251. Cobbett died in 1835; the English edition of Brigham's work (note 35) with notes by Robert Macnish was brought out by Chambers in 1836. See also: Simpson, "On Elementary Education," *Analyst*, 6 (1837), 7–8.

38. Vol. 7 (1835), 290. See also: Epps's *Diary*, p. 293. The SDUK immediately appreciated the value of Combe's physiology; see: *Quart. J. Educ.*, 8 (1834), 326–32; and *Educ. Mag.*, 1 (Mar. 1835), 183–90.

39. Preface to Fowler's "Amativeness," p. 1. See also: Holyoake, *The Origin and Nature of Secularism* (1896), p. 106.

40. Sidney Smith, *Principles of Phrenology* (Edin., 1838; 2nd ed., 1849), p. 15.

41. See: John Fletcher, *Discourse on Physiology* (Edin., 1836), p. 24; and J. Blackman, "Popular Theories of Generation: the evolution of *Aristotle's Works*: the study of an anachronism," in Woodward and Richards, eds., *Health Care and Popular Medicine*, 56–88 at p. 88.

Holyoake was summing up the attitude of many artisans when he wrote, "He may be an enthusiast who expects to reform mankind, but he fails in his first and most important duty who neglects to reform himself": "The Healthian," *Oracle of Reason*, 8 Oct. 1842, p. 352. See also: *Reasoner*, 7 (1 Aug. 1849), 65.

42. *The Life and Adventures of Valentine Vox, the Ventriloquist* (1840), chap. 23 "Valentine Attends a Phrenological Lecture," p. 165. See also: David M. Reese, "Of Phrenology," in his *Humbugs of New York* (Boston, 1838), 75–76; and M. Ryan,

"Physiology, Phrenology, and Materialism," p. 49. Ryan felt that the poor could gain no real comfort from so excusing themselves from guilt.

43. See, for example: "Principles of Phrenology, IV: objections considered," *Moral Reformer*, 1 (May 1838), 114–15. See also: C. Rosenberg, "The Bitter Fruit: heredity, disease, and social thought in nineteenth-century America," *Persp. Amer. Hist.* 8 (1974), 189–235, esp. at pp. 199–200, 208.

44. Combe, q. in Gibbon, *Life of Combe*, I, p. 148. On phrenology as extending Christian forebearance, see: John Elliotson, "An Account of the Head of Rush, the Norfolk Murderer," *Zoist*, 8 (July 1849), 107–21 at p. 120; Robert Macnish, *Introduction to Phrenology* p. 204; William Wildsmith, *An Inquiry Concerning the Relative Connexion Which Subsists between the Mind and the Brain: with remarks on phrenology and materialism* (Leeds, 1828), p. 44; J. D. Burn, *The Autobiography of a Beggar Boy* p., 20; *Phren. J.*, 9 (1834/6), 381.

45. "On Human Capability of Improvement," *Phren. J.*, 7 (1831/2), 197–212. Cf. the original theory in Gall's "How Far Is the Human Species Perfectible?" in his *On the Functions of the Brain*, vol. 6, pp. 218–87.

46. On the likening of Marxism to Calvinism, see: Isaac Deutscher, *The Prophet Armed: Trotsky, 1879–1921* (N.Y., 1965), I, p. 27n.; and to the religion of Comtean positivism: Royden Harrison, *Before the Socialist* (1965), pp. 270–71.

47. See, for example: the letter from W. Cookson to Joseph Barker, 24 Oct. 1848, in "Combe's Work," *The People*, 1 (1848), 199.

48. Martineau on the *Constitution of Man* in "Representative Men: Pestalozzi, the Combes, Roland Hill," *Once a Week*, 6 (18 May 1861), 575–80 at p. 579.

49. *Phrenology: its evidences and inferences, with criticisms upon Mr Grant's recent lectures* (2nd ed., Sheffield, 1858), p. 14; see also: James Freeman Clarke, *Autobiography, Diary, and Correspondence* (Boston, 1891), p. 49, q. in J. D. Davies, *Phrenology: fad and science*, p. 169.

50. The Rev. Henry Clarke[‡] was one of many authors to find the double roles confusing: "Thus, one has maintained that phrenology annihilates the idea of Deity, and another affirms that it annihilates atheism. By Calvinist believers in Phrenology, I have been solemnly assured that it puts beyond all controversy and doubt the truth of Calvinism; while, by others, I have been as earnestly certified that it wars to the death with the dogmata of Calvin": "Party Phrenologists," pp. 239–40.

51. Turner, *Phrenology*, p. 13; A. Taylor, "Dundee Mechanics' Phrenological Society," p. 456.

52. "Phrenology," *The People*, 1 (1848), 280.

53. Cited in David Bakan, "The Influence of Phrenology on American Psychology," *J. Hist. Behav. Sci.*, 2 (July 1966), 200–220 at p. 201.

54. *Phil. Mag.*, 45 (Jan. 1815), 62; Chenevix, *Phrenology Article*, pp. 37–9; Paul Rogers letter to the editor, *Phreno-Magnet*, 1 (May 1843), 104; cf. Uwins, *Eclectic Rev.*, 3 (Apr. 1815), 329.

55. "Book of the Week: phrenology and physiology," *Aldine Mag.*, 1 (19 Jan. 1839), 120–22 at p. 121, in the course of extolling the *Constitution of Man* as "one of the most important and invaluable books, as conducive to the improvement and happiness of the human race, that ever emanated from the mind and pen of man." To the frequent remark that had Combe removed the phrenology from his lectures on education the lectures would have seemed founded purely on common sense, Combe replied that his lectures "make a deeper and more permanent impression on the understanding than if based on mere Common Sense, and can be more certainly and successfully carried into practice." Cited in Jolly, *Education Developed by Combe*, p. 1. Accused of monopolizing "all the *good sense* current in the world to themselves, and allow[ing] to no one else a particle of natural sagacity," phrenologists responded: "Our science, by discovering and ascertaining the primitive faculties of the human mind, and the relation of these to external nature, has given us the means of *testing* good sense, and reducing it to a regular harmonious means of human happiness; while the merely sagacious writers had no such standard, and neither themselves nor thier readers could

have perfect confidence in the soundness of their views": *Phren. J.*, 10 (1836/7), 674. It was the "natural and self-evident manner" in which man was represented, said *Human Nature* in an article on phrenology in Aug. 1868 (p. 345), "which at once recommends itself to the experience and common-sense of mankind."

56. Luke Burke in his lectures at the London Mechanics' Institute, q. in *People's Phren. J.*, 1 (1843), 180; "Introduction," ibid., 1 (1843), 2. See also: "Equality," *Reasoner*, 5 (13 Sept. 1848), 241–4, legitimating inequality on the basis of natural law. The cerebral superiority of the respectable classes was supposedly justified via: "On the Size of Hats Used by Different Classes of Society; by a hat-maker of Dundee," *Phren. J.*, 5 (1828/9), repr. in Cox, *Selections*, pp. 170–4; or "Size of Head, National and Provincial; observed by an experienced hat-maker of London," *Phren. J.*, 4 (1826/7), 539–52. Cf. D. G. Goyder, "The Duties of Masters and Servants" in his *Sermons to My Household* (1861), p. 19: Calling the relationship a necessary one requiring submission on the one hand and kindness on the other, he argued (as he did secularly in his phrenology lectures), "*All men are equal* in the eye of the Lord; with Him there is no respect of persons. . . . But the truth, *all men are equal*, is an abstract one, which requires to be properly understood; for it is very certain that it has been used to defend very improper conduct. . . . equality in actual situations seems by the Creator never to have been intended. . . . in mental and physical constitution, the various races of men are widely different." Clearly the "logic" of this was in need of some scientific backing.

57. Ralph Waldo Emerson, *Journals and Miscellaneous Notebooks*, vol. 8 (1841–3), ed. William H. Gilman and J. E. Parsons (Cambridge, Mass., 1970), entry for Mar. 1843, p. 341.

58. M. Ryan, *Manual of Medical Jurisprudence* (1831), pp. 16–18 as q. and condemned in *Lon. Med. & Phys. J.*, n.s., 11 (1831), 494; William Pyper, *Edin. Advertiser*, 24 Dec. 1833 (attribution and citation in Shapin, "Phrenological Knowledge," p. 228); and Sam Sly, *Keene's Bath J.*, 28 Feb. 1843, n.p. The fear that the science would be an easy means of leavening the masses is evident in, among others, Hazlitt's writings on phrenology; see: Howe, *Works*, vol. 20, esp. pp. 248–55. The accusation of antiphrenologists that the science "sprang from the wrong people, those of the *lower orders*" would have been reason enough for many of the militant in the working class to endorse the science. See Brewin Grant, in *Discussion on Phrenology [with] Charles [sic] Donovan* (Birm., 1849), p. 3.

59. See: *Constitution of Man*, p. 220; Combe, "Condition of the Labouring Classes," *Phren. J.*, 6 (1829/30), 630–4; idem, "Commercial Distress," *Phren. J.*, 3 (1825/6), 313–22; Andrew Combe, "Factories Regulation Bill," *Phren. J.*, 8 (1832/4), 231–7; "Hints to the Operative Classes in Britain," ibid., 7 (1831/2), 276–80. The Dundee phrenologists supported a petition to Parliament in 1832 to limit to ten the hours of labor for persons under the age of eighteen: G. Combe to A. Combe, 19 July 1832, Combe Papers, NLS 7385. For Combe's reaction to working-class rejection of the Factory Act limiting the hours of child labor, see: Gibbon, *Life of Combe*, I, p. 307.

60. In his fifth lecture to the Liverpool Medical Institution, q. in *Liverpool Standard*, 6 Feb. 1838, p. 4.

61. Arguing for the Charter in "The Campsall Society and Universal Suffrage," *Sheffield Iris*, 9 Oct. 1838, n.p.

62. Watson, *Public Opinion; or safe revolution, through self representation* (1848), suggests the formation of a national association to give machinery for a correct census of public opinion and for complete suffrage. Most phrenologists were not among the ultraradical wing of what Mill called the "natural Radical party" but were among the ultraliberals, critical of Whigs if only because (as pointed out in an editorial in the *Halifax Express* of 21 Nov. 1840, p. 2) the Whigs had cheated so many members of the middle classes from the vote. Epps, with Chartist backing, stood unsuccessfully for Northampton in 1847: *Diary*, pp. 449–50; John Foster, *Class Struggle*, p. 104; R. C. Gammage, *History of the Chartist Movement* (1894), pp. 283, 285.

63. Hodgson to Combe, 1842, q. in Gibbon, *Life of Combe*, II, p. 118.
64. *Religion and Science*, p. 30n.; cf. the Peoples' edition of 1857, p. 174n., where the note is amended to utilization of physical force only as a *last resort*; note also the following change in the *Constitution of Man* between the 6th edition of 1836 (pp. 211–12) and the People's edition of 1855 (p. 63): "If the supremacy of the moral sentiments and intellect be the natural law, then, as often observed, every circumstance connected with human life must be in harmony with it ..."; *to* "If the harmonious action of the whole faculties, and in cases of conflict the supremacy of the moral sentiments and intellect, be the natural law."
65. "Mr W. J. Vernon," *Reynold's Political Instructor*, 1 (26 Jan. 1850), 89–90: "was pounced upon as a fitting individual to expiate by two years' imprisonment the alarm caused to the illustrious field marshall of Osborn [i.e., Prince Albert], and to the aristocratic and money vicinities of Belgrave Square and Lombard Street. Mr Vernon was arrested, tried, and as a matter of course, found guilty; in the judge's disturbed brain our harmless peaceable lecturer on phrenology was converted into a Marat, a Couthon, or a Robespierre, and his lordship forthwith sentenced him to undergo two years' imprisonment." I am grateful to Dorothy Thompson for this reference.
66. Willoughby Wood, "Lectures on Political Economy," *Star in the East*, 25 Aug. & 1 Sept. 1838, pp. 386, 397; "Mr W. Wood's Lecture on Political Economy," *Sheffield Iris*, 5 Feb. 1839; "Campsall Society," ibid., 9 Oct. 1838. In his lecture "On the Position of the Cerebral Organs in the Human Head" in the Doncaster Lyceum in 1838, Charles Wood broke the rules by speaking of fatalism and materialism; defending himself against an attack in the *Doncaster Chronicle*, he pointed out that all phrenologists were actually materialists but were "too cowardly" to admit it and were thus forced by the pressure of religious opinion into "moral swindling": "Knowledge versus Ignorance, or Science versus Religion: the Woods and the would-nots," *Star in the East*, 22 Dec. 1838, p. 113. Cf. "Phrenology and Political Economy," *Phren. J.*, 11 (1837/8), where Hewett Watson argues in far more typical phrenological fashion that he was not at all in agreement with renegade phrenologists such as Wood or Joshua Toumlin Smith that "phrenology in any way demonstrates the erroneousness of most of the principles of [orthodox] political economy" (p. 201).
67. *Sheffield Iris*, 9 Oct. 1838. On cultural exploitation through anticlericalism, see: Foster, *Class Struggle*, p. 104; and on the need to distinguish between secularist and anticlerical traditions in working class history, see: Eric Hobsbawm, *Age of Capital, 1848–1875* (N.Y., 1975), pp. 271–2.
68. S. T. Hall, *Mesmeric Experiences* (1845), p. 24. Hall was particularly bitter at the way the polite middle class had rejected him with his mesmerism, whereas certain sections of the working class had greeted him with enthusiasm (pp. 21–22).
69. [John Minter Morgan], *Hampden in the Nineteenth Century* (1834), I, p. 241n.; (for other examples of reactionary views on education and the popularization of science, and examples of the use of these straw men for liberalism, see: J. Twist, *The Policy of Educating the Poor* [1822]; J. B. Summer and S. T. Coleridge, "Mechanics' Institutes and Infant Schools," *Quart. Rev.*, 32 [Oct. 1825], 410–28, esp. at p. 415; D. Robinson, "Education of the People," esp. p. 534; Country Gentleman, *The Consequences of a Scientific Education to the Working Classes* [1826]); T.S. Prideaux, *Gall's Organology*, repr. *from Anthropol. Rev.*, 7 (Jan. 1869), 76–92 at p. 11; Brewster, "On the Characteristics of the Age," p. 7; J. L. Levison, *Mental Culture; or the means of developing the human faculties* (1833), p. 207; S. Smith, *Principles of Phrenology*, p. 24.
70. Cited in Brian Simon, *History of Education*, p. 338.
71. [Engledue], "Physical Well-being: a necessary preliminary to moral and intellectual progression," *Zoist*, 5 (1847), 82–101 at p. 85; see also: J. Forbes, *Of Happiness in Its Relations to Work and Knowledge*, pp. 31–2.
72. The opening sentences of the preface to the 7th edition (c. 1840) of Spurzheim's [*A Sketch of*] *The Natural Laws of Man: a philosophical catechism* [1st ed., 1825], published in a cheap edition by John Heywood of Manchester, were: "Men have

long been treated as children. They have been taught that ignorance and credulity are virtues and that fear is wisdom – that they may glorify God by flattery rather than by moral excellency. Arbitrary regulations of all sorts have been imposed upon them, and blind and unconditional obedience to these required.... Sensual gratifications have proved sufficient inducements for them willingly to follow the good pleasure of their masters. Even religion, in one or other form, has been an engine to crush the human mind." The rhetoric was typical: see: the dedication to Combe in Joshua T. Smith's *A Popular View of the Progress of Philosophy* (1836); cf. the evident *dis*parity between political opinion on the franchise and "radical" views on state education in a person such as Robert Lowe: Simon, *History of Education*, p. 355.

73. Combe's Glasgow speech on national education, *North Briton Daily Mail*, q. in Jolly, *Education Developed by Combe*, pp. 531–2; review of S. Smith's *Principles of Phrenology*, *Tait's Mag.*, 5 (Sept. 1838), 555–8.

74. A. J. Peacock, *Bradford Chartism, 1838–1840*, Borthwick Papers no. 36 (York, 1969), p. 15. Similar complaints against diversion and mystification were to be heard later in the century when socialists quarrelled with freethinkers, claiming that the latter were pursuing a peripheral and anachronistic religious issue; see: S. Budd, "The Loss of Faith, Reason for Unbelief among Members of the Secularist Movement in England, 1850–1950," *Past and Present*, no. 36 (1967), 106–25 at p. 125; F. B. Smith, "Atheist Mission, 1840–1900," in Robert Robson, ed., *Ideas and Institutions of Victorian Britain* (1962), 205–35 at p. 222; and Frank Harris on Bradlaugh's tremendous waste of energy on the wrong issue in *My Life and Loves* (1925; new ed., 1966), I, pp. 179, 183.

75. Compare, for instance, the deliberateness of Cobden in 1848 asserting that "our aristocracy must be made to submit again" in order to win workers' sympathies to liberalism, to Combe asserting (as late as 1854) that Britain was "ruled by the upper and middle classes, who keep the people in obedience by means of standing armies of soldiers and clergymen; and the State can thus afford to indulge them in the glorious privilege of ignorance," in an appeal for the political rights of all. Cobden is quoted in J. T. Ward, *Chartism* (1973), p. 202, Combe in "Notes on a Visit to Germany in 1854," *Scotsman*, 9 Sept. 1854, n.p. (Admittedly, to many working people by the 1840s "antiaristocracy" was a general term for antiauthoritarianism of any kind against bad masters of any sort.) On the actualities of aristocratic power after the Reform Bill (mistakenly equated with the ideological realities of power), see: W. L. Guttsman, *The British Political Elite* (1963); Norman Gash, *Politics in the Age of Peel* (1953); idem, *Reaction and Reconstruction in English Politics, 1832–52* (Oxford, 1965); F. M. L. Thompson, *English Landed Society in th Nineteenth Century* (1963); G. Kitson Clark, *Peel and the Conservative Party* (new ed., 1964); W. L. Arnstein, "The Myth of the Triumphant Victorian Middle Class," *Historian*, 27 (1975), 205–21; and R. S. Neale, " 'The Bourgeoisie, Historically, Has Played a Most Revolutionary Part,' " in Neale and Eugene Kamenka, eds., *Feudalism, Capitalism, and Beyond* (1975), 85–102, esp. at pp. 101–2. Cf. R. Q. Gray, "Bourgeois Hegemony," 73–93.

76. Engledue, *Cerebral Physiology* (1842), p. 5; the rest of the passage indicates clearly that from his point of view the bourgeois revolution was by no means over.

77. Hodgson, for example, wrote to Bray in July 1879 that the cure for society's religious and social blindness "is slow and distant, and you and I shall turn our toes to the daisies ere the happy time comes when superstition will flee away before knowledge and free thought": *Life and Letters*, p. 356. Hodgson was then sixty-four years old, Bray sixty-eight.

78. Engledue, *Cerebral Physiology*, p. 6; and see: idem, "Education as It Is and as It Ought to Be," *Zoist*, 1 (1844), 351–69, & 2 (1844), 1–20; and G. Mackenzie, *Principles of Education* (Edin., 1836).

79. *Diary of Epps*, p. 322.

80. Marx, "The Chartists," *New York Daily Tribune*, 25 Aug. 1852, in *Marx and Engels on Britain* (Moscow, 1962), p. 360; *Leeds Times*, 16 Nov. 1844, q. in A. Tyrrell, "Smiles," p. 112. Martineau was fully aware that had the Combe broth-

ers ever understood that their key *failed* to unlock the secrets of human nature and that their proposals were *inadequate*, "they would not have been the zealous and happy and confident apostles that they were, and could hardly have led forward the middle and working-classes to the point of improvement which they have reached": "Representative Men ... the Combes," p. 579.

81. Combe, *Moral Philosophy; or, the Duties of Man* (1840; rev. ed., 1893), p. 97.

82. Engledue, "Physical Well-being," p. 85; *Constitution of Man*, p. 335 et passim.

83. Thompson, *The Making*, p. 839. Cf. John Doherty, trades union leader, who in 1830 attacked the "aristocratic order" that tried to halt the march of the school-masters abroad: R.G. Kirby and A.E. Musson, *The Voice of the People: John Doherty, 1798–1854* (1975), pp. 333–4.

84. For an illustration of the burning, see: frontispiece to Philip Jones, *The Constitution of Man: his soul, mind, and brain. Popular phrenology tried by the word of God and proved to be Antichrist and injurious to individuals and families* (1845). That the works of Paine and Combe were read and regarded in the same light receives some qualification from the uniform binding of a 6th edition of the *Constitution of Man* with the *Political Works of Thomas Paine* (Chartist Co-operative Land Society, n.p., n.d.) in a volume once belonging to J. Peacock of Nottingham and now in the collection of phrenological works housed in the library of the Subdepartment of the History of Medicine, University College, London. For Combe as the epitome of what Mrs. Butler called the "Joseph Hume Nation," see: [J.G. Lockhart] "[James Silk] Buckingham and Combe on the United States," *Quart. Rev.*, 68 (Sept. 1841), 281–312 at p. 284.

85. "Next to religion, find who can / A system so befitting man / His mind t'exalt, delight his sense, / Or teach him pure benevolence": lines from a Southampton mechanic's "Eulogy on Phrenology," q. in *Phren. J.*, 9 (1834/6), 381.

86. According to the definition provided by Clifford Geertz, religion is "(1) a system of symbols which acts to (2) establish powerful, pervasive, and long-lasting moods and motivations in men by (3) formulating conceptions of a general order of existence and (4) clothing these conceptions with such an aura of factuality that (5) the moods and motivations seem uniquely realistic": "Religion as a Cultural System," in Michael Benton, ed., *Anthropological Approaches to the Study of Religion* (1966), 1–46 at pp. 4, 13. See also: Raymond Firth, "Problems and Assumptions in an Anthropological Study of Religion," in his *Essays*, 225–56, esp. at pp. 229, 232.

87. Frank Parkin, *Class Inequality and Political Order: social stratification in capitalist and communist societies* (1972), p. 82, cited in G. Crossick, "The Labour Aristocracy and Its Values: a study of mid-Victorian Kentish London," *Vict. Stud.*, 19 (1976), 301–28 at p. 320. Cf. Douglas, "Deciphering a Meal," in her *Implicit Meanings*, p. 249; *Natural Symbols*, p. 137; and Roland Barthes, "The Photographic Message," in his *Image–Music–Text*, essays selected and trans. Stephen Heath (Glasgow, 1977), 15–31 at pp. 15–16.

88. Mrs. John S. D. Pugh, *Phrenology Considered in a Religious Light; or thoughts and readings consequent on the perusal of "Combe's Constitution of Man"* (1846), p. 6. For very similar, see: Harriet Hunt (after hearing Combe's lectures in Boston in 1838) in her *Glances and Glimpses; or, fifty years social, including twenty years professional life* (Boston, 1856), pp. 142–4. For other female responses to phrenology, see: Jane Loudon, "Remarks on 'The Constitution of Man,' " *Monthly Repository*, 10 (1836), 153–8; Mrs. Thomas Spurr, "On the Brain as the Organ of Intellect," in her *Course of Lectures on the Physical, Intellectual, and Religious Education of Infant Children; delivered before the ladies of Sheffield* (Sheffield, 1836); [Emily G. S. Saunders], *Christian Phrenology* (1881); "Thoughts on Phrenology," *Christian Lady's Mag.*, 15 (1841), 369–71; "Dr Spurzheim," *Ladies Mag. & Lit. Gaz.*, 5 (1832), 570–2. A Mrs. L. Miles produced a package of forty cards illustrating the science entitled *Phrenology and the Moral Influence of Phrenology* [1836].

89. Combe was presented with a pair of silver calipers by a number of women in 1838 in token appreciation for his letting them attend his class (Gibbon, *Life of Combe*, I, p. 208); women were frequently admitted to phrenological societies

on special evenings, partly as a radical gesture, partly for bumping up attendance figures. A correspondent to the *London Med. Gaz.* observed that where the bluestockings had not been admitted to the proceedings they were "not idle at home with their mapped casts of heads": "Phrenology," 5 (27 March 1830), 826–7 at p. 827. In the presence of his wife Spurzheim told the EPS on 25 Jan. 1828, "There can be no doubt among phrenologists, that minds of ladies should be cultivated as well as ours, to fit them for their social relations and duties": q. in Carmichael, *Memoir on Spurzheim*, pp. 32–3. See also: "On the Female Character," *Phren. J.*, 2 (1824/5), 275–88; Combe, "Female Education," in his *Lectures on Popular Education* (3rd ed., Edin., 1848), lect. 3; J. Wilson, *Phrenology Consistent with Reason and Revelation* (Cheltenham, 1843), I, p. xiv; Edouard Guillot, "The Phrenological Constitution of Woman," *J. Health*, 6 [1857], 193–4; J. W. Jackson, "On the Superiority of the Male Element in the Plan of Nature," *Future*, 1 (1860–1), serially 62–135; and B. Hollander, *The Female Mind* (repr. from *Ethol. J.*, Oct. 1927). For other C19 literature on the female brain in relation to the male, see: B. Kanner, "The Women of England in a Century of Social Change, 1815–1914: a select bibliography," pt. II, in M. Vicinus, ed., *A Widening Sphere: changing roles of Victorian women* (Bloomington, Ind., 1977), 199–270 at pp. 257–8.

90. See: Flora Tristan, "English Women," in her *London Journal* 244–61, esp. p. 249; Donald Meyer, "The Troubled Souls of Females," in his *The Positive Thinkers* (N.Y., 1980), 46–59; see also: S. A. Shields, "Functionalism, Darwinism, and the Psychology of Women: a study in social myth," *Amer. Psychologist*, 30 (1975), 739–54.

91. "Religion as Cultural System," pp. 15, 19.

92. See: Peter L. Berger, *The Social Reality of Religion* (1969); on diagrams and pictures as assemblages of symbols or "culturally meaningful components" preclassifying what we perceive, see: Barry Barnes, *Interests and the Growth of Knowledge* (1977), esp. pp. 4–10; see also: Barthes, *Mythologies*.

93. "Burke and the Edinburgh Phrenologists," *Atlas*, 4 (15 Feb. 1829), 105, in Howe, *Works of Hazlitt*, vol. 20, pp. 200–4.

94. By Feuchtwang, "Investigating Religion," p. 67, citing Louis Dumont, *Homo Hierarchicus* (1970).

95. See: Raymond Firth, "The Sceptical Anthropologist? Social anthropology and Marxist views on society," in M. Bloch, *Marxist Analysis*, 29–60, esp. p. 32; M. Rosenberg, "Perceptual Obstacles to Class Consciousness," *Social Forces*, 32 (1953), 22–7; and H. C. Greisman and S. S. Mayes, "The Social Construction of Unreality: the real American dilemma," *Dialectical Anthropology*, 2 (1977), 57–67.

96. Combe, *Science and Religion* (Edin. 4th ed., 1857), p. xvii.

97. "Base and Superstructure," p. 9 (or a nearly identical statement in his *Marxism and Literature*, p. 110)(emphasis added); see also: Thompson, "Peculiarities of the English," pp. 72 ff.; M. Fellman, "Approaching Popular Ideology in Nineteenth Century America," *Hist. Reflections*, 6 (1979), 321–33; J. Femia, "Hegemony and Consciousness in the Thought of Antonio Gramsci," *Political Studies*, 23 (1975), 29–48. On the Gramsci industry, see: K. Nield and J. Seed, "Waiting for Gramsci," *Social Hist.*, 6 (1981), 209–27.

98. Joshua Toulmin Smith, *Phrenology Vindicated* (1836), p. 13 (emphasis added); for similar, see: below, note 110.

99. Thomas Wakley's first toast to the electors of Finsbury after his election victory of 1837: *London Mercury*, 3 Sept. 1837, p. 705.

100. Ure, *Philosophy of Manufactures*, pp. 424–5, he was not, however, unaware of science's role from a technological point of view: "When capital enlists science in her service, the refractory hand of labour will always be taught docility": q. in D. Dickson, "Science and Political Hegemony," p. 33. On the insufficiency of the policeman and the workhouse in winning the "hearts and minds" of the working class, see: G. Stedman Jones, "Working-Class Culture and Working-Class Politics in London, 1870–1900: notes on the remaking of a working class," *J. Soc. Hist.*, 7 (1974), 460–508 at p. 466.

101. See: Bernard Semmel, *The Methodist Revolution* (1973), p. 12; Gertrude Himmelfarb, *Victorian Minds* (1968), pp. 279–80; [A. Smith], "Phrenological Ethics," p. 390.
102. Wesley, q. in Keith Thomas, *Religion and the Decline of Magic* (Harmondsworth, 1973), p. 765.
103. See: James Deville, "Account of a Number of Cases in Which a Change Had Been Produced on the Form of the Head by Education and Moral Training," *Phren. J.*, 14 (1841), 32–8; and Andrew Combe, "Remarks on the Possibility of Increasing the Development of the Cerebral Organs by Adequate Exercise of the Mental Faculties," *Phren. J.*, 10 (1836/7), 414–26.
104. Cited in T. Tholfsen, "The Intellectual Origins of Mid-Victorian Stability," *Pol. Sci. Q.*, 86 (1971), 57–91 at pp. 82–3.
105. On the Methodist, see: E. R. Wickham, *Church and People in an Industrial City* (1957), p. 85 et passim; Henry Pelling, review of K. S. Inglis, *Churches and the Working Classes in Victorian England* (1963) in *Past & Present*, no. 27 (1964), 128–33 at p. 129; Alan Gilbert, *Religion and Society in Industrial England* (1976), p. 92; Robert Moore, *Pit-Men, Preachers, and Politics*; for class and occupational statistics on Methodists and changes over time, see: C. D. Field, "The Social Structure of English Methodism: eighteenth–twentieth centuries," *Br. J. Sociol.*, 28 (1977), 199–225.
106. *Methodist Revolution*, pp. 8–9 and conclusions.
107. Cited in Richard Garnett, *The Life of W. J. Fox, Public Teacher and Social Reformer, 1786–1864* (1910), p. 215.
108. Holyoake, *Sixty Years of an Agitator's Life* (1892; 3rd ed., 1906), I, p. 60; Wilberforce, *Practical View of the Prevailing Religious System of Professed Christians, in the Higher and Middle Classes in This Country, Contrasted with Real Christianity* (1797). Wilberforce's book was notable for its matter-of-factness, certitude, puritan attack on the past, individuality, and energetic optimism for worldly perfection.
109. G. M. Young, after commenting on the extent to which phrenology was an exception in being regularly taught in the mechanics' institutes, noted that the science probably helped to "keep the idea of personality alive under the steamroller of respectability": *Portrait of an Age* (1936; new ed. 1960), p. 26n.
110. Combe might be seen as revealing an awareness of this need–dependency on the science in the conclusions to the *Constitution of Man*, where he wrote: "The doctrine before unfolded, if true, authorizes us to predicate that the most successful method of ameliorating the condition of mankind will be that which appeals most directly to their moral sentiments and intellect; and I may add from experience and observation, that, in proportion as any individual becomes acquainted with the real constitution of the human mind, will his conviction of the efficacy of this method increase" (p. 339).
111. "Representative Men ... the Combes," p. 579. In perceiving Combe's phrenology in this way, Martineau was foreshadowing Durkheim's view of liberalism as the secular religion of industrial society (see: Steven Lukes, "Political Ritual and Social Integration," in his *Essays in Social Theory* [1977], 52–73). On the surrogate religious function of the organized freethought movement in Britain in the C19, see J. Eros, "The Rise of Organized Freethought in Mid-Victorian England," *Sociol. Rev.*, n.s. 2 (1954), 98–120.
112. Cf. Webb, *Working Class Reader*, p. 160.

CHAPTER 7: *Richard Carlile and infidel science*

1. Jacob, *Radical Enlightenment*, esp. at pp. 137, 263. On social Darwinism and its abundant secondary literature, see: Gretta Jones, *Social Darwinism and English Thought: the interaction between biological and social theory* (Brighton, 1980); and Alfred Kelly, *The Descent of Darwin* (1981). On mesmerism and the French radicals, see: Darnton, *Mesmerism*.
2. William Thompson, *An Inquiry into the Principles of the Distribution of Wealth Most*

Conducive to Human Happiness (1824), p. 274 (a new edition of the work was issued in 1850 by the Owenite William Pare). On the view of science as a cultural antidote to the division of labor, see also: Maxine Berg, *The Machinery Question*, p. 150.

3. Frank Harris, *Life and Loves*, p. 309.
4. See, for instance, William Aitken, introducing his weekly "Scientific Information" to the readers of *McDouall's Chartist and Republican Journal*, 10 Apr. 1841, pp. 14–15; and J. F. Bray, *Labour's Wrongs and Labour's Remedy; or, the age of might and the age of right* (Leeds, 1839), esp. at pp. 25, 29–34.
5. Cited in Shapin and Barnes, "Head and Hand," p. 253n.; for similar statements, centered largely on the SDUK, see *Poor Man's Guardian*, 31 Mar. 14 Apr. 1832, pp. 334, 359.
6. *Man: a rational advocate for universal liberty, free discussion, and equality of conditions*, 1 (7 July 1833), p. 1. Earlier politically militant journals such as William Rogers's *The People* (1817), *The Medusa; or, Penny Politician* (1819), or Cobbett's *Political Register* seldom ever referred to science, partly as a consequence of time and space, but partly as well it seems, from either an instinctive distrust or the feeling that for all intents and purposes science was irrelevant to the real needs of working people.
7. William Devonshire Saull in a lecture in the Rotunda, *Isis*, 1 (3 Mar. 1832), 60.
8. Quoted in Tholfsen, *Working Class Radicalism*, p. 64.
9. For an excellent example of this critique see: the Owenite condemnation of the BAAS editorial in *New Moral World* (hereafter *NMW*), 10 (28 Aug. 1841), 68–9. Similarly, George Orwell's major objection to scientists was that they were more subject to totalitarian habits of thought than writers, yet they had all the prestige: "What is Science?" *Tribune*, 26 Oct. 1945, repr. in *Collected Essays*, vol. IV (Harmondsworth, 1970), p. 29.
10. See: Gillispie, "Jacobin Philosophy of Science"; and, for the argument that not all Jacobins thought science either irrelevant or a threat to liberation, see: L. Pearce Williams, "The Politics of Science in the French Revolution," in Clagett, *Critical Problems*, 291–308. Henry Guerlac rehearses the conventional history of science view of the Jacobins as hooligans and of Lavoisier as "the outstanding martyr to the excesses of the Reign of Terror during the French Revolution" in his entry on Lavoisier in *DSB*, 69–91 at p. 67.
11. The "principle of vitality" is referred to in the editorial in the *NMW* (note 9). See also: the views of the Concordians cited below, Chapter 8. On Winstanley, see: Christopher Hill, ed., *Winstanley: the love of freedom and other writings* (Harmondsworth, 1973), pp. 42–59; and idem, "Forerunners of Socialism in the Seventeenth Century English Revolution," *Marxism Today*, 21 (1977), 270–6 at p. 274. Vitalist views were of course also expressed within the orthodox scientific community and in bourgeois society by such persons as Carlyle, Coleridge, and Julian Hare (see: R. Yeo, "Image of Science," p. 76). In general, the difference between these persons' interest in vitalism and that of working-class radicals lay in the latter's more or less direct association of the principle with amending the socioeconomic relations of industrial capitalism.
12. See: Stanley Diamond, "Anthropology in Question," in Dell Hymes, ed., *Reinventing Anthropology* (N.Y., 1974), 401–29 at p. 410; and Barbara Goodwin, *Social Science and Utopia: nineteenth-century models of social harmony* (Hassocks, Sussex, 1978), pp. 162–3.
13. Jacob, *Radical Enlightenment*, p. 96. Consider also the role assigned to artisans by Edgar Zilsel, "The Genesis of the Concept of Scientific Progress," repr. in P. Wiener and A. Noland, eds., *The Roots of Scientific Thought* (N.Y., 1957), 251–75.
14. Cf. Michael Polanyi, *Knowing and Being* (Chicago, 1974), p. 81: "Laymen normally accept the teachings of science not because they share its conception of reality, but because they submit to the authority of science."
15. Cf. Paul Feyerabend, *Science in a Free Society*, p. 75.
16. Anthony Wedgewood Benn at a Northwestern University Colloquium, "The

Control of Science for Civil Needs," Apr. 1971, q. in Morris Goran, *Science and Anti-Science* (Ann Arbor, Mich., 1974), p. 11. But cf. the view of Saint-Simon that the scientists were "a free floating elite with no natural class alignments": q. in Frank Manuel, "Henri Saint-Simon on the Role of the Scientist" in his *Freedom from History*, p. 207.

17. *Anti-Dühring (Herr Eugen Dühring's Revolution in Science)* (Peking, 1976), p. 33.

18. The appearance is deceptive, however, in that phrenology might be excepted only in that it was conducive to political and social discussion.

19. On Lysenko, see: R. M. Young, "Lysenkoism." Popular phrenology and Lysenkoism are indeed consanguineous in that Lysenko took up the ideas of Lamarck, and that Lamarck took up phrenology partly in his rebellion against the late-C18 scientific elitism of Buffon.

20. Carlile, *An Address to Men of Science; calling upon them to stand forward and vindicate the truth from the foul grasp and persecution of superstition* (1821), p. 23; William Wickwar, *The Struggle for the Freedom of the Press, 1819–32* (1928), p. 90, q. in Weindling, "Science and Sedition," p. 150. This chapter was written and revised without benefit of Joel Wiener, *Radicalism and Freethought in Nineteenth Century Britain: the life of Richard Carlile* (Westport, Conn., 1983), the first full biography. It supercedes the main biographical sources consulted here: Edward Royle, *Victorian Infidels* (Manch., 1974), pp. 31–43; and John W. Nott, "The Artisan as Agitator: Richard Carlile, 1816–43," Ph.D. thesis, Wisconsin, 1970.

21. *Republican*, 7 (25 Apr. 1823), p. 543. This admission followed upon his reading of the only full account of the science he had seen up to that time: a "small periodical work." Very likely this was the ambivalent essay review of William Scott's *Observations on Phrenology*, which was offprinted from *Medico-Chirurgical Rev.* of Mar. 1823. If so, Scott's aligning of phrenology with orthodox religion, on the one hand, and the reviewer's medico-physiological objections against phrenology, on the other, could hardly have left Carlile other than in doubt. Carlile reflected on his acquisition of phrenology in "Mania of Religion, Phrenologically Illustrated," *Lion*, 3 (8 May 1829), 586–8.

22. *Republican*, 11 (22 Apr. 1825), 487. On the visit to Deville (who was to credit Carlile with having a "religious" character), "Phrenology," *Republican*, 13 (14 Apr. 1826), 449–51; and "Physiognomy and Phrenology Essential to the Establishment of a Correct Moral Philosophy," *Lion*, 1 (20 June 1828), 769–72 at p. 771; see also: "What Is Love?" *Republican*, 11 (6 May 1825), 545–53 at p. 549. Carlile's thinking on phrenology was likely influenced by the respectful attentions paid the science by Lawrence in his *Lectures*, which Carlile republished; and by the fact that his gifted atheist friend and patron Julien Hibbert joined the LPS in Apr. 1824 (never to waver in his conviction). For Lawrence's association with Carlile, see: W. F. Bynum, "Time's Noblest Offspring," pp. 135, 139, 150, 162–3; on Hibbert (1800–34), see: entry by J. Wiener in *Biographical Dictionary of Modern British Radicals*, vol. 1 (1979), pp. 221–2. In accordance with his will, Hibbert's head was secured for phrenological study by his and Carlile's friend and fellow Rotundist Pierre Henri Baume and deposited in the private phrenological museum of W. Devonshire Saull: "Extract from the Will of Julien Hibbert," *Scourge*, 21 Feb. 1834, copied in Baume, *Autobiography* (MS, Wellcome Institute, London), pp. 641–2; see also: ibid., p. 480; and Holyoake, *History of Co-operation*, II, p. 405.

23. "Mania of Religion," p. 588; "Physiognomy and Phrenology," p. 771.

24. *Lion*, 4 (17 July 1829), 65: "I treated but cursorily on that class of organs, immediately over the eye, which are called *perceptive*. On the *intellectual*, the *moral*, the *superstitious*, and the *energetic* organs, I treated more at large, and I flatter myself, that I satisfied the audience as to their immediate bearing against the validity of religion and the too common custom of mankind." He had an audience of "about fifty."

25. Thelwall is cited in Ian Inkster, "Studies in the Social History of Science in England during the Industrial Revolution, c. 1790–1850," Ph.D., Sheffield, 1977, vol. II, p. 70.

26. "Phrenology," *Republican*, p. 451.
27. "Phrenology," *Lion*, 2 (3 Oct. 1828), p. 433 (for Welsh's views, see: *Phren. J.*, 5 (1828/9), 109–12); "Dr Spurzheim and Phrenology," *Prompter*, 1 (11 June 1831), 497–500 at p. 497. See also: [Carlile], "Craniology," *Newgate Monthly Mag.*, 2 (Sept. 1825), 10–18, 127–30.
28. E.g., James Parkinson, pamphleteer and author of the *Organic Remains of a Former World* (1804–11), and John Thelwall, itinerant political preacher, medical writer, and author of the *Rights of Nature* (1796). Like the constitutional radical James Montgomery of Sheffield, Thelwall had become thoroughly tame by 1825. Government suppression of the London Corresponding Society resulted in large part from their republication and distribution of the works of Paine.
29. See: J. Ann Hone, *For the Cause of Truth: radicalism in London, 1796–1821* (Oxford, 1982), esp. at pp. 285, 336 ff.
30. Ibid., pp. 355, 285.
31. Peter Linebaugh, "Labour History without the Labour Process: a note on John Gast and his times," *Social Hist.*, 7 (1982), 319–28 at p. 323.
32. Quoted in Tholfsen, *Working Class Radicalism*, p. 567; see also: ibid., p. 59. Although under certain conditions, as Foster has shown (*Class Struggle*), working-class consciousness was able to develop, from this we cannot jump to the conclusion that there was in the early C19 a *real* working-class radicalism based on industry and an *artisan* radicalism that was somehow more liberal and ideological in outlook. For the most part the radical press remained in the hands of the "superior artisans," and while the sentiments of the fustian cutter, the factory hand, or the pitman might be expressed more frequently, the control voice behind them remained that of – as Thompson describes the voice of Carlile – "the Shoreditch hatter or the Birmingham toymaker and his audience," aficionadoes of Enlightenment rationalism with a practical edge. *The Making*, p. 84.
33. *Fact versus Fiction; an essay on the functions of the brain, selected from Lawrence's lectures* (1832; 2nd ed., 1840); cf. anon., *Thought NOT a Function of the Brain: a reply to the arguments for materialism advanced by Mr Lawrence, in his lectures on physiology* (1827).
34. *The Works of George Petrie: comprising Equality and other poems. Select extracts from the letters of Agrarius: with a biographical memoir of the author* (n.d.), p. 6. Petrie's death in Feb. 1836, after he had spent some time in Hanwell Lunatic Asylum, was popularly attributed to Baume, who cohabited with Petrie's wife. Baume, a former spy in the service of the Sicilian government who had earned considerable fortune thereby, had already acquired his reputation in the press and in popular ballad as "The Islington Monster" for having cohabited with his sister and, upon her death in childbirth in 1830, having sold her body and that of her stillborn baby to a London hospital. See: *Autobiography*. Petrie's radical views may be found in *Man*, e.g. 8 Dec. 1830, p. 173. "Equality" was dedicated to Robert Owen.
35. Cited in Petrie, *Works*, p. 29.
36. See: Gwyn Williams, *Rowland Detrosier: a working class infidel, 1800–34*, Borthwick Papers no. 28 (York, 1965), p. 15.
37. *Movement*, 2 (8 Jan. 1845), 9–12; and Chilton, " 'Materialism' and the Author of the 'Vestiges,' " *Reasoner*, 1 (3 June 1846), 7–8. Chilton felt that Chambers had expropriated his and Charles Southwell's "Theory of Gradation."
38. "Dr Spurzheim and Phrenology," pp. 497–8. The regard for Paley in the Zetetic tradition is captured in Holyoake, *Paley Refuted in His Own Words* (1847).
39. Wallace, *The Revolt of Democracy* (1913), p. 5. For his Owenite background: *My Life* (1905), I, pp. 87–9, 104.
40. George Eliot, *Felix Holt the Radical*, chap. 30, cited in R. M. Young, "Man's Place in Nature," p. 378.
41. In his comments on "Phrenological Exhibition of the Reforming Optimist [i.e., Baume]," *Lion*, 3 (8 May 1829), 588.
42. However, it should be borne in mind that prior to and during the passage of

the Reform Bill *political individualism* was to reformers and antireformers alike synonymous with anarchy. See: D. C. Moore, "Concession or Cure: the sociological premises of the first Reform Act," *Hist. J.*, 9 (1966), 39–59, at p. 43.

43. Thompson, *The Making*, pp. 845–51.

44. "Co-operative Competition against Competitive Co-operation," *Lion*, 1 (29 Feb. 1828), 260; "Co-operation," *Lion*, 3 (9 Jan. 1829), 39. (Carlile recognized that in holding the opinion that cooperation could only produce a mediocre state of society, he was of the same opinion as Ricardo.) See also: T. W. Mercer, *Richard Carlile on Co-operation: a century old criticism. Reprinted from the Co-operative Review* (1929). Similar criticisms of Owenism werre voiced by Carlile's first employer in London, Thomas Wooler, the Painite editor of the *Black Dwarf*; see: R. Hendrix, "Popular Humour and 'The Black Dwarf,' " *J. Brit. Stud.*, 16 (1976), 108–28 at pp. 112–13.

45. *Lion*, 1 (11 Apr. 1828), 465–6; for Thompson on economic individualism, see: his *Inquiry*, Pare edition, pp. 391–4.

46. "Co-operative Competition against Competitive Co-operation" (note 44) p. 260. Ernest Jones argued for the nationalization of cooperatives in order to undermine capitalism and establish social equality: "A Letter to the Advocates of the Co-operative Principle, and to Members of Co-operative Societies," *Notes to the People*, 1 (1851), 27–31. Far closer to Carlile was the Chartist Feargus O'Connor, who claimed that socialism "is at variance with the ruling instinct of man, which is selfishness, self-interest, self-reliance, and individuality": *Northern Star*, 23 Sept. 1848, n.p. Holyoake and James Linton held similar individualist antisocialist views; see: Holyoake, "The Disease of State Socialism," a new chapter in the 2nd edition of his *History of Co-operation* (1879), II, 479–88; and Linton, *The English Republic*, ed. K. Parkes (1891), pp. 141–4. For the conservative workingman's view, see: Charles Manby Smith, "A Working-Man's Notions on Socialism," in app. to his *The Working-Man's Way in the World: being the autobiography of a journeyman printer* [1851], pp. 337–47.

47. "Competitive Co-operation versus Co-operative Competition," *Lion*, 2 (4 July 1828), 12.

48. "Co-operation" (note 44), p. 38.

49. "Physiognomy and Phrenology," p. 771; see also: Carlile, "Moral Philosophy Necessarily Founded on the Animal Nature of Man; that animal nature various in its degrees and qualities, phrenologically or organically and chemically constituted and physiognomically indicated," *Lion*, 2 (4 July 1828), 1–5.

50. For his encouragement to mechanics to form institutes for mutual instruction, see: "Philosophical Institutions for the Improvement of Mechanics," *Republican*, 8 (26 Dec. 1823), 767; and Holyoake, *The Life and Character of Richard Carlile* [1870], p. 23. For Carlile, unlike Brougham and Co., "Halls or temples of science" were to be places for the popularization of Paine's works; cf. "Mechanics' Institutions and Tom Paine's Works," *London Mechanics' Reg.*, 3 (4 Feb. 1826), 255–6.

51. "Physiognomy and Phrenology," p. 771. See also: "The Creed of Richard Carlile," *Prompter*, 1 (12 Feb. 1831), 235; Carlile, *A New View of Insanity* (1831), p. 29; idem, "Discussion with the Sect of Owenites," *Political Reg.*, no. 8 (7 Dec. 1839), 127–8; "Mr Carlile and the Socialists" [editorial], *New Moral World* 4 (23 Dec. 1837), 67–70; and Nott, "Carlile," pp. 37, 158–9.

52. "Physiognomy and Phrenology," p. 771.

53. "New Plan of Reform," *Lion*, 1 (11 Jan. 1828), 33–6 at p. 33.

54. *Lion*, 1 (11 Apr. 1828), 466; *Phren. J.*, 6 (1829/30), 623.

55. On the function of liberal bourgeois education, see: André Gorz, "Technology, Technicians, and Class Struggle," in Gorz, ed., *The Division of Labour: the labour process and class-struggle in modern capitalism* (Hassocks, 1978), 159–89 at p. 178.

56. "Notebook VII [1858]," *Grundrisse*, trans. M. Nicolaus (Harmondsworth, 1973), p. 706.

57. *The Autobiography of William Cobbett*, ed. W. Reitzel (1967), p. 218. Cobbett saw Owen's educational system at New Lanark as fashioning the rising generation

"to habits of implicit submission." On New Lanark, see: Chapter 8. Cf. Marx and Engels: From the moment a division of material and mental labor appears, "consciousness *can* really flatter itself that it is something other than consciousness of existing practice, that it *really* represents something without representing something real; from now on consciousness is in a position to emancipate itself from the world and to proceed to the formation of 'pure' theory, theology, philosophy, morality, etc.": *The German Ideology*, in *Collected Works*, vol. 5 (1976), 44–6. As Ernst Bloch has pointed out: "For Marx ... the fundamental subject is never mind but man, economic and social ... man as a totality of social relationships, changing through history ... in the social realm of interests, not in the celestial realm of ideas": *On Karl Marx*, trans. J. Maxwell (N.Y., 1968), p. 111. Phrenology was the "celestial realm" cerebrally reified.

58. *Lion*, 1 (11 Apr. 1828), 466; and on utopian thought in general, see: Goodwin, *Social Science and Utopia*, pp. 150, 162–3 ff.; and Frank Manuel and Fritzie Manuel, *Utopian Thought in the Western World* (Oxford, 1979).

59. On Carlile's various journals and their circulations and readerships, see: Patricia Hollis, *The Pauper Press: a study in working-class radicalism of the 1830s* (Oxford, 1970), pp. 117–20, 211; and Wickwar, *Struggle for the Press*, p. 95 et passim. On Carlile's waning popularity, see: Royle, *Victorian Infidels*, pp. 37–8.

60. See: *Lion* 4 (10 July 1829), 37.

61. On Taylor (whom Hibbert and Baume also followed), see: Guy A. Aldred, *The Devil's Chaplain: the story of the Rev. Robert Taylor, MA, MRCS (1784–1844)* (Glasgow, 1942); on Carlile's adoption of Taylor's views, see: Royle, *Victorian Infidels*, p. 38. For the C18 pantheistic materialists, see: Jacob, *Radical Enlightenment*, esp. pp. 22, 263.

62. *Isis*, 1 (23 June 1832), 307. That she regarded phrenology as a means of improving on Owenism, see: ibid., 17 Mar. 1832, p. 81 (As the mistress of the Warner Street Temperance Hall in the late 1840s and 1850s, Sharples became something of a foster mother to Charles Bradlaugh; see: Royle, *Victorian Infidels*, p. 308.)

63. Owen correspondence, letter 262, 13 June 1830, q. in Nott, "Carlile," p. 133.

64. Manuel and Manuel, *Utopian Thought*, pp. 720 ff.

65. *The Lectures of Mr Richard Carlile to the Inhabitants of Brighton with a Syllabus of his Course of Seven Lectures* [1836]. The lectures were to be delivered in the Hall of Science, City Road, London, on 16 and 23 Dec. 1839, admission 3d: *Political Register*, no. 8 (7 Dec. 1839), 128.

66. Carlile, *Manuel of Freemasonry* [1860], first part published in 1825, 4th ed. of all 3 parts c. 1845. Toland is referred to in Carlile, *The Gospel According to Richard Carlile; showing the true parentage, birth, and life, of our Allegorical Lord and Saviour, Jesus Christ* (1827), p. 6. See: Sophia Elizabeth De Morgan, *Threescore Years and Ten* (1895), pp. 46–7 (p. 53: "The Duke of Sussex used to say that Godfrey Higgins, Richard Carlile, and he himself, were the only persons who knew anything of the matter [of Freemasonry]."). See also: J. Harrison, *Second Coming*, pp. 155–6. Carlile's Allegorical Christianity has mostly been dismissed or ignored by historians; Nott, "Carlile," p. 11, essentially agrees with G. D. H. Cole in his *Richard Carlile* (1943), p. 3, that it was simply a changing of means for the same radical republican ends. Carlile's daughter, Theophilia Carlile Campbell, in *The Battle for the Freedom of the Press as Told in the Story of the Life of Richard Carlile* (1899), refers to the subject but offers no commentary on it.

67. On Paine's Newtonianism and his assertion that "motion is *not a property* of matter," see: Royle, *Victorian Infidels*, p. 27; and John Derry, "Tom Paine: an international radical," in his *The Radical Tradition: Tom Paine to Lloyd George* (1977), 1–45 at p. 12. (According to C18 freethinkers, if motion is inherent in matter, then God, who, according to Newton, puts things in motion, is rendered impotent and therefore nonexistent. See: Jacob, *Radical Enlightenment*, p. 240. On plebeian spiritualists and phreno-mesmerism, see: Barrow, "Socialism in Eternity."

68. Quoted in *Lion*, 4 (25 Sept. 1829), 395.

69. "Dr Spurzheim and Phrenology," p. 499.

70. "Phrenology," *Lion*, 1 (18 Apr. 1828), 481.
71. *Lion*, 2 (4 July 1829), 3.
72. *Lion*, 3 (6 Feb. 1829), 164.
73. Thomas Turton, letter to editor, *Lion*, 1 (18 Apr. 1828), 483; and idem, "A Paper Read before a Small Society in Sheffield, on the Properties of Mind," *Lion*, 1 (25 Apr. 1828), 508–12. For Montgomery's contribution to antiphrenology, see: his *An Essay on the Phrenology of the Hindoos and Negroes; showing that the actual character of nations as well as of individuals, may be modified by moral, political, and other circumstances, in direct contradiction to their cerebral developments* [read before the Sheffield Lit & Phil, 7 Feb. 1827] *together with strictures thereon by Cordon Thompson* (1829); but see: J. Wigley, "James Montgomery and the 'Sheffield Iris,' 1792–1825: a study in the weakness of provincial radicalism," *Trans. Hunter Arch. Soc.*, 10 (1975), 173–81; and Donnelly and Baxter, "Sheffield and the English Revolutionary Tradition, 1791–1820," pp. 412–13. On Godwin's veiws, see: "Of Phrenology," in his *Thoughts on Man, His Nature, Productions, and Discoveries* (1831), 357–75; and the extended reply, by a slightly embarrassed Elliotson, in *Lancet*, 10 Dec. 1831, pp. 357–63.
74. See: [Baume], "Phrenological Exhibition of the Reforming Optimist," *Lion*, 3 (24 Apr. 1829), 541–4; ibid., (8 May), 603–8. Though Baume took phrenology seriously, believing that it "must be the saviour of the world" and also, that "the most clever phrenologists were to be found among government spys" (*Autobiography*, pp. 60–1, 410), he was not adverse to lampooning it in the manner that Carlile had in the *Republican* in the early 1820s (e.g., vol. 10, 19 Aug. 1824, 194); see: for example: [Baume], "Sambo's Lecture on Craniology," *New John Bull and Penny Satirist*, 17 Jan. 1835, copied in *Autobiography*, pp. 682–7.
75. "On the Science of God. Chapter IX: " 'God as a spirit,' " *Political Register*, no. 7 (Nov. 1839), 105.
76. On socialism seriously considered as a cause of insanity, see: James Copland, *A Dictionary of Practical Medicine* (1858), II, p. 588, sec. 597. On radicalism as the pathological consequence of an average endowment of "Veneration" plus large "Self-Esteem," see: *Tait's Mag.*, 5 (Sept. 1838), 557–8.
77. "Uses of Phrenology," *Phren. J.*, 6 (1829/30), 623.
78. Vol. 1 (10 Nov. 1833), 142.
79. See: T. Travers, "Samuel Smiles," p. 173; Lloyd Jones, *A Reply to Mr R. Carlile's Objections to the Five Fundamental Facts as Laid Down by Mr Owen* (Manch., 1837).
80. James Hill, *Star in the East*, 2 (23 June 1838), 214. See also: "Mr Carlile on Equality of Condition," *Man*, 1 (22 Dec. 1833), 190; for the middle-class press's exploitation of Carlile's religiosity in an effort to tar all radicals as "touched," see: *The Printing Machine or Companion to the Library and Register of Progressive Knowledge*, 1 (June 1834), 186. For Carlile's own awareness by 1840 that "being neither a Tory, Whig, Radical, Socialist, or Chartist, I find I am nothing and nobody," see: Campbell, *Carlile*, p. 217.
81. *Science in a Free Society*, p. 75. See also: Noel Annan, *The Curious Strength of Positivism in English Political Thought* (1959), esp. pp. 10–11: "The battle between rationalism and religion was fought by both sides almost entirely on positivist ground – on the verification of evidence and the credibility of hypotheses – very different ground from that which in Germany the Idealist historian, David Strauss, had chosen in his *Leben Jusus*, which related religious belief to the changing structure of society."
82. A. L. Morton, *The English Utopia* (1952), p. 137n.
83. Roy Porter summarizing the views of Chris Green's manuscript on natural history as ideology in Britain, 1820–60, in "The Politics of Geology: the case of George Hoggart Toulmin," *J. Hist. Ideas*, 39 (1978), 435–50 at p. 450n.
84. *Lion*, 2 (4 July 1828), 1. The trek to the Anti-Corn Law League is referred to in Hollis, *Pauper Press*, p. 308 (his application was declined).
85. Cited in G. Williams, *Detrosier*, p. 16. O'Brien, like other "proto-Marxists," scientific socialists, and secularists, was not only unaware of the snag in rational scientific thought, but, unlike Carlile, was not personally bothered by it. Ex-

cluded from his attack on the bourgeoisie and the bourgeois-minded were physicians and surgeons, engineers, architects and other professionals, along with artists, mechanics, and artisans and all others who had, or whose knowledge had, no direct connection with the socioeconomic structure. Cited in Stan Shipley, *Club Life and Socialism in Mid-Victorian London*, History Workshop Pamphlet no. 5 (1972), p. 12.

86. Marx to P. Annenkov, 28 Dec. 1848, in *The Letters of Karl Marx*, selected and trans. Saul K. Padover (Englewood Cliffs, N.J., 1979), p. 53. See also: *Communist Manifesto*, p. 494.

CHAPTER 8: *On standing socialism on its head*

1. John Epps was thus solicited by Owenites anxious to hear his phrenology lectures at Bermondsey: *Diary*, entry for 13 Mar. 1835, p. 251. "All nature cries with one voice," Holyoake wrote in *Reasoner*, 4 (1 Dec. 1847), 4; "man, look to thyself – there is no Providence but Science." See also: his *History of Co-operation* I, p. 217.

2. Tholfsen, *Working Class Radicalism*, p. 118; J. F. C. Harrison, *Robert Owen and the Owenites in Britain and America* (1969), p. 235.

3. The Owenite interest in phrenology has been noted in passing in Harrison, ibid., pp. 239–43; idem, "A New View of Mr Owen," in Pollard and Salt, *Owen: prophet of the poor*, 1–12 at p. 8; Eileen M. Yeo, "Social Science and Social Change: a social history of some aspects of social science and social investigation in Britain, 1830–1890," Ph.D. thesis, Sussex, 1972, p. 42 et passim; McLaren, "Phrenology: medium and message," p. 88; De Giustino, *Conquest of Mind*, pp. 140–5; and A. C. Grant, "New Light on an Old View," *J. Hist. Ideas*, 29 (1968), 293–301.

4. J. C. Prichard explained the popularity of Gall as resulting from the general lack of complete satisfaction with Locke's doctrine of human understanding (despite the impressive work of Hartley, Condillac, and Helvetius), since innateness always seemed to be present no matter how a child was raised: "The first writer who should reduce these observations into a connected form was sure to make many proselytes. This, in fact, was done by Dr Gall, who stated in a more distinct and systematic way than any preceding writer, the doctrine of the innateness of particular talents and intellectual and moral propensities": *Treatise on Insanity* (1835), p. 465.

5. Lamarck, "Systeme de Gall" [unpublished lecture, c. 1800], in William M. Wheeler and Thomas Barbour, eds., *The Lamarck Manuscripts at Harvard* (Cambridge, Mass., 1933), 3–38. For Gall's views on Lamarck, see: Hilts, "Phrenological Views on Inheritance and Eugenics," p. 64.

6. Owenites drew in particular from Helvetius, as popularized by Godwin, Priestley, Thomas Hodgskin, and others; see: introduction to Harold Silver, ed., *Robert Owen on Education* (Cambridge, 1969), p. 15.

7. Spurzheim, *A View of the Elementary Principles of Education* (Edin., 1821; trans. into French, 1822), retitled *Education: its elementary principles founded on the nature of man* (Manch., n.d.), pp. 14, 9. Cf. the fatalistic antiperfectibility comments on phrenology by Honoré Balzac, *A Harlot's Progress* (Paris, 1838–47), trans. J. Waring (1896), I, p. 69; and [H. C. Robinson], *Account of Gall's New Theory*, p. 135.

8. Owen, *A Dialogue in Three Parts* (Manch., 1838), p. 11.

9. See, for example: *Elements of Phrenology* (7th ed., Edin., 1850), pp. 23–4. Combe considered Gall as lacking "the analytic spirit and talent which is necessary to reach first principles or primitive faculties in mental philosophy": Gibbon, *Life of Combe*, II, pp. 15–16.

10. S. Smith, *Principles of Phrenology*, p. v. The essentially environmentalist educational ideas of Pestalozzi were as widely endorsed by phrenologists as by Owenites. See for example: J. L. Levison, *Mental Culture* (1833), pp. 177, 240, et passim. The phrenologist D. G. Goyder‡ visited New Lanark in his capacity as an organizer of Pestalozzian schools in Britain (*Autobiography*, pp. 187–90) and

. James P. Greaves (on whom see: below) studied under Pestalozzi in Yvedon before returning to England in 1825 to establish the London Infant School.

11. *Report of Proceedings at Several Public Meetings Held in Dublin; preceded by an introductory statement of his opinions and arrangements at New Lanark extracted from his "Essays on the formation of Human Character"* (Dublin, 1823), p. iv.

12. Quoted in De Morgan, *Threescore Years and Ten*, p. 156.

13. Quoted in Harrison, *Owen and the Owenites*, p. 79. For the "Five Fundamental Facts," see: *Crisis*, 1 (13 Oct. 1832), 126.

14. *Co-operative Mag.*, 3 (July 1828), 104 and repr. in *New Moral World* [hereafter *NMW*], serially, 1 (3–25 Apr. 1835), 180–208.

15. Barbee-Sue Rodman, "Bentham and the Paradox of Penal Reform," *J. Hist. Ideas*, 29 (1968) 197–210 at p. 202.

16. Hazlitt, review of Farington's *Life of Sir Joshua Reynolds*, *Edin. Rev.*, 34 (Aug. 1820), repr. in *Works*, vol. 16, p. 189.

17. "K" [Catherine Barmby], "Phrenology," *Co-op. Mag.*, 2 (Sept. 1826), 278–81 at pp. 279–80. On Barmby, see: entry by A. L. Morton and J. Saville in *Dictionary of Labour Biography*, vol. 6 (1982) 10–18; and Barbara Taylor, *Eve and the New Jerusalem: socialism and feminism in the nineteenth century* (1983), esp. pp. 172 ff., 386 ff.

18. William Hawkes Smith, "Remarks on the Application of Phrenology as a Test of the Practicability of Socialism," *Phren. J.*, 13 (1840), 119–28 at p. 129. On Hawkes Smith‡ see: Harrison, *Owen and the Owenites*, p. 74; E. Yeo, "Social Science and Social Change," pp. 21–5; Holyoake, *Life*, pp. 48–50. Also see: obituaries in *Phren. J.*, 13 (1840), 284; and *NMW* 7 (25 Apr. 1840), 1260–1, vol. 8 (25 July 1840), 59. His interest in phrenology, which was acquired simultaneously with his interest in Owenism, was akin to Carlile's insofar as it was a revalidation of his relevance among a younger generation of radicals. Phrenology and Owenism essentially updated the role that Unitarianism had played during his earlier career as a constitutional radical.

19. Thus the Rev. Henry Clarke on the contrary uses of phrenology could claim that "Owenites have urged Phrenology on me as demonstrative evidence of man's entire irresponsibility, until reminded that if that be true, no man is responsible for believing in, and contending for human responsibility, and opposing this principle of Owenism": "Party Phrenologists," p. 239.

20. *On Human Responsibility as Affected by Phrenology* (privately printed, Edin., 1826), pp. 6, 1; cf. his comments in *Essays on Phrenology* (Edin., 1819), p. 142.

21. Owen, "Formation of Character," *Crisis*, 1 (26 May 1832), p. 33.

22. Bray first comes to notice in 1836 in Watson, *Statistics of Phrenology*, p. 121, in a report from Coventry on "a young man ... giving a course of lectures on phrenology to the Mechanics' Institutions ... respectably attended by, perhaps, about two hundred persons." For the story of Bray shaving off his hair and hurrying to London to have his bumps cast by Deville (and to purchase a hundred of Deville's famous casts), for the lessons on organology that he encouraged Marian Evans to pursue, and for the occasion on which he asked for a cast of J. W. Cross's head to check his suitability as a husband for Evans, see: Bray, "Phrenology and the Natural Laws of Man," in his *Autobiography*, pp. 20–47; Gordon S. Haight, *George Eliot* (Oxford, 1968), p. 51; Lawrence Hanson and Elizabeth Hanson, *Marian Evans and George Eliot: a biography* (1952), pp. 316–17. See also: Gibbon, *Life of Combe*, II, p. 312; J. M. Robertson, *History of Freethought*, pp. 338–9; Bray, "Phrenology and Its Applications," *Union*, 1 (June 1842), 75–77; and J. F. C. Harrison, "From the Margins: a view of the social history of George Eliot's England," paper delivered to the Eliot conference at Rutgers University, Nov. 1980.

23. For the Owenite reception of the book, see: *Union*, 1 (Apr./May 1842), 21–8, 55–60; see also: *Reasoner*, 4 (12 Apr. 1848), 39. For the phrenologists' view, see: *Phren. J.*, 15 (1842), 161–74 (only phrenologists could really appreciate the work, they said).

24. See: *The Philosophy of Necessity; or, the law of consequences, as applicable to mental,*

moral, and social science (1841), I, p. 64; and Bray's introduction to Mary Hennell, *An Outline of the Various Social Systems and Communities Which Have Been Founded on the Principle of Co-operation* (1844; [first published as app. to *The Philosophy of Necessity*]), pp. cvii–cviii.

25. See: Peel, *Spencer*, p. 222 et passim.
26. *Philosophy of Necessity*, I, p. 44; II, pp. 464–5. See also: Bray, *Psychological and Ethical Definitions on a Psychological Basis* (1879), p. 31.
27. Quoted in the notices on the 2nd ed. of Epps, *Horae Phrenologicae* [1834], p. 92.
28. Catherine Barmby, "Phrenology," p. 281. Hugh Doherty, the editor of the Fourierist *London Phalanx*, in response to a letter on "The Philosophy of Phrenology" by E. J. Hytche, the phrenology class leader at the London Mechanics' Institute, dissented from the view that "some passions and propensities [are] . . . innately evil in themselves, and quite incapable of moral unity in action," while agreeing that there was a collective harmony in the head as (ideally there ought to be) in society: 1 (11 Dec. 1841), 586.
29. Hawkes Smith, "Application of Phrenology," p. 119; "Address to Phrenologists," *Co-op. Mag.*, 3 (July 1828), 99. Holyoake, a student of phrenology under Hawkes Smith, called the science "a natural corollary of Owenism": *Logbook of Self-Education*, Bishopsgate Institute, cited in Budd, *Varieties of Unbelief* p. 24.
30. *NMW*, 1 (17 Oct. 1835), 406.
31. *Morning Chron.*, 22 July 1839, q. in Hawkes Smith, "Chartism and Socialism – to editor. *Morning Chron.* [29 July]," *NMW*, 4 (10 Aug. 1839), 670.
32. Holyoake, *Life*, I, p. 255. Hollick and Holyoake were both pupils of Hawkes Smith and acquired their knowledge of phrenology in the Birmingham Mechanics' Institute: ibid., pp. 47–9, 60–8. See also: handbill for Holyoake's "Eclectic Lectures," in the Rationalist Institution, Gt. Hamilton St., Sunday morning, 10 Feb. 1846: "The Phrenological Philosophy of George Combe and Dr Engledue; including our unsettled personal reminiscence," NLS 6.1699(3). Cooper discusses his introduction to phrenology (through Combe's lectures in Manchester) in "An Autobiographical Sketch," *Nat. Reformer*, 11 (14 June 1868), 373–4; see also: his eulogy on Engledue in *Investigator* 5 (Feb. 1859), 172. For Southwell's reliance on phrenology, see, for example: his *Socialism Made Easy; or, a plain exposition of Mr Owen's Views* (1840), esp. pp. 7–8; idem, *Superstition Unveiled* (1854), pp. 31, 33; idem, "The Philosophy of the Human Mind," *NMW*, 8 (15 Aug. 1840), 109; and the response to his lectures in Bristol in *Keene's Bath J.*, 14 Feb. 1842, n.p. For Clarke's deployment of phrenology, see: his *The Christian's Looking-Glass; or, a reply to the animadversions of the Rev Dr Redford LLD of Worcester, and the clergy of all denominations, who attempt to oppose the religion of charity as propounded by Robert Owen, being a lecture delivered in the Social Institution, Manchester* (Hulm, 1836). Clarke announces himself on the title page as "Lecturer on phrenology."
33. William Lowe, "Lecture VI: Phrenology in Relation to Religion" (Dec. 1839), in his *Lectures*, p. 189; for Goyder's attack on the socialists, see: *NMW*, 7 (22 Feb. 1840), 1123 (thereafter his works ceased to be advertised in the *NMW*); Rumball's attack on the Owenite S. Rowbotham in Worcester led to the latter's debate with the antiphrenologist and antisocialist Rev. John Brindley (though Rumball had earlier vanquished Brindley in debate on phrenology in Worcester): *NMW*, 5 (2 Mar. 1839), 302; ibid., 7 (11 Jan. 1840), 1018. For Cowan's attack, see: "Dr Cowan and the Christians of Reading," *NMW*, 7 (2 May 1840), 273–5; Dewhurst, who was apparently accompanied at his lectures by "a raving wild Irish Parson, a Rev. D. Delaney," denounced Owen in 1840: *NMW*, 7 (30 May 1840), 1263. In reference to the antisocialist Rev. T. Dalton, see also: *NMW*, 4 (3 Feb. 1838), 124. On Bushea's "Sheffield Phrenological Institution and Anti-Socialist Society" see: Inkster, "Phrenology in Sheffield," pp. 277–8. In *Socialism: public discussion between Mr Alexander Campbell, socialist missionary, and the Rev. J. T. Bannister of Coventry* (Coventry, 1839), it is Bannister who introduces phrenology and Combe's classification system, and supremacy of the intellectual faculties in particular, to ascertain "what is human nature" (pp. 19–20).

34. Hall, *Phreno-Magnet*, 1 (May 1843), 98.
35. See: John Brindley and J. Barber, "Phrenology Discussion between Mr Brindley and Mr Barber, at Bristol," [Brindley's] *Anti-Socialist Gaz.*, 1 (Feb. 1842), 91, repr. in *Phren. J.*, 15 (1842), 185–6, 280–3; see also: *Keene's Bath J.*, 17, 21, 24 Jan. 1842; *Midland Counties Advert.*, 10 Jan. 1839; Brindley, "Dr Andrew Combe and Phrenology," *Birmingham J.*, 8 Dec. 1838, p. 7; ibid., 10 Nov. 1838, p. 5; *Liverpool Standard*, 24 June 1842; *NMW*, 5 (26 Jan. 1839), 218; ibid., 5 (2 Mar. 1839), 302; ibid., 7 (11 Jan. 1840), 1018. On Brindley, see: Holyoake, *Life*, I, pp. 48–50; Royle, *Victorian Infidels*, p. 64; and Thomas Frost, *Forty Years Recollections* (1880), p. 18. On Grant, see: Henry Turner, *Phrenology*; Grant, *Discussion with Donovan*; and Royle, *Victorian Infidels*, pp. 203–7 et passim.
36. Contained in a speech on moral accountability at the London Co-operative Society's Rooms, Red Lion Square, May 1826, *Co-op. Mag.*, 1 (Aug. 1826), 264.
37. "Phrenology," *London Mag.*, 8 (Nov. 1823), 541–4 at p. 541: "We thenceforth became prepared, – scoffers as we had previously been at Phrenology – to look into it with candour, if not with some little prepossession in its favour." On Owen's enthusiasm, see: Gibbon, *Life of Combe*, I, p. 132. Owen's purchase of at least one phrenological bust is confirmed by M. Browning, "Owen as an Educator," in John Butt, ed., *Robert Owen: prince of cotton spinners* (1971), 67.
38. Owen, description of his psychography and psychography in the introduction to James Jennings, *The Family Cyclopedia; being a manual of useful and necessary knowledge* (1821), I, p. xxiv, together with an illustration of the psychograph (among the faculties listed by Owen were Strength, Courage, Sensibility, Perception, Reflection, Memory, Imagination, Judgment, Affection, and Self-Attachment, labels that, compared to those of the phrenologists, have more of a romantic and socially reflective quality); and Jennings, *An Inquiry into Phrenology* pp. 19–20 (the *Inquiry* was dedicated to Owen).
39. Cited in Alexander Cullen, *Adventures in Socialism: New Lanark Establishment and Orbiston Community* (Glasgow, 1910), p. 196.
40. After Combe's 1820 visit to New Lanark, William Ballantyne, one of Owen's schoolteachers, began seriously to pursue phrenology and, after six months of study, wrote to Combe that he had acquired more valuable knowledge of human nature "than I have been able to acquire in the six years precedings (during which I have been in Mr Owen's schools) without such assistance." The letter was proudly reprinted in "Spurzheim on Education," *New Edin. Rev.*, 1 (1821), 321–2n.

    On the failure of the Orbiston community, for example, Hamilton expressed regret that "selection by phrenological principles had not been applied": q. in Harrison, *Owen and the Owenites*, p. 184; see also: Cullen, *Adventures in Socialism*, pp. 181, 197.
41. Robert Dale Owen (1801–77) recorded his "Visit to Spurzheim: sketch of the phrenological theory," *Free Inquirer*, 3 (1 Jan. 1831), 79–80, and further details of his phrenological delineations (by Spurzheim and Deville) in his autobiography *Threading My Way: twenty seven years of autobiography* (1874), pp. 296–301. He claimed to have first met Spurzheim in November 1827, but the month previous he had written to Combe: "I attach to the Science of phrenology generally a much greater importance than I did, my attention has been much attracted to it of late; and I intend to study it for myself until I become convinced either of the truth or error of the *craniological* part of the science": Combe papers, NLS 7220/35 6. S. T. Hall recorded that Robert Owen visited him in Birmingham in the autumn of 1843 and "asked me if I would give him my opinion of his head." Hall found one side of the head to be larger than the other, for which Owen accounted "that the lesser half might perhaps belong to the old world going out, and the larger to the 'new moral world' which he believed was beginning to grow": "Robert Owen," in Hall, *Biographical Sketches of Remarkable People* (1873), 276. For Combe's delineation of Owen's head, see: *Phren. J.*, 1 (1823/4), 235; cf. the delineation given by the LPS on 6 Mar. 1844 after a Mr Hands had brought forward a cast of Owen's head: *Zoist*, 2 (July 1844), 162.

42. *NMW*, 2 (13 Aug. 1836), 335 and (15 Oct. 1836), 406. By this mode of publication, it was claimed, the author has "done his utmost to give his favourite subject an additional appearance of attraction, and to pourtray the outlines of the elaborate state in which the science is now brought by its very numerous and talented supporters." On another occasion the *NMW* praised a new phrenological "divisional bust" as but one of the "numberless inventions that have been made in mechanism, by which the various sciences have been brought to their present state of perfection": 2 (23 Jan. 1836), 102–3.

43. Reported in *People's Phren. J.*, 1 (1843), 216; the proposal was first made in Aug. 1841: "The Uses of Phrenology," *NMW*, 10 (28 Aug. 1841), 67.

44. "Lecture of Mr Saull in Bristol," *Crisis*, 3 (5 Oct. 1833), 38. On Saull, see: *DNB*; and J. M. Wheeler, *Dictionary of Freethinkers*, pp. 290–1. On Cabet, see: A. McLaren, "A Prehistory of the Social Sciences: phrenology in France," *Comp. Stud. in Soc. & Hist.*, 23 (1981), 3–22 at p. 18.

45. See: R. G. Garnett, "E. T. Craig: communitarian, educator, phrenologist," *Vocational Aspect*, 15 (1963), 135–50; Craig, *An Irish Commune: the history of Ralahine* (Dublin [1920]); E. T. Craig, *Educationalist and Social Reformer: a biographical sketch with phrenological delineation* [repr. from *Phren. Mag.*, 4 (Dec. 1883), 56–61]; "Memoir of E. T. Craig," *Republican*, 9 (July/Sept. 1883), serially.

46. *Work and Wages; or, capital, currency, and production* (1865), cited in Garnett, "Craig," p. 150n. See also: A. E. Musson, "The Ideology of Early Co-operation in Lancashire and Cheshire," in his *Trade Unions and Social History* (1974), 173–94; Holyoake, *Self-Help by the People* (1858); Philip Backstom, *Christian Socialism and Co-operation in Victorian England* (1974); S. Pollard, "Nineteenth-Century Co-operation: from community building to shopkeeping," in Asa Briggs and John Saville, eds., *Essays in Labour History* (1967), 74–112, esp. pp. 108–9; and G. D. H. Cole, *A Century of Co-operation* (1947).

47. Wallace, "Ralahine and Its Teaching," in his *Studies Scientific and Social* (1900), II, 455–77 at p. 474. For Wallace's definition of socialism, see: his *My Life* (1905), II, pp. 266–7; and for his faith in phrenology: "The Neglect of Phrenology," in his *The Wonderful Century* (3rd ed., 1899), 159–93.

48. See: Craig, *Star in the East*, 3 (8 Dec. 1838), cited in Garnett, "Ralahine, 1831–33," in his *Co-operation and the Owenite Socialist Communities in Britain 1825–45* (Manch., 1972), 110.

49. Holyoake, *History of Co-operation*, II, p. 405.

50. See: Thompson, *The Making*, pp. 858–64; H. Silver, *Popular Education* p. 130; Arthur E. Bestor, *Backwoods Utopias: the sectarian and Owenite phase of communitarian socialism in America, 1663–1829* (Phila., 1950), p. 140; Owen, *Life of Robert Owen by Himself* (1857), pp. 151–2; Elie Halévy, *Thomas Hodgskin*, ed. A. J. Taylor (1956), p. 38. Like Hodgskin and Cobbett, the Regency radical Thomas Wooler criticized Owen for reducing workers to "mere automata" by rules and regulations: *Black Dwarf*, 20 Aug. 1817, q. in Patricia Hollis, *Class and Conflict in Nineteenth Century England, 1815–1850* (1973), pp. 31–3.

51. Gibbon, *Life of Combe*, I, p. 131; and Grant, "New Light on an Old View," p. 294.

52. Combe to the Rev. David Welsh, 4 Oct. 1823, q. in Gibbon, *Life of Combe*, I, p. 165.

53. Combe to the Rev. David Welsh (after 4 Oct. 1823), q. in ibid., p. 165.

54. [G. Combe], *The Life and Dying Testimony of Abram Combe in Favour of Robert Owen's New Views of Man and Society*, ed. Alexander Campbell (1844), p. 8; Grant, "New Light on an Old View," p. 294. Abram initially called his community "The First Society of Adherents to Divine Revelation": Harrison, *Owen and the Owenites*, p. 104.

55. See: Abram Combe to Robert Owen, 29 Oct. 1823, printed in *NMW*, 2 (19 Dec. 1835), pp. 60–1; and Harrison, *Owen and the Owenites*, p. 105.

56. [Combe], "Phrenological Analysis of Mr Owen's New Views of Society," *Phren. J.*, 1 (1823–24), 218–37, esp. pp. 226, 232 (the essay had been submitted to an advocate of the New Views – probably Abram – whose comments were foot-

noted); "Phrenology and Mr Owen" [containing Owen's letter to the *Edinburgh Advertiser* of 2 Mar. 1824 protesting against Combe's smear], *Phren. J.*, 1 (1823/4), 463–6; and Owen to Combe, 26 Feb. 1821, Combe Papers, NLS 7213/156. Combe was not allowed to forget the differences between himself and his brother: in a letter of 14 May 1848 Bray told him, "of the three brothers in my opinion he [Abram] took the highest favour, but then he was a century or *two* before his time. But Christ was 20 centuries." Combe Papers, NLS 7289/108–9.

57. A. J. Hamilton to Combe, 16 May 1824, Combe Papers, NLS 7213/46–7.
58. G. D. H. Cole, *The Life of Robert Owen* (1930), p. 222; the quotation from the *Report from the County of Lanark* is given in Tholfsen, *Working Class Radicalism*, p. 55; Combe, "Phrenological Analysis of Mr Owen's New Views," p. 235.
59. "Phrenological Criticism on Ballads of the Olden-times," *Edin. Mag. & Lit. Misc.*, 93 (May 1824), 543–51 at p. 544.
60. Combe et al., "Orbiston: meeting of the proprietors," *Co-op. Mag.*, 1 (Nov. 1826), 345 (Combe was replacing Abram, who was ill). Noticeably, the biography of Abram that Combe wrote for *Co-op. Mag.* (2 [Nov. & Dec. 1827], 517–20, 560–9) contained no aspersions on Owen, though it is likely that any such aspersions would have been expunged by the editors. Together with extracts from Abram's *Orbiston Reg.*, the biography in *Co-op. Mag.* makes up the *Life and Dying Testimony of Abram Combe* edited by Campbell.
61. Alexander Paul to A. J. Hamilton, 17 Aug. 1829, q. in Cullen, *Adventures in Socialism*, p. 312.
62. Combe, "Parliamentary Reform," pp. 120, 127.
63. Hawkes Smith to Combe, 7 Apr. 1837, Combe Papers, NLS 7244/21; and Combe to Hawkes Smith, 28 Aug. 1838, Combe Papers, NLS 7288/82. See also: Combe, *Life of Andrew Combe* pp. 143–5; and Gibbon, *Life of Combe*, II, pp. 64–5, where it is also lamented that the £36,000 Abram had raised for Orbiston had been wasted. Although it was well within Combe's financial means to alleviate the poverty into which Abram's family were thrown, it was characteristic of him not to.
64. Karl Bernhard [Duke of Saxe-Weimar-Eisenach], *Travels* (1828), q. in Bestor, *Backwoods Utopias*, p. 81n. On the shift in Owenism see also: ibid., pp. 82–8; and Thompson, *The Making*, pp. 859 ff.
65. As in Harriet Martineau's story "For Each and for All"; see: her *Autobiography* I, p. 232.
66. Owen, *A Development of the Principles and Plans on Which to Establish Self-Supporting Home Colonies* (2nd ed., 1841), p. 31, q. in Bestor, *Backwoods Utopias*, p. 81; "Mechanics' Institutes and Socialism," *NMW*, 5 (24 Nov. 1838), 72.
67. Owen, *NMW*, 1 (25 Apr. 1835), 204.
68. The "realization" by phrenologists is hard to date and obviously differed among them; papers such as that on the "Exposure of Socialism" presented by R. J. Reid, A.M., to the Aberdeen Phren. Soc. in 1845 were rare before c. 1838: *Phren. J.*, 18 (1845), 187.
69. Combe to William Ellis, 10 Apr. 1848, q. in A. C. Grant, "Combe and his Circle," p. 290.
70. Combe to C. Bray, 20 Apr. 1848, Combe Papers, NLS 7391/425–7. See also: Combe's enthusiastic response to Mill's *Political Economy* in his letter to Ellis, 27 Oct. 1848, cited in Grant, "Combe and his Circle," p. 292.
71. William Newham, *The Reciprocal Influence of Body and Mind Considered* (Religious Tract Society, 1842), pp. 47–8: "Certain it is ... that the doctrines of phrenology are appealed to in evidence of the truth of these abominable [socialist] conclusions."
72. George Fleming (then secretary of the Social Institution, Manchester, and a member of Owen's Central Board), open letter to Combe, *NMW*, 3 (27 May 1837), 245.
73. Isaac Ironside, secretary of the Sheffield Hall of Science, report to *NMW*, 11 (10 Dec. 1842), 194.
74. Cited in H. C. Watson, "Political Economy," p. 201.
75. For the classic expression of this view, see: Henry M'Cormac, *On the Best Means*

of Improving the Moral and Physical Condition of the Working Classes; being an address, delivered on the opening of the first monthly scientific meetings, of the Belfast Mechanics' Institution (1830), pp. 22–4.

76. *Phren. J.*, 15 (1842), 173. Though Combe would have been the likely reviewer of this work, his travels in Germany at this time possibly prevented the task. The review, signed "Z" bears little to identify it as Combe's.

77. And was duly praised in *NMW*, 3 (7 Oct. 1837), 405.

78. Ironside, *NMW*, 11 (10 Dec. 1842), 194.

79. "Combe's Constitution of Man," *Br. & For. Rev.*, p. 145; and see: above, note 19.

80. Ibid., pp. 179–80; *Constitution of Man*, pp. 219–26.

81. Bestor, *Backwoods Utopias*, p. 140; Thompson, *The Making*, pp. 857–87; J. F. C. Harrison, "The Poor Man's Advocate," *Times Higher Education Supplement*, 30 Apr. 1976, p. 530.

82. *Proceedings of the Third Co-operative Congress; held in London on the 23rd of April 1832*, ed. William Carpenter (1832), pp. 56–57, 19. On Marriott, see: Holyoake, *History of Co-operation*, I, p. 221; *Reasoner*, 4 (10 May 1848), 47; ibid., 5 (26 July 1848), 142; *Baptist Messenger*, no. 26 (Jan. 1861), 23; and idem, *Catechism on Circumstances; or, the foundation stone of a community* (Salford, [183?]), and *Community: a drama* [Manch., 1841].

83. T. Parssinen and I. Prothero have observed that very few Owenite trade unionists followed James Morrison and "Shepherd" Smith into a theory of class conflict, finding the theory irrelevant to their interest in higher wages: "The London Tailor's Strike of 1834," *Int. Rev. Soc. Hist.*, 22 (1977), 65–107 at pp. 74–5. Moreover, it has been observed by Foster that in Oldham there were many small employers who suddenly turned to Owenism in the mid-1830s as an ideological outlet for the somewhat forced alliance with working-class radicals in which they found themselves: *Class Struggle*, p. 136. See also: Eileen Yeo, "Robert Owen and Radical Culture," in Pollard and Salt, *Owen: prophet of the poor*, 84–114, esp. at pp. 89–94.

84. See: "Phrenological aphorisms," *New Age, Concordium Gazette: a Temperance Advocate*, 1 (May/June 1844), 214, 251, later extended into ninety-three aphorisms and published as *Phrenology* (n.d.); see also: Greaves, *Three Hundred Maxims for the Consideration of Parents in Relation to the Education of Their Children* (1837); *Letters and Extracts from the M.S. Writings of James Pierrepont Greaves*. 2 vols., ed. Alexander Campbell (Ham Common, 1843); *The Healthian: a Journal of Human Physiology, Diet, and Regimen* (1842–3). The best source for Greaves and his philosophy is A. F. Barham, *A Memoir of the Late James Pierrepont Greaves, Esq.*, p. II of his *An Odd Medley of Literary Curiosities, Original and Selected* [1845]. See also: W. H. G. Armytage, *Heavens Below: utopian experiments in England, 1560–1960* (1961), pp. 171–83; and Harrison, *Second Coming*, p. 159. On Ham Common, see: D. Hardy, *Alternative Communities in Nineteenth Century England* (1979), pp. 58–62.

85. In his prospectus for the "London Aesthetic Institution" (c. 1835) Greaves fulminated against Sedgwick's 1834 BAAS address against the study of sentient matter (q. above, Chapter 3), decrying the prescriptively dehumanized brand of science promoted by men of Sedgwick's ilk: "Prospectus," printed in Barham, *Memoir of Greaves*, pp. 16–19. Greaves therefore proposed "The British Association for the Advancement of Astral and Other Sciences, Phrenology, Magnetism, &c, and for the Protection of Students": prospectus printed in *New Age*, 1 (1 Feb. 1844), 169–70. Goodwyn Barmby (1820–81) was the Spinozist author of "The book of Platonopolis," published serially in the *Communist Chronicle* (1843); see: *Dictionary of Labour Biography*, vol. 6 (1982), 10–18.

86. T. Campbell, *Carlile*, pp. 219, 253, et passim. The Ham Common School was largely financed by the same two Gloucestershire widows who gave a great deal of financial aid to Carlile, and Carlile himself had some involvement in the community. On the Commonwealthmen and the radical tradition of dissent from Newtonian science since the 1690s, see: Jacob, *Radical Enlightenment*, esp.

p. 93; and Christopher Hill, *The World Turned Upside Down* (Harmondsworth, 1975).

87. See: "The Development of Human Intelligence," *NMW*, 5 (22 Dec. 1838), p. 143; and the review of "Positive Philosophy," *NMW*, 5 (25 May 1839), pp. 493–4, in which "Comte" is consistently spelt "Combe."

88. E. P. Thompson, *William Morris: romantic to revolutionary* (1955), p. 316: see also: J. F. C. Harrison, *Learning and Living*, p. 116.

89. See, for example: Harrison on the Owenite Thomas Dudgeon, who believed that the millennium would be hastened by the adopting of small communities, phrenology, and "modern science," especially hydrostatics: *Second Coming*, p. 159. In light of the "millennarian current" in Owenism, Owen's own phreno-mesmerically assisted "conversion" to spiritualism in 1853 should not be seen as a weird "irrational" departure from his rationalist views, but rather, as a logical extension of them. Whether or not we regard phreno-mesmerism as a kind of positivist means to the occult for some Owenites, it is clear that the distinction made in hindsight between the "rational" and the "irrational" is meaningless when applied to the early C19 and prior.

90. *NMW*, 4 (24 Mar. 1838), p. 175.

91. *Co-op. Mag.*, 3 (July 1828), p. 111.

92. Frances Wright, "Phrenology," *Free Enquirer*, 3 (25 Dec. 1830), pp. 69–70. On Wright, see: Margaret Lane, *Frances Wright and the "Great Experiment"* (Manch., 1974); and Taylor, *Eve and the New Jerusalem*, pp. 65 ff.

93. R. D. Owen to Combe, 27 Oct. 1827, Combe Papers, NLS 7220/35–6. Combe also sent a copy of his book to Owen senior; see: Owen to Combe, 15 Nov. 1827, Combe Papers, NLS 7220/33.

94. *NMW*, 1 (21 Mar. – 3 Apr. 1835), 166–80. The second dialog, which was mainly concerned with phrenology (pp. 169–72) had been read on 26 Mar. 1835 by Owen at the lecture room of the phrenologist J. D. Holm‡ of Bedford Square. Holm, who was clearly on good terms with socialists (Flora Tristan stayed with him on one of her visits to London), replied in the "Answer to the Dialogues Touching on Phrenology," *NMW*, 1 (18 Apr. 1835), 197–8; and ibid. (25 Apr. 1835), 205 (reprinted as "Owenism and Phrenology," *Phren. J.*, 9 [1834/6], 492–4, along with a summary of Owen's views, pp. 489–92). He insisted that "education is only second to organization, but it *is* second" (thus allowing social deviancy to be traced to pathology). The "dialog" was reprinted as a pamphlet in Manchester in 1838 and is reproduced in part in A. L. Morton, *The Life and Ideas of Robert Owen* (1962), pp. 223–4. See also: Owen's speech before the phrenologists meeting in Newcastle (where he was hooted off the stage): "The Phrenological Association and Meeting," *Newcastle Courant*, 7 September 1838, pt. II, p. 3.

95. "Mr Combe's Lectures at Birmingham," *NMW*, 4 (23 June 1838), 273–4, full text in *Birm. J.*, 26 May–23 June 1838 (following upon these lectures the Birmingham Phren. Soc. was formed, largely of medical men). A possible further source of Owenite annoyance with Combe was the revelation of his shoddy handling of the Orbiston affairs: "Facts about New Lanark, Motherwell, and Orbiston," *NMW*, 7 (4 Jan. 1840), p. 995: "Orbiston was righting itself of its idlers and its unsuitable members – it was gradually consolidating and would, but for the forcible legal interference of the great phrenologist [G. Combe], have righted itself, and been at this day a flourishing establishment." They were mistaken, however, as Harrison has pointed out, it was William Combe (one of the major subscribers to the community) who "succeeded the management of Orbiston when Abram died and when the mortgage began to press for payment in 1827 it was William who ordered the members to quit": *Owen and the Owenites*, p. 169. In the *Life and Dying Testimony of Abram Combe*, Campbell claimed that George Combe, acting as the legal agent of the community, took the "most effectual steps to bring the community ... to a speedy termination."

96. *NMW*, 8 (4 July 1840), 1–3.

97. According to Holyoake, Murphy was a respectable member of Birmingham

society whose skill as a dentist gave him "sufficient position [that] no social persecution could reach him": History of Co-operation, I, p. 222.

98. Holyoake, "Fourteen Nights with George Combe," in his Life, I, 60–65; idem, "Reminiscences," Reasoner, 1 (16 Sept. 1846), 225–6 and (with the dates wrong) in Life, I, 48–49. See also: Holyoake to Combe, 24 Jan. 1846, Combe Papers, NLS 7280 f 69 (Combe called him "a wrong-headed radical").

99. Murphy, "Phrenology," in his Science of Consciousness, 213–21. In its review, NMW called this section on phrenology the most exciting part of the book: 5 (3 Nov. 1838), 28–30. Cf. one of the rare attacks on phrenology from the left in France: Dr. D. Cerise, Exposé et examen critique du système phrenologique (Paris, 1836), cited in McLaren, "Phrenology in France," p. 12.

100. Murphy, Science of Consciousness, pp. 220, 221. For an example of ignominy befalling a person whose head reading had not been favorable, see: "Specimen of Antiphrenological Facts: correspondence between Mr G. Combe and Mr David Dunn, teacher at New Lanark," Phren. J., 10 (1836/7), 267–70. For condemnation of this use of phrenology, especially as applied to servants (written sympathetically from the servant's point of view), see: "Phrenology," Dublin Penny J., 1 (July 1832), 39–40 at p. 39; and "Craniology," Olla Podrida, [1] (June 1825), 178–82.

101. R. D. Owen to Combe, 27 Oct. 1827, Combe Papers, NLS 7220/35–6; Murphy, Science of Consciousness, pp. 200, 221.

102. Ibid., pp. 219–20. On Mill's Essay on Nature, see: Chapter 4.

103. As a promoter of materialism who had previously debated with Brindley (see: Garnett, Co-operation, p. 175), Murphy welcomed the phrenological proof of the brain as the organ of the mind, though he disclaimed the phrenological novelty of the idea.

104. Ironside NMW, 11 (10 Dec. 1842), 194.

105. NMW, 11 (17 Dec. 1842), 202.

106. "Phrenology versus Murphy," NMW, 5 (22 Dec. 1838), 130–1. See also: an earlier debate in NMW, 5 (12 Jan. 1839), 190.

107. "George Combe's Visit to the United States" [review], NMW, 9 (8 May 1841), 288. Such preaching the journal considered to be the "grand and essential object" of Combe's volume. A decade later when James Linton met Combe he was to hear from him "an amusing account of Robert Owen's impracticability at his American colony 'New Harmony' ": Linton, Memories (1897), p. 123.

108. Ironside, NMW, 11 (10 Dec. 1842), 194. Engledue, Cerebral Physiology; published by James Watson, the edition of 1842 sold at 4d. It was also reproduced serially as "The Philosophy of Phrenology and Animal Magnetism" in NMW, 11 (17 Sept. – 8 Oct. 1842), a reprint of the original printing in Medical Times, 6 (2 July 1842), 209–14. For NMW, this was the first substantial article on phrenology since the debacle with Combe in 1838. Thereafter appeared a number of enthusiasms, including a front page leader; "On the Applicability of Phrenology to the General Affairs and Management of the Rational Society," NMW, 11 (26 Nov. 1842), 173–4; and "Materialism and Phrenology," (8 & 15 Oct. 1842).

109. Isaac Vale, letter to the editor, People's Phren. J., 1 (1843), 167.

110. E.g.: M. Q. Ryall, "Science and Religion," Movement, 2 June 1844, pp. 196–7; [Robert Buchannan], "Mrs Pugh on Phrenology," Reasoner 1 (20 Aug. 1846), 184–6; T. Paterson, "Cerebral Physiology," Oracle of Reason 1 (8 Oct. 1842), 345–6.

111. NMW, 11 (20 May 1843), 337. See also: reports from the branches of the Rational Society in Leeds and Derby: NMW 11 (17 Dec. 1842), 202–3; Ironside's comments in his report the following week; ibid. (31 Dec. 1842), 218; and the report from Newcastle, ibid. (27 May 1843), 389. See also: "Animal Magnetism," NMW, 11 (25 Feb. 1843), 278–9; and R. D. Owen, Neurology: an account of some experiments in cerebral physiology. By Dr Buchanan of Louisville (1842); idem, Autobiography, p. 240n. He ranked Buchanan's discovery "not with those of Gall and Spurzheim alone, but hardly second to that of any philosopher or philanthropist,

who ever devoted his life to the cause of science and the benefit of the human race" (p. 11).

112. See, in particular: Ironside's report *NMW*, 11 (7 Jan. 1843), 228. In the John Street Institute J. N. Bailey[‡] lectured continuously on phreno-mesmerism in 1843, and John Ellis[‡] gave demonstrations in the Stockport Hall of Science. See also: *New Age*, 1 (10 June 1843), 44–5; *Mesmerist*, 1 (27 May 1843), 23; *NMW*, 12 (13 Apr. 1844), 335; ibid. (11 May 1844), 366.

113. *NMW*, 11 (10 Dec. 1842), 194.

114. *Cerebral Physiology* (as offprinted from *Med. Times*), p. 5. See also: report from Ipswich, *NMW*, 11 (24 Dec. 1842), 212.

115. *NMW*, 11 (17 Dec. 1842), 202. A similar, and similarly isolated, caution appeared in the long review of Engeldue and Elliotson's *Zoist: NMW*, 12 (29 July 1843), 37–9. Cf. J. L. Hammond and Barbara Hammond, *The Skilled Labourer* (1936), p. 381: "In an age of such rapid invention and development it was easy to slip into the belief that the one task of the human race was to wrest her secrets from nature, and to forget how much of the history of mankind is the history of the effort to find a tolerable basis for a common life."

116. See: Royle, *Victorian Infidels*, pp. 70–71 ff.; on Lovett, see: *Life and Struggles of William Lovett in His Pursuit of Bread, Knowledge, and Freedom* (1876; repr. 1967), p. 48. On Hetherington, see: his "Mr Owen and the Working Classes," *Poor Man's Guardian*, 14 Jan. 1832, p. 245; and ibid., 24 Dec. 1831, p. 221. Cf. G. D. H. Cole, *Robert Owen* (Boston, 1925), p. 225.

117. Engels, *Anti-Dühring*, p. 341, who added that "I myself was acquainted with several former members of this communist, model experiment."

118. Among the anti-phreno-mesmerists helping to fan the flames of Owenite interest in phreno-mesmerism was the great "No-Popery" campaigner Rev. Hugh M'Neile; see: "Satanic Agency and Mesmerism," *NMW*, 11 (11 Feb. 1843), 263.

119. *NMW*, 11 (4 Mar. 1843), 292. The remark is all the more noteworthy in being made in response to the demonstrations on phreno-mesmerism by S. T. Hall (cf. Engels' remarks cited above, Chapter 5, note 58).

120. *Phren. J.*, 15 (1842), 86–7. (Arguing that Christian socialism was absurd and that phrenology and physiology demonstrated that religion should have no place in schools, Redburn supported the amendment to the rules for Harmony Hall that the words "god" and "religion" be struck out and replaced by "nature" and "morality": *Movement*, 2 March 1844, p. 93. A few years later he led the campaign for the release from prison of the infidel Charles Southwell.) For Epps's lectures at the John Street Institute, see: *NMW*, 7 (18 Apr. 1840), 1253; and ibid. (6 June 1840), 1286–7. The Phrenology Class at the institute met on Sunday afternoons and cost 2s per quarter or 4s for seven months except in summer, although some members paid extra to make "good use of the books during that space." See also: *Movement*, 1 (25 Sept. 1844), 360; *Reasoner*, 1 (July–Oct. 1846), 142; 270, 288, 296, 304, 308. For an account of the John Street Institute, see: Wallace, *My Life*, I, p. 87.

121. *Phren. J.*, 15 (1842), 87.

122. See: Nicholas Abercrombie and B. S. Turner, "The Dominant Ideology Thesis," *Br. J. Sociol.*, 29 (1978), 149–70, esp. at p. 161; Thompson, "Peculiarities of the English"; R. Q. Gray, "Styles of Life," esp. pp. 437–8.

123. Report to Congress, May 1843, *NMW*, 11 (10 June 1843), 410. The comment came at the same congress at which Walter Newall of the A1 Branch (John Street) made his proposal for phrenological screening of applicants to Harmony Hall and at which it was claimed that the Phrenology Class at the A1 was now "possessing property, in books, casts etc., to the amount of £22, which had been accumulated by the *subscription* of the class." Since A1 subscriptions to the community fund for Harmony Hall had fallen from 105 to 69 between May 1842 and May 1843, it is little wonder that Lloyd Jones complained. *NMW*, 11 (20 May 1843), 377–8. On Jones's reputation as a critic of Combean phrenology, see also: *Movement*, 2 (19 Feb. 1845), 62n.

124. *William Morris*, p. 356.

125. Craig, "Owen in Ireland," *American Socialist*, 1 Nov. 1877, cited in Garnett, "Craig," p. 136; repeated in Craig, *Memoir and in Memorium of Henry Travis, M.D.* (Manch., n.d.), p. 10. Similarly, in 1840, Hawkes Smith had accused Owen of rejecting phrenology out of an impatience and misunderstanding that was ill-founded: *Phren. J.*, 13 (1840), 124. For Smith, "socialism" was "the intended realization of the logical deductions of George Combe": *Letters on the State and Prospects of Society* (Birm., 1838), pp. 19–20, 32. On Arthur George O'Neill, who gained an interest in phrenology while a medical student in Glasgow and who partly financed his studies by lecturing on the science, see: A. Wilson, "Chartism in Glasgow," in Asa Briggs, ed., *Chartist Studies* (1959), 249–87; and Mark Hovell, *The Chartist Movement* (Manch., 1918, repr. 1966), pp. 200–3. For phrenology in O'Neill's Christian Chartist Church, see: R. Alun Jones, "Knowledge Chartism," M.A. thesis, Birmingham, 1938, p. 206. On Cooper, see: *Life*, p. 169; G. D. H. Cole, *Chartist Portraits* (1941; repr. 1965), pp. 187–217; and Robert J. Conklin, *Thomas Cooper the Chartist (1805–1892)* (Manila, 1935). Kingsley's portrayal of Chartism in *Alton Locke*, in which there is much discussion of phrenology, is largely based on Cooper, with whom Kingsley was intimate. Another leading Chartist involved with dissenting science (and in all likelihood phrenology) was Henry Vincent, who presided over the Christian Chartist Church in Bath after his release from prison in 1841. He adopted Lovett and John Collin's plans for halls where Chartists could acquire "Political, Moral and Scientific Information." See: Brian Harrison's entry on Vincent in *Dictionary of Labour Biography*, vol. 2, 326–34.
126. Lovett to G. Combe, 22 Nov. 1849; and *The Charter*, 3 Feb. 1839, both cited in R. A. Jones, "Knowledge Chartism," pp. 57–8. The *Constitution of Man* was one of the books that Lovett urged his wife to supply him with while he was in Warwick Gaol writing *Chartism: a new organization of the people* (1840), which acknowledges its debts to Combe.
127. Lovett, *Life and Struggles* (1876; repr. 1967), pp. 238, 279; *People's Phren. J.*, 1843, p. 166; Jolly, *Education as Developed by Combe*, p. 230. Lovett was reproached in *McDouall's Chartist & Repub. J.*, 1 May 1841, p. 35; and in the *Northern Star*, 8 May 1841, p. 2 (which also scorned Hetherington, Holyoake, and O'Neill as birds of a feather). Other feather friends included James Linton and George Howell, the latter coming from a Methodist background similar to Lovett's and who read the *Constitution of Man* upon the suggestion of the *British Controversialist*; see: F. B. Smith, *Linton*, esp. p. 34; and F. M. Leventhal, *Respectable Radical: George Howell and Victorian working class politics* (1971), pp. 12, 23. On Lovett's typicality as a early Victorian working-class radical, see: R. H. Tawney's preface to the 1920 reprint edition of Lovett's *Life*, p. vi.
128. On Charles Southwell's faith in competitiveness as lying at the root of earnestness and improvement, see: F. B. Smith, "The Atheist Mission," p. 219; and Royle, *Victorian Infidels*, p. 70.
129. As early as 1842 Holyoake wrote on Richard Carlile in the *Oracle of Reason* claiming that "Reformers of every grade owe much to Carlile – for their honour may their regard ever be commensurate with his merit": 1 (30 July 1842), 257. Shortly before he died Carlile wrote, "The more I see and hear of Holyoake the more I like him," and his daughter added that he "often wished that Holyoake had been his son, and Holyoake as often wished too, that he had been": q. in Campbell, *Carlile*, p. 257. Southwell also eulogized Carlile in lectures on the "Life and Times of Richard Carlile" at the Paragon Hall coffeehouse: *Reasoner*, 2 (23 Dec. 1847), 8.
130. Carlile's Allegorical Christianity tended to be quietly forgotten by such men, while Greaves was regarded by Holyoake as next to mad: *Reasoner*, 1 (21 Oct. 1846), 265–6. Rejecting pantheism, William Chilton in his review of *Vestiges* wrote, "It is true that the materialist and [Chambers] . . . are agreed upon one point – they both believe that the properties of matter are sufficient for the production of the phenomena of the universe": *Reasoner*, 1 (3 June 1846), 8.
131. In 1858, the year that Bradlaugh replaced Holyoake as president of the Secular

Society, the *London Investigator* declared, "More converts have been made this last quarter of a century by the *Constitution of Man* to freethought than any other agency": 5 (1858), 93. See also: "Phrenology as It Affects Free Will and Immaterialism," *London Investigator*, 1 (July 1854), 49; T. Paterson, "Phrenology and Materialism," *Oracle of Reason*, 1 (10 Sept. 1842), 313–14; idem, "Cerebral Physiology and Materialism," ibid., (8 Oct. 1842), 345–6; *Free-Thinkers Information for the People*, 2 [1843], 20; and M. Q. Ryall, "Science and Religion," *Movement*, 2 June 1844, pp. 196–7. "It cannot be denied," wrote Samuel Brown in his article on "Physical Puritanism," 419, that "Owen and his disciples have long been working in the same direction [as the brothers Combe; and] that the very atheism of the times, among the illuminated artisans of our great cities, is all in favour of the bodily virtues now under discussion. Cleanliness and temperance are the very religion of the materialist, and should be the complement of religion for all."

132. Craig, *History of Ralahine*, p. 145. Cf. H. G. Atkinson and H. Martineau: "We do not war against ... the rights of men and of property in any sense; but only against lies, hypocrisy, and delusions of every sort. We desire real freedom, – the freedom of the mind to perceive clearly what is true, and to reason justly on all questions": *Laws of Man's Nature and Development*, p. 190.

133. Holyoake, "Socialism," *Movement*, 1 (20 Jan. 1844), 41. On Combe and the origins of the term *secularism*, see: Jolly, *Education as Developed by Combe*, p. 718; Holyoake, *Life*, II, pp. 254–5, 293; and idem, *Origins and Nature of Secularism* (1896).

134. Such was William Bateson's description of the reaction of a First World War soldier who perceived Darwinism to be nothing but "scientific Calvinism": q. in Arthur Koestler, *The Case of the Midwife Toad* (1971), p. 31.

Conclusion

1. James Hunt [founder and president of the London Anthropol. Soc.], "On Physio-Anthropology: its aim and method," *J. Anthropol. Soc.*, 5 (June 1867), ccxvii. Hence E. W. Cox[‡] at the fifth meeting of the Psychol. Soc. of Great Britain in Nov. 1878 proposed changing the organization's name to the "Pneumatological Society": *Proceedings of the Psychological Society, 1875–1879* (1880), p. 8.

2. Lewes, "Phrenology in France," *Blackwoods Mag.*, 82 (Dec. 1857), 665–74, esp. at p. 673; idem, "Phrenology," in his *Biographical Dictionary of Philosophy* (1857), 629–45; Spencer, *The Principles of Psychology* (1855), p. 607; Hunt, "Physio-Anthropology," p. ccxiv; and see: B. Hollander, "Herbert Spencer as a Phrenologist," *Westminster Rev.*, 139 (1893), 142–54.

3. Bray, *Autobiography*, p. 23.

4. E.g.: James Carson, *The Fundamental Principles of Phrenology Are the Only Principles Capable of Being Reconciled with the Immateriality and Immortality of the Soul* (1868), pp. 63–4; A. R. Wallace, "Neglect of Phrenology," p. 179; Bernard Hollander, *In Search of the Soul and the Mechanism of Thought, Emotion, and Conduct* [c. 1920], I, pp. 359–63; J. M. Robertson, "The Revival of Phrenology".

5. Ibid., pp. 250, 255. For the opinions of the medical profession, see: *J. Psychol. Med.*, 6 (1853), 344; Hollander, *The Revival of Phrenology* (1901), p. 393.

6. See, in particular: William Mattieu Williams, *A Vindication of Phrenology* (1894), p. 307.

7. On Paracelsianism, see: Charles Webster, *From Paracelsus to Newton*: (Cambridge, 1982); idem, "Paracelsus and Paracelsianism: basic data," *Bull. Soc. Social Hist. Med.*, no. 30–31 (1982), 47–50. On astrology, see: K. Thomas, *Religion and the Decline of Magic*, pp. 341 ff.; and Capp, *English Almanacs*, chap. 8, "The Eighteenth Century."

8. See: S. Smith, *Principles of Phrenology* (2nd ed., 1849), p. iii; W. B. Hodgson, letter of 18 July 1859, in *Life and Letters*, p. 22; H. Martineau, "Representative Men ... the Combes," p. 579; Gibbon, *Life of Combe*, I, p. xi; Nicholas Morgan, *The Skull and Brain: their indications of character and anatomical relations* (1875), p. 201.

9. As reprinted in *On the Study of Character; including an estimate of phrenology* (1861), preface. See also: H. C. Bastian, "Phrenology: old and new," p. 520. On Fowler and Wells, see: M. B. Stern, *Phrenological Fowlers*; and J. Millott Severn, "The Late Professor L. N. Fowler," *Popular Phrenologist*, 1 (Oct. 1896), 148. On the hiatus in phrenology's popularization in the 1850s, see: Gibbon, *Life of Combe*, II, p. 360; "Death of George Combe," *J. Health & Phren. Mag.*, 7 (July 1858), 142–3 (after two years with no articles on phrenology, this journal changed its title in 1860 to *Journal of Health and Vegetarian Messenger*); "Phrenology," *Human Nature*, 2 (1868), 346.

10. W. H. Thomson, *Brain and Personality*, p. 20.

11. "Professor Bridges' Manipulation of Viscount Palmerston," *J. Health & Phren. Mag.*, 7 (Apr. 1858), 58–9; and see: Bridges, *Criminals, Crimes, and Their Governing Laws as Demonstrated by the Sciences of Physiology and Mental Geometry* (Liverpool, 1860), preface. A. McLaren notes that Bishop Wilberforce had his head read in 1852: "Medium and Message," p. 90.

12. Exceptions to decline in serious phrenological discussion of insanity, crime, and education include James G. Davey, "Paper on the Relations between Crime and Insanity," *J. Mental Sci.*, 5 (1858), 82–94; John P. Brown, *Phrenology and Its Application to Education, Insanity, and Prison Discipline* (1860). On phrenology and ethnology and anthropology, see: J. W. Jackson, *Ethnology and Phrenology as an Aid to the Historian* (1863); P. A. Erickson, "Phrenology and Physical Anthropology: the George Combe connection," *Current Anthropology*, 18 (1977), 92–3; Marvin Harris, "Raciology, Phrenology, and the Cephalic Index," in his *The Rise of Anthropological Theory* (1968), 99; and Nancy Stepan, *The Idea of Race in Science: Great Britain, 1800–1960* (1982), esp. pp. 20–8.

13. William Osler, "On the Brain of Criminals: with a description of the brains of two murderers," *Canadian Med. & Surg. J.*, 10 (1881/2), 385–98; and "Report on the Brains of Richards and O'Rouke," ibid., 11 (1882/3), 461–6. For Conan Doyle and phrenology, see: Madeleine B. Stern, *The Game's A Head: a phrenological case-study of Sherlock Holmes and Arthur Conan Doyle* (Rockville Center, N.Y., 1983).

14. On the links with eugenics, see: Hilts, "Hereditary Descent"; Pearson, the first Galton Professor of Eugenics at the University of London, delivered the fifth of the lectures of the Henderson Trust (for the propagation of phrenology): *On the Skull and Portraits of George Buchanan* (Edin., 1926). I am indebted to Charles Webster and Joan Austoker for the reference to Leonard Darwin. On pre–First World War craniometrics in schools, see: William L. Mackenzie and Edwin Matthew, *The Medical Inspection of School Children* (Edin., 1904), pt. III: "School Anthropometry."

15. See: A. L. Vago, *Phrenology Vindicated* [1879], p. 9; cf. F. G. Mandley, *A Few Words on Popular Phrenology* (Manch., 1862), esp. p. 3; and J. P. Catlow, "On the Fallacy of Phreno-Magnetism, or Mesmero-Phrenology," *North of Eng. Mag.*, 2 (May 1843), 428–36.

16. As tallied from the phrenological journals published between 1848 and 1911.

17. Charles Shaw (b. 1832), *When I Was a Child*, p. 65.

18. On J. D. Burns, a leading plebeian spiritualist and the editor of *Human Nature*, see: *Human Nature*, 1 (1867), 51; and Barrow, "Socialism in Eternity," pp. 41–2, 54–5, 67n. On Wright, see: the handbill to his lectures in Johnson Collection in the Bodleian Library, box on "Phrenology & Chirology." On Bridges, see: Appendix. Taylor referred to himself as a "Hygienic Physician and Consulting Phrenologist and Specialist on the Brain, Lungs and Stomach"; see: "Directory of Phrenologists," in *Popular Phrenologist* (1896), and his *Applied Psychology* (Morcambe, [1912]); Fowler's Phrenological Institute in Ludgate Circus opened in 1873, and Jazeb Inwards's‡ Phrenological Museum in Oxford St., London (formerly William Horsell's Phrenological Depot and Homoeopathic Medical Dispensary) opened in 1880.

19. "Directory of Phrenologists," 1896. See also: "Some Notes at Starmouth" *Punch*, 17 Sept. 1887, p. 132.

20. *The Pelican Papers* (1873), p. 47. On Chartists turning their attention to rationalist intellectual pursuits upon the collapse of the movement, see: Ben Brierley [the Oldam Chartist], *Home Memories* (Manch., [1886]), p. 49. See also: Prothero, *Artisans and Politics*, p. 338.

21. Stan Shipley, *Club Life and Socialism*, p. 45. Shipley observes (p. 42) that in the clubs physiology was "the single most popular science subject." As previously, secularists had no monopoly in phrenology: The Rev. John H. Howshall of Oldham chose his profession on the basis of a phrenological delineation by Fowler in 1861; in 1882 he and his church committee sponsored two courses of lectures on phrenology by Fowler: *Phren. Mag.*, 4 (Jan. 1883), 40–1. For the defining of plebeian culture, see: L. Barrow, "Determinism and Environmentalism in Socialist Thought," in Raphael Samuel and Gareth Stedman Jones, eds., *Culture, Ideology, and Politics* (1983), 193–213 at p. 194.

22. Page 308. See also: his *The Intellectual Destiny of the Working Man; an address delivered on the 28th May, 1863 to the members of the "Institute Chemical Society"* (Birm., 1863); for his lectures on the "Elements of Phrenology," see: London Mechanics' Institute Prospectus of Courses for June–Sept. 1848: NLS 6.1697(23), and "The Study of Phrenology," *J. of Health*, 13 (1864), 7–8. Williams was the headmaster of the secular school in Edinburgh set up by Combe; see: *Annual Reports of Mr. William's Secular School* (Edin., 1850–4). He named his son George Combe Williams.

23. "Farewell Entertainment to Mr and Mrs Fowler, and Presentation to Mrs Fowler," *Dundee Advertiser*, 4 Apr. 1863.

24. *Diary of Epps*, p. 578, entry for 10 Nov. 1860.

25. "Bitter Fruit," p. 214.

26. Holyoake, *Reasoner*, 6 (14 Mar. 1849), 161. On Barker's phrenological publications, see: Chapter 5, note 108.

27. *First Impressions of England and Its People* (Edin., 1889), p. 106.

28. F. B. Smith, "The Atheist Mission," p. 220. See also: Gay Weber, "Degeneration and Progress in early C19th Social Theory," paper presented to the British Society for the History of Science, Cambridge, 1976.

29. Joshua T. Woodhead [M.D.–"Anatomical Museum," Liverpool], *The Golden Referee; a guide to health, and the causes that prevent it . . . with the duties and obligations of marriage: practical observations on the nature, origin, and cause of local weakness and general debility; the injurious effects of solitary and sexual indulgence, etc.* (Liverpool [1874]), pp. 27–8; for similar statements, see: John Stevens, *Man-Midwifery Exposed* (1849), p. 16.

30. Advertisement on the flyleaf of the first number of *Zadkiel's Mag., or Record and Rev. of Astrol., Phrenol., Mesmerism, and Other Sci.* (Jan. 1849). On antiintellectualism among bourgeois groupings in the late C19, see: Christopher Kent, *Brains and Numbers: elitism, Comtism, and democracy in mid-Victorian England* (Toronto, 1978), pp. 139 ff.

31. *A Vindication of Phrenology*, pp. 46, 308.

32. For examples of the latter, see: David Brewster, "Characteristics of the Age," pp. 7–13; Andrew Wilson, "The Old Phrenology and the New," *Gents. Mag.*, 244 (Jan. 1879), 68–85. For the phrenological response to Brewster, see: above, Chapter 3, note 80; and to Wilson, C. Donovan, *A Reply to Dr Andrew Wilson's Attack on Phrenology* (1879).

33. Cf. Pierre Bourdieu and Jean-Claude Passeron, *Reproduction in Education, Society, and Culture*, trans. R. Nice with a forward by Tom Bottomore (1977), p. 210 et passim; and Paul Feyerabend, "How to Defend Society against Science," *Radical Philosophy*, 2 (1975), 4–8.

34. See: Barrow, "Socialism in Eternity"; idem, "Determinism"; idem, "Anti-Establishment Healing: spiritualism in Britain," in W. J. Sheils, ed., *The Church and Healing*, vol. 19 of *Studies in Church History* (Oxford, 1982), 225–47; idem, "Democratic Epistemology: mid-19th-century plebeian medicine," *Bull. Soc. Social Hist. Med.* no. 29 (1981), 25–9; J. V. Pickstone, "Medical Botany (Self-Help Medicine in Victorian England)," *Memoirs of the Manchester Literary and*

Philosophical Society, 119 (1976/7), 85–95; idem, "Establishment and Dissent in Nineteenth-Century Medicine," in *Church and Healing*, pp. 165–89; R. J. Cooter, "Interpreting the Fringe," *Bull. Soc. Social Hist. Med.*, no. 29 (1981), 32–6.

35. *Elements of Psychological Medicine* (1853), pp. 52–3.
36. See, for example: J. L. McIntyre [lecturer in psychology and ethics at Edinburgh], "Phrenology," in *Encyclopedia of Religion and Ethics*, vol. 9 (1917), 897–900. Cf. Frederick Bridges, *Phrenology Made Practical and Popularly Explained* (Liverpool, 1861), p. 1.
37. Gibbon, *Life of Combe*, II, pp. 365 ff.
38. See: Henry Steel Olcott, *Old Diary Leaves: the only authentic history of the Theosophical Society*, 5th ser., Jan. 1893–Apr. 1896 (Madras, India, 1932), p. 370; and Barrow, "Socialism in Eternity," p. 67.
39. *Chart of Spiritual Gifts and Mediumistic Capabilities* (Sunderland, c. 1890). In addition to Burns's *Human Nature*, see: William Carpenter's one-penny *The Spiritual Messenger* (1858–9) published by the phrenologist, hydropathist, temperance advocate, and vegetarian William Horsell (1807–63), which was devoted, in addition to spiritualism, mesmerism, and psychology, to phrenology, "the noblest Science that can engage the attention of man."
40. On Bergson, see: H. Stuart Hughes, *Consciousness and Society* (Brighton, Sussex, 1979), pp. 113 ff.; and for related reflections on this theme: R. J. Cooter, "Medicinae Cultura e Alternativa," *Prometeo*, 1 (Dec. 1983), 22–31.
41. Leaflet on the "Spiritual and Reform Literary Depot" in Johnson Collection, Bodleian Lib., Oxford, "Supernatural" Box 1. L. N. Fowler: *Phrenological Character of Mr Charles Bradlaugh, M.P. ... marvellously verified by his career up to the present time* [1880] was sold in London in J. Martin's "Anti-Ritualistic Depot," Strand.
42. *Scarbro' Gaz.*, 27 Aug. 1874, q. in R. B. D. Wells, ed., *Phrenological Messenger* (Leeds, 1878), p. 3. See also: James Webb, "Phrenology in the Schoolroom," *Phren. Mag.*, 5 (1884), 321–31; *Phrenology Made Easy; or, the art of studying character in relation to love, courtship, and marriage, showing the best means of cultivating character so as to arrive at early wealth, position, and happiness, being a complete guide to fortune* (1874), cost 1d. On phrenology as an antidote to Darwinism, see: Ambrose L. Vago, *The Alphabet of Phrenology* [1883], p. 4.
43. *The Ragged Trousered Philanthropists* (St. Albans, Herts., 1965), chap. 22, pp. 214–23.
44. Levison, *Mental Culture*, p. 102.
45. James Garth Wilkinson, letter to Henry James, Sr., q. in Clement J. Wilkinson, *James John Garth Wilkinson: a memoir of his life* (1911), p. 89.
46. John Cleland [professor of anatomy at Glasgow], "The Lingering Admirers of Phrenology," *Popular Sci. Rev.*, 8 (1869), 378–88 at p. 379; see also: William James, "The Phrenological Conception," in his *The Principles of Psychology* (1910), I, 26–30 at p. 28.
47. J. J. Spark, *Confessions of a Phrenologist; or, facts stranger than fiction* (1891), p. 3.
48. Bourdieu and Passeron, *Reproduction*, p. 9.
49. Chorover, *Genesis to Genocide*, p. 148. See also: Pierre Bourdieu, *Outline of a Theory of Practice*, trans. R. Price (Cambridge, 1977), at pp. 79 and 218n.
50. See: G. B. Risse, "Vocational Guidance during the Depression: phrenology versus applied psychology," *J. Hist. Behav. Sci.*, 12 (1976), 130–40; and Brian Evans and Bernard Waites, *IQ and Mental Testing: an unnatural science and its social history* (1981).
51. See: Chorover, *Genesis to Genocide*; Edward Yoxen, "The Social Impact of Molecular Biology," Ph.D. thesis, Cambridge, 1978; and J. Crocker, "Sociobiology: the capitalist synthesis," *Rad. Sci. J.*, 13 (1983), 55–72.
52. Marx to Ludwig Kuglemann, 11 Jan. 1868, *Letters*, p. 242. Needless to say, the remark was gratuitous and made tongue in cheek, although it is interesting that Marx was referring to "one of my friends here [in London] who dabbles a lot in phrenology."

MANUSCRIPT SOURCES AND PUBLIC DOCUMENTS

National Library of Scotland
Combe papers.

Edinburgh University Library
Letter book of the Phrenological Society, 1820–40. Gen. 608/1.
Minute book of the Phrenological Society. Vol. I, 1820–40; Vol. II, 1841–70. Gen 608/2.
Names of members and visitors, inspecting the casts etc. belonging to the Phrenological Society, 1822–46. Gen. 608 x (iii).
Catalog 2: unbound, marked "superceded, much corrected and annotated, etc."
Catalog 3: in four parts; n.d., watermark 1828. Compiled by Robert Cox. Gen 608/5.
Catalog of skulls, busts, masks, etc. in the Edinburgh Phrenological Society's collection, arranged alphabetically; n.d. Gen. 608/4
Cash book of the Edinburgh Phrenological Society, 1820–70. Gen. 608/3
Phrenological scrapbook [1858–61]. Gen. 608 x (iii)
Goyder, David George, *Heads of the People, 1843: measurements and manipulations of heads* [365 deliniations]. Gen. 608 x (v).

Bodleian Library
John Johnson Collection (Box of ephemera on "Phrenology and Chirology").
Forster Papers. MS Eng. Letters c.200 f.181.
J.G. Spurzheim. MS Autog. f.181–2.
J.G. Spurzheim. MS Top. Oxf. b.23., f.301(d).

Guildhall Library
London Institution. Collection of managers' and auditors' reports of lectures and other miscellanea, 1805–94, 4 vols. AN.16.8.
London Institution. Syllabuses of Lecture Courses, 1819–74. SL 50-2.

British Library
Collection of reports and private letters by W. J. Roberts on the Liverpool Mechanics' Institute, 1826–40, 2 vols. 1866e.7.
MS papers relating to Liverpool Mechanics Institution, 1777–1850 8364. b. 24.

Swedenborg Society of London
Charles Augustus Tulk, *Aphorisms on the Laws of Creation as Displayed in the Correspondences That Subsist between Mind and Matter* (n.d.). A/83.

Wellcome Institute, London
Pierre Henri Joseph Baume, *Autobiography*, 1838–55.
Phrenology: Spurzheim Lecture (watermark, 1827). MS 4685.

Unpublished theses and papers
Baxter, P. "Combe, the Constitution of Man, and the Churches." Paper delivered to the
    British Society for the History of Science, Durham, 1979.
Baxter, P. "Natural Laws and Divine Judgments: some reflections on Scottish natural
    theology." Paper delivered to the British Society for the History of Science, Bath,
    1980.
Corsi, Pietro. "Natural Theology, the Methodology of Science, and the Question of Species
    in the Works of the Reverend Baden Powell." D.Phil. thesis, Oxford, 1980.
Grant, Alastair Cameron. "George Combe and His Circle: with particular reference to his
    relations with the United States of America." Ph.D. thesis, Edinburgh, 1960.
Harrison, J. F. C. "From the Margins: a view of the social history of George Eliot's
    England." Paper delivered to the George Eliot Conference at Rutgers University,
    November 1980.
Hinton, D. A. "Popular Science in England, 1830–1870." Ph.D. thesis, Bath, 1979.
Inkster, Ian. "Studies in the Social History of Science in England during the Industrial
    Revolution, c. 1790–1850." Ph.D. thesis, Sheffield, 1977. 2 vols.
Jones, R. Alun. "'Knowledge Chartism': a study of the influence of Chartism on nineteenth
    century educational development in Great Britain." M.A. thesis, Birmingham, 1938.
Lineham, Peter J. "The English Swedenborgians, 1770–1840: a study in the social dimen-
    sions of religious sectarianism." Ph.D. thesis, Sussex, 1978.
Nott, John William. "The Artisan as Agitator: Richard Carlile, 1816–1843." Ph.D. thesis,
    Wisconsin, 1970.
Porter, Roy. "Charles Lyell: the public and private faces of science." Typescript, 1980.
Pyenson, Susan Sheets. "Low Scientific Culture in London and Paris, 1820–1875." Ph.D.
    thesis, Pennsylvania, 1976.
Salt, John. "Isaac Ironside and Education in the Sheffield Region in the First Half of the
    Nineteenth Century." M.A. thesis, Sheffield, 1960.
Waddell, Margot. "Scientific Naturalism and Philosophies of Nature and Man in the Novels
    of George Eliot." Paper presented to the British Society for the History of Science,
    London, 1972.
Weber, Gay. "Degeneration and Progress in Early Nineteenth-Century Social Theory."
    Paper presented to the British Society for the History of Science, Cambridge, 1976.
Yeo, Eileen M. "Social Science and Social Change: a social history of some aspects of
    social investigation in Britain, 1830–1890." Ph.D. thesis, Sussex, 1972.
Young, Robert M. "Functionalism." Typescript, 1971.
Young, Robert M. "Who Cares about Objectivity? – And Why?" Paper presented to the
    Imperial College of Science and Technology, London, 1976.
Yoxen, Edward. "The Social Impact of Molecular Biology." Ph.D. thesis, Cambridge,
    1978.

Parliamentary Papers
Census of Great Britain, 1851: education, England and Wales
Report from the Select Committee on:
    *The Extent, Causes, and Consequences of the Prevailing Vice of Intoxication among the Labouring
        Classes of the United Kingdom, 1834*
    Foundation Schools and Education in Ireland, 1835
    Education in England and Wales, 1835
    Arts and Manufactures, 1835
Education of the Poorer Classes in England and Wales, 1838
    Public Libraries, 1849
    Newspaper Stamps, 1851

PHRENOLOGICAL JOURNALS

1823. *Transactions of the* [Edinburgh] *Phrenological Society:* Edinburgh, 1 vol. only, ed. George Combe and others; continued as:

1823–47. *Phrenological Journal and Miscellany:* Edinburgh, quarterly, Dec. 1823–Oct. 1847, 20 vols.; ed. Richard Poole, 1824, then George Combe, Andrew Combe, James Simpson, Robert Cox, and others, 1825–Sept. 1837 (4s); n.s. London, ed. Hewett Cottrell Watson, 1838–40 (2s 6d); Edinburgh, ed. Robert Cox, 1841–47.

1833. *Phrenologist:* London, 16 Feb. 1833–?, 1 vol. only, ed. Louis Henry Ehn (2d, unstamped).

1835–8. *Christian Physician and Anthropological Magazine:* London, Sept. 1835–Oct. 1838, ed. John Epps, Charles Loosely; continued as:

1838–9. *Phrenological (Anthropological) Magazine and Christian Physician:* London, Nov. 1838–Feb. 1839, ed. John Epps and Charles Loosely, organ of the Finsbury Discussion Society and of the Anthropological Society.

1841. *Illustrations of Phrenology: Comprising Accounts of the Lives of Persons Remarkable in Some Mental Respect, Whether Intellect or Feeling, and Accurate Delineations of Their Heads; Together with a Statement of the Various Measurements and the Development of the Individual Organs:* London, 1 issue only, ed. George R. Lewis (2s 6d).

1842–4. *Phrenological Almanac; or, Annual Journal of Mental and Moral Science:* Glasgow, ed. D. G. Goyder, published under the auspices of the Glasgow Phrenological Society; continued as *Phrenological Almanac and Psychological Annual* (below).

1843. *Phreno-Magnet and Mirror of Nature: A Record of Facts, Experiments, and Discoveries in Phrenology, Magnetism, etc.:* London, 1 vol. only, ed. Spencer Timothy Hall.

1843–4. *Peoples Phrenological Journal and Compendium of Mental and Moral Science:* London, weekly, 2 vols., ed. W. John Vernon, 1843, then Luke Burke, 1844.

1843–56. *Zoist: A Journal of Cerebral Physiology and Mesmerism and Their Application to Human Welfare:* London, Mar. 1843–Jan. 1856, ed. John Elliotson and William Collins Engledue.

1845. *Phrenological Almanac and Psychological Annual:* Glasgow, 1 vol. only, ed. D. G. Goyder; continued as:

1846. *Phrenological Annual and Psychological Almanac for the Year 1846:* Glasgow, 1 vol. only, ed. D. G. Goyder.

1846–52. *Journal of Health and Disease:* London, 1846–9, ed. Walter Johnson and others (2s 6d); about one-quarter devoted to phrenology; continued as *Monthly Journal of Homoeopathy and Journal of Health and Disease* but with diminished phrenological content, 1850–2.

1848–53. *Ethnological Journal: A Magazine of Ethnography, Phrenology, and Archaeology, Considered as Elements of the Science of Races: With the Applications of This Science to Education, Legislation, and Social Progress:* London, June 1848–Mar. 1849, then n.s. (without "Phrenology" in title) to Jan. 1854, ed. Luke Burke.

1848–67. *Journal of Health: A Monthly Magazine:* London, Aug. 1848–Aug. 1850, ed. R. B. Grindrod, 1849–?; not issued Sept. 1850–Apr. 1851; n.s. May 1851–5; then became *Journal of Health and Phrenological Magazine* to Jan. 1860, ed. Frederic Towgood; then became *Journal of Health and Vegetarian Magazine* to 1867, ed. Jacob Dixon, June 1862–7.

1849. *Zadkiel's Magazine; or, Record and Review of Astrology, Phrenology, Mesmerism, and Other Sciences:* Jan.–Feb. 1849, ed. Richard James Morrison (1d).

1858–9. *Spiritual Messenger: A Magazine Devoted to Spiritualism, Mesmerism, and Other Branches of Psychological Science* [including phrenology]: London, Sept. 1858–Mar. 1859, ed. William Carpenter (1d).

1867–78. *Human Nature: A Monthly Record of Zoistic Science and Intelligence, Embodying Physiology, Phrenology, Psychology, Spiritualism, Philosophy, the Laws of Health, and Sociology: An Educational and Family Magazine:* London, monthly, Apr. 1867–July 1878, ed. J. D. Burns.

1878. *Phrenological Messenger:* Leeds, 1 issue only, ed. R. B. D. Wells (2d).

1880–9. *Phrenological Magazine: A Journal of Education and Mental Science:* London, 5 vols., ed. Alfred T. Story, issued by L. N. Fowler; later ed. Jessie Fowler.

1888. *Phrenological Annual and Record for 1888:* London, ed. Alfred T. Story (4d).

1891–3. *Know Thyself: A Monthly Magazine Devoted to Phrenology, Physiology, Pathology, Pathognomy, Physiognomy, Pleasure, and Profit:* 1 Sept. 1891–Dec. 1892, ed. Prof. Ida Ellis (1d, then 2s 6d); continued as *Phrenological Review*: Leeds, monthly, Jan. 1893–Nov. 1893, then Blackpoool, quarterly, 1893, 1 isssue only; ed. Ellis Family (1d); official organ of the Universal Phrenological Society.

1892–3. *Phrenological Record; Being the Quarterly Abstract of the Proceedings of the British Phrenological Association:* London, 1 Jan. 1892–1 July 1893, ed. Bernard Hollander (3d).

1893. *British Phrenological Journal and Christian Worker:* Sheffield, May 1893 issue only, ed. Eli Ward (1d). [John Johnson Collection, Bodleian Library, Oxford]

1896–7. *British Phrenological Year Book:* London.

1896–1904. *The Popular Phrenologist:* London.

1898. *Phrenologist and Physiological Register:* London.

1905–6. *Phrenological Review* [of the British Phrenological Society Inc.]: London, Apr. 1905–July 1906, ed. Bernard Hollander.

1905–22. *Ethological Journal*; London, Jan. 1905–June 1914; resumed Jan. 1922–Oct. 1922, ed. Bernard Hollander.

1907. *Phrenologist.*

1909–11. *Gall Journal: A Resume of Lectures Delivered Before the Gall Society:* London, 3 vols.

1920–1. *British Phrenological Annual:* Morecambe, ed. Taylor family.

BIBLIOGRAPHICAL INDEX

The following list gives the page and note where the first full citation of a source referred to in the notes may be found. Works are listed according to author name, except in the cases of anonymous works, for which short titles are given, and in the cases of unsigned articles (on phrenology only) in encyclopedias, dictionaries, and nonphrenological journals, all of which are entered under the volume title. Where more than one work by an author has been cited in different notes, separate sources are indicated by key words from the short titles (or, in the case of journals, by dates).

GENERAL INDEX

For reference or additional reference to people whose published works have been cited and to all twentieth-century authors referred to in the text, see the Bibliographical Index.